"Compelling, grounded, and utterly human. Susan and Kathleen present the mindful parenting program that has emerged out of their sustained engagement with their mindfulness practice, with their daily lives as parents, and with the lives of the parents who have participated in their classes. The result is a personal, practical, and informative description of the program and its background.

A parent training program that focuses on enabling participants to parent their children from the place they and their children are in moment-by-moment, rather than striving towards some idea of how things could or should be. What a relief!"

Rebecca Crane
Director, Centre for Mindfulness Research and Practice,
Bangor University
Author of *Mindfulness-Based Cognitive Therapy, Distinctive Features*

"A brilliant book with enormous practical implications for all parents. Written with great skill and clarity, Susan Bögels and Kathleen Restifo bring together insights from the evolution of parenting with the latest psychological science on compassion, attachment, and schemas. But then they go further, giving us a step-by-step guide through their unique and evidence-based mindful parenting program.

This book is a must-read for child and family practitioners but it will also be on the shelves of all mindfulness teachers who wish to understand how to recollect and explore their own experience as a parent or a child, and in doing so, to understand more deeply the entanglements of those who come to them for help."

Mark Williams
Professor of Clinical Psychology, University of Oxford
Author of *Mindfulness-Based Cognitive Therapy for*
Preventing Relapse in Depression

MINDFUL PARENTING

MINDFUL PARENTING

A GUIDE FOR MENTAL HEALTH PRACTITIONERS

SUSAN BÖGELS
KATHLEEN RESTIFO

Foreword by Jon and Myla Kabat-Zin

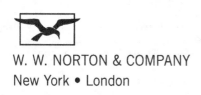

W. W. NORTON & COMPANY
New York • London

English paperback edition:
Mindful Parenting
by Susan Bögels and Kathleen Restifo
Copyright © 2014
Springer New York
Springer New York is a part of Springer Science+Business Media
All Rights Reserved

First published as a Norton paperback 2015

Printed in the United States of America

For information about special discounts for bulk purchases, please contact W. W. Norton
Special Sales at specialsales@wwnorton.com or 800-233-4830

Manufacturing by Lakeside Book Company
Book design by Bytheway Publishing Services
Production manager: Christine Critelli

Library of Congress Cataloging-in-Publication Data

Bögels, Susan M. (Susan Maria), 1960–
    Mindful parenting : a guide for mental health practitioners / Susan
Bogels and Kathleen Restifo.
        pages cm. — (A Norton professional book)
    Includes bibliographical references and index.
    ISBN 978-0-393-70992-6 (pbk.)
    1. Parents—Mental health.   2. Parenting—Psychological aspects.
3. Meditation—Therapeutic use.   4. Stress management.   5. Family
psychotherapy.   I. Restifo, Kathleen.   II. Title.
    RC488.5.B636 2015
    616.89'156—dc23
                        2014049384

ISBN: 978-0-393-70992-6 (pbk.)

W. W. Norton & Company, Inc., 500 Fifth Avenue, New York, N.Y. 10110
www.wwnorton.com
W. W. Norton & Company Ltd., Castle House, 15 Carlisle Street, London W1D 3BS

2   3   4   5   6   7   8   9   0

CONTENTS

ACKNOWLEDGMENTS

SUSAN'S ACKNOWLEDGMENTS

First of all, I'm grateful to Mark Williams who was my first teacher in mindfulness, gave me the freedom to adapt the MBCT program to groups I wanted to use it with, and always supported me in my clinical and research steps in this area. Guido Sijbers taught me the basics of Vipassana meditation, and it was a joy to run the first mindfulness groups in the adult clinic with him, and in the child clinic with Bert Hoogstad. Nirbhay Singh, Jon Kabat-Zinn, and Myla Kabat-Zinn have been of great inspiration and support in our work in Mindful Parenting. Christopher Germer gave more recent inspiration in self-compassion practice. I have learned tremendously from the teachings and retreats of Martine Batchelor, Stephan Batchelor, Trish Bartley, Susan Woods, and Ferris Urbanowski.

I have benefited much from the wisdom and long experience in mindfulness of Joke Hellemans, who has run many Mindful Parenting groups, taking on her side new mindfulness trainers who were curious to learn about Mindful Parenting. Joke and I developed a teacher training program for mindfulness teachers who wanted to specialize in Mindful Parenting, and I've learned so much from the participants of that program and from participants in workshops on Mindful Parenting, professionals who often were the first to try out new practices that we considered to build into the Mindful Parenting program. I thank Kathleen Restifo for teaching me the patience to write and deepen my thinking.

I am very grateful to the team of the academic treatment center for parent and child *UvA minds*. Sacha Lucassen, the team leader of *UvA minds*, who through her energy and enthusiasm created the flexible and dynamic infrastructure of our clinic so that parents could find their way to the Mindful Parenting course. I am thankful to mindfulness trainers Dorreke Peijnenburg, Rachel van der Meulen, Anne Formsma, Eva van de Weijer-Bergsma, and Eva Potharst, who co-led the Mindful Parenting groups; Esther de Bruin for the energy, enthusiasm, and ideas she put in the research; Nynke Wagenaar and the many master students that have supported the research on Mindful Parenting. Saskia Wessels, the office manager of *UvA minds*, who is the first person parents talk to when they call our center and makes families feel at home in our clinic, has been crucial in offering the Mindful Parenting program to parents.

The University of Amsterdam supports our research in Mindful Parenting in many ways. My thanks go to the rector magnificus and the dean, Dymph van der Boom and Edward de Haan, for their support in setting up the academic clinic; to Jan Randsdorp and Piet Scholten from UvA Holding for their support of *UvA minds*; Frans Oort in his role of research director and for his statistical support; and the whole team of Rearing and Developmental Problems for their passion for research and teaching.

My gratitude goes to my parents, for having facilitated my creative and intellectual development, to become a free mind. Their examples have helped me to become who I am. I am grateful to my siblings, Paul, Gert, Corien, and Ceciel, for their love and companionship.

My children, Thomas, Renate, and Leyla, thank you for the happiness you bring in my life, and for reminding me each and every day that there is more to life than work. Sofia, thanks for your trust when you were growing up.

I thank the fathers of my children, Rudolf and Enrico, and their partners, Ingrid and Ingrid, and our child minders, Annie and Margreet, for sharing the task of raising our children to maturity. And Jelle, we met when I was writing this book. Thanks for distracting and supporting me.

KATHLEEN'S ACKNOWLEDGMENTS

I want to thank Susan Bögels, for giving me the chance to collaborate with her on the Mindful Parenting course, and for her creativity in applying mindfulness to parents and children at a time when many were skeptical. I want to thank Joke Hellemans for her deep embodiment of mindfulness, and for her generosity in sharing the depth of her experience with me.

One of the unexpected pleasures of writing this book was the correspondence with the many readers, all of whom had no time, and all of whom nonetheless managed to read through earlier versions of this manuscript. In particular, I want to thank Myla Kabat-Zinn, Jon Kabat-Zinn, Mark Williams, and Nirbhay Singh for their thoughtful comments on two versions of the manuscript. I want to thank Franca Warmenhoven and Rebecca Crane for their detailed comments on two difficult chapters.

Christopher Germer and Paul Gilbert helped me to understand how to work with strong emotional reactions to loving-kindness practice. Joke Hellemans tried out many of the newer practices in this program and provided valuable feedback on them. I would like to thank Sarah Hrdy for clarifying her ideas about evolution of parenting, and Paul Gilbert for helping me put evolutionary processes in the context of mindfulness. Marisol Voncken helped me to write about the neuroendocrine basis of attachment from a more personal point of view.

I am thankful for all of my meditations teachers. I want to thank Mark Williams for presenting mindfulness in a way that made me curious, and Rob Vincken for teaching me mindfulness, and then showing me how to teach others. I have benefited from retreats with meditation teachers whose words and practices continue to inspire my own practice: Martine and Stephen Batchelor, who helped me understand and feel the power of Buddhist concepts in mindfulness; Christina Feldman and John Teasdale, who helped me to deepen my mindfulness practice, and Christopher Germer and Sylvia Boorstein for deepening my understanding of compassion. I am grateful to Megan Cowan for showing me that mindfulness is really child's play. I am thankful to Thich Nhat Hanh, and the community of nuns at Lower Hamlet, for teaching me how to bring mindfulness into my family (and for playing a mean game of soccer!).

Reading about our evolution as cooperative breeders made me reminisce about my Brooklyn days, when my children were very young. I am so thankful for the Brooklyn moms and other friends, especially Rachel, Pam, Christiane, Nina, Karen, Susan, Judith, Meryl, and Laura—who mothered me, and helped me to realize that I had what it took to mother my own children. I also want to thank Lori for helping me to create a home away from home here in Maastricht and Reina, Ariane, Kaat and Joos for welcoming me into their circle with open arms. I am grateful to my sisters, Linda and Diana, for their support from far away. I want to thank Cristel Achterberg, for teaching me how to be a good mother to myself. I am grateful to the wonderful allomothers who helped me to care for my children: Litza, Rosita, Ada and Maria.

I want to thank my mother, for everything she has done for me— both the things I know about, and the many things I will never know about. I am grateful to my father, for encouraging my intellectual development and my humor. I am grateful to my stepfather, for being the best alloparent a teenager could ever have hoped for.

And finally, I want to thank my children, Gabriella and Max. Without them, this book would not have been conceivable. I am so grateful for their presence in my life. They have had to put up with many moments of distraction as this book was being finished, and they did so with patience and humor, and when necessary, pulled me out of my work to be with them. I am grateful for their dogged insistence on meeting me with beginner's mind, each and every day, ready to begin with me anew with love, despite whatever ways I may have floundered the day before.

And to David, for being a father in the tradition of the best Aka fathers: warm, sensitive, and caring. His love and support sustain me.

TOGETHER

We are grateful to all parents who have attended the Mindful Parenting courses, who have shared their stories and experiences, and have participated in the research. We are grateful to their children and partners who have experienced their attempts to become more mindful in their relations to family members, and have responded to that in ways that reinforced their first steps in Mindful Parenting.

We want to thank Nirbhay Singh for his support and guidance throughout the process of writing this book. We are grateful to Judy Jones, for providing support and advice, and for helping us to get to the finish line.

Most thanks go to our Buddha teachers in the first place: our children. Thank you for your temperament, your tantrums, your sleeping problems, your fears and avoidance, your social difficulties, your not doing your homework, your failing to win a sport match, your restlessness and hyperactivity, your lack of eye contact, your not coming home in time at night, your drinking too much (we can go on). In sum, thank you for not being what we had fancied you to be, a better version of ourselves, but for being what you are: yourselves. Thank you for teaching us that we are evolved parents, for teaching us to recognize our punitive or demanding parent modes, or angry or vulnerable child modes, that we can take a breathing space when we are losing it or have lost it, that we can use self-compassion in difficult parenting times, and that we can repair our conflicts. Thank you for your patience, your trust, your love, so that we can go on with our mindful parenting process for the rest of our lives.

FOREWORD

THIS BOOK and the program it offers the world are a pioneering effort to bring mindfulness into the domain of parenting and the mental health care of stressed families, for the benefit of both the children and their parents.

When we wrote the first edition of our book on mindful parenting, published in 1997, it did not include a formal program for parents, nor a curriculum for training health professionals to teach parents. Such a curriculum is long overdue. We are grateful to the authors for bringing it to life in this form. Their program is both profoundly practical and, at the same time, potentially transformative and healing. One of its main virtues is that it spans and unifies two different ways of knowing: that of empirical scientific understanding, in this case clinical and behavioral psychology research, and that of contemplative mindfulness-based programs and practices, which are themselves increasingly resting on a firm scientific foundation. At the same time, these mindfulness-based programs tap into an orthogonal dimension of wisdom and compassion going back several thousand years, mostly derived from the universal elements underlying Buddhist meditation, of which mindfulness is often said to be the heart.

The authors and their colleagues have done research in the field of stress and parenting and have conducted a number of studies to validate their clinical program in mindful parenting. The curriculum is presented here in a remarkably accessible, clear, and detailed way. It builds on other mindfulness-based clinical approaches such as MBSR (mindfulness-based stress reduction) and MBCT (mindfulness-based cognitive therapy) and broadens their reach to the complex realm of family interactions and the particular challenges of parenting children with psychiatric diagnoses. Here you will find both the formal and informal mindfulness practices utilized by MBSR and MBCT, adapted and extended in imaginative ways to the domain of parenting.

This work rests on a powerful foundation of compassion and kindness, for both parents and children, essential in the face of the inevitable suffering of families. These qualities of heart are not some kind of super-ficial window-dressing or façade, but in fact constitute the ground of all mindfulness practices and their clinical applications. For the word *mind-fulness* equally implies *heartfulness*. Without that visceral understanding and embodiment, the power of this approach would be lost. Happily, the authors emphasize this critical point throughout the book, as they do the fact that to really understand mindfulness and be able to use it creatively to help others, one must actually cultivate it in one's own life as a way of being. In both these critical regards, the author's own lived experience and wisdom are evident and palpable. Their articulation of this way of being called mindful parenting will be an inspiration to those seeking to adapt this curriculum in their own settings and in their own lives.

We are delighted that Susan Bögels and Kathleen Restifo have brought this profound and nuanced curriculum into the world in this way. Admittedly, it asks a lot of all involved. Mindfulness always does. But you will find, through actual practice, that it does not ask more of parents than they are capable of giving for the sake of their children and themselves.

We hope that this book, with its refined perspective and skillful guidance, benefits families of all kinds, far and wide.

Jon and Myla Kabat-Zinn
Lexington, Massachusetts

MINDFUL PARENTING

PART I

THEORETICAL AND EMPIRICAL BACKGROUND

CHAPTER 1

INTRODUCTION TO MINDFUL PARENTING

Every baby can be seen as a little Buddha or Zen Master; your own private mindful teacher . . .

> Jon Kabat-Zinn, *Wherever You Go, There You Are*
> (1994), pg. 248

WHY PARENTING CAN BE STRESSFUL

PARENTING IS one of the most consuming and responsible tasks in a lifetime for many parents, yet parents do it with love, joy, pride, and a sense of fulfillment. In fact, raising children and having grandchildren may be the most fulfilling "job" that we ever have, and being a good father or a good mother our highest ambition in life. If we would be asked what we want people to say about us at our funeral, having been a good parent (and grandparent) is what comes up for most of us who have had the fortune to be a parent (and have grandchildren).

Wanting to do it so well—to be the best parent possible—may in itself be a source of stress. Many other challenges and obstacles on the way may make parenting stressful. To start with, the transition in adult life of taking care of our own lives, to giving birth to children and taking care of their lives as well, requires an enormous change in how we divide our time, attention, energy, and resources (e.g., Bardacke. 2012). Life will never be the same after having children. In taking care of children and organizing family life, and balancing that with our working lives, we may forget to take care of ourselves. When inner resources get depleted, this may result in irritable or depressed mood, fatigue, somatic complaints, and eventually in mental or physical disorders, interfering with parenting qualities.

Children's, as well as parents', possible behavior problems or psychopathology symptoms represent a challenge or obstacle that can make parenting more stressful, and these are the families for which the Mindful Parenting course as described in this book is developed. A child who, for example, becomes highly stressed or oppositional when confronted with novelty, who cannot play on his or her own or cannot organize school work, who cannot be left alone with siblings because of aggressive behavior, or who cannot sleep at night, can represent an extra burden for parenting. Parents' own symptoms of psychopathology may also add stress to the parenting task. For example: a parent who is suffering from depression may experience the parenting task as too heavy and himself or herself as a bad parent; a parent suffering from anxieties may be overly concerned and overprotective with the child; a parent suffering from obsessive–compulsive traits may not be able to let go of or share the parenting task; and a parent with problems in executive functioning may react impulsively and inconsistently to the child.

Even if no specific psychopathology in children or parents is present, parents encounter many sources of stress. Children develop, and therefore constantly change, challenging parents to keep adapting to these ongoing changes: a baby that starts to walk, an adolescent that does not obey the family rules anymore, and an adult child leaving home. Parents, even when the children are long grown up, feel a strong sense of responsibility for the safety and well-being of their children, and may worry and feel stressed in phases when their children meet new challenges on their own.

Stress in parenting may also arise from unexpected family changes such as divorce. Nowadays, the majority of children live in a situation with stepparents or stepchildren, in which issues about boundaries and loyalties are likely to arise. Stepparents and stepchildren can be a source of support and joy but may also add stress to parenting. Moreover, many parents raise children as a single parent, and the lack of support of another parent who is co-responsible for the parenting task can be a source of stress.

Marital problems, and problems in the co-parental relationship, are another source of stress related to parenting. While the reliance on social communities has decreased in Western, individualistic cultures, marital relationships have become more and more important as a source of social connectedness and support, and the expectations of marital relationships have become higher (Johnson, 2008). As a result, problems in the marital relationship form an important source of stress for parents. This stress has been found to negatively affect parenting, in fathers even more so than in mothers (Bögels, Lehtonen, & Restifo, 2010).

WHY MINDFUL PARENTING CAN HELP

When under stress, parenting skills are found to collapse (e.g., Belsky, 1984; Webster-Stratton, 1990a). Parents may have learned parenting skills from parenting courses, parenting books, or television programs on parenting. However, when under stress or other intense emotions, parents of all socioeconomical levels will tend to yell at their children, threat, and even beat them. Courses and knowledge about how a good parent should handle difficulties may even have the effect of parents being more harsh with themselves for having lost it.

Not only may parents forget to apply skills they have learned in parenting courses when under stress, parental psychopathology may also hinder parents, and their children, in benefiting from such courses. To illustrate, Parent Management Training is an effective training for parents of children with ADHD, decreasing children's behavior problems. However, children of parents who themselves have ADHD do not benefit as well from such parent training (e.g., Sonuga-Barke, Daley, Thompson, 2002). Interestingly, specifically in families in which child and parent share symptoms of psychopathology, such as inattentive or impulsive behavior, children are at the highest risk of developing mental health disorders such as ADHD (Sonuga-Barke, 2010). In a similar vein, children of depressed mothers are found to benefit less from parent training (Forehand, Furey, & McMahon, 1984; Owens et al., 2003; Reyno & McGrath, 2006; Webster-Stratton, 1990b). Also, parents with marital problems may benefit less from parent training (Reisinger, Frangia, & Hoffman, 1976; Webster-Stratton, 1985), although other studies failed to find an association between marital distress/dissatisfaction and parent training outcomes (Brody & Forehand, 1985; Firestone & Witt, 1982). Therefore, there is a need for parent training in which parents' own stress, suffering, and symptoms of psychopathology have an important place in the process of improving family functioning.

Mindful Parenting offers another way of approaching parenting in high stress times, and for parents with psychopathology themselves. In Mindful Parenting, parents' own stress, suffering, and, if present, psychopathology are the primary focus of the training rather than the problem behavior of the child. Clearly, the problem behavior of the child can be the major source of stress in the family, but the resulting stress in the parent is what we work with. Dealing differently with stress, or stress reduction, is at the heart of the Mindfulness-Based Stress Reduction program.

Mindfulness is a form of meditation based on the Buddhist tradition and involves being present in the moment, focusing on the reality and accepting it for what it is. Jon Kabat-Zinn developed the Mindfulness-Based Stress Reduction (MBSR) program to address the unmet needs of chronically ill people to participate in their own healing, cope with their illness, and for dealing with life stress in general. Zindel Segal, Mark Williams, and John Teasdale, based on this work, developed the Mindfulness-Based Cognitive Therapy (MBCT), an approach specifically for depressed patients. Over the last two decades, mindfulness-based interventions have been used to successfully bring change in a multitude of physical, stress-related, and mental health problems. Bringing mindfulness into the situation of parenting, children, and family life ("Mindful Parenting") is one of the newer applications of mindfulness.

This book is about Mindful Parenting in the context of mental health care, that is, when parents seek or are advised help with their parenting because their child or they themselves have a mental health problem. In the following, we will describe the evolution of the Mindful Parenting program, as outlined in this book, from the start more than 10 years ago until now.

THE EVOLUTION OF THE MINDFUL PARENTING COURSE

THE FIRST STEPS: MINDFUL PARENTING FOR PARENTS WHO TAKE A MINDFULNESS COURSE—SUSAN'S STORY

As an attention researcher, I had gotten interested in task concentration training for people with social anxiety disorder, particularly, a fear of blushing. Scientific research had shown that individuals with social anxiety disorder suffer from heightened self-focused attention during social situations and as a result they have little attention for their environment and other people (Bögels & Mansell, 2006). This was found to have many negative consequences for their social behavior, how they would come across, and heighten their negative emotions, thoughts, and physiological arousal. The idea behind this training was that if we could train people to focus their attention outside, on the task at hand, at moments of social fear when their attention naturally would go to themselves, their social anxiety would reduce. When we published our first paper on task concentration training back in 1997 (Bögels, Mulkens, & de Jong, 1997, later papers Bögels, 2006; Mulkens, Bögels, Louwers, & de Jong, 2001), Isaac Marks, a well-known anxiety researcher, e-mailed me: "Isn't this the same as mindfulness?" No, it was not the same, but we did observe the positive effects that task concentration training practices, like walking in a forest while paying attention to all senses, had on getting people out of their (anxious) head and into experiencing life from moment to moment and how it helped them to be more present with other people rather than self-absorbed in their social fears, which is the same as mindfulness. The seed of mindfulness was planted, at least in my research head.

In 2000, I invited Mark Williams to provide our adult and child mental health center teams in Maastricht with an introductory training in MBCT. We were very impressed by the mindfulness approach to mental health problems, which was so different from what we were used to, being trained as cognitive-behavior therapists. We immediately planned a randomized clinical trial to compare mindfulness with cognitive-behavior therapy for adults suffering from social anxiety disorder. However, inspired by Mark Williams' training, my colleagues from the child mental health care center asked if I could start a mindfulness course for anxious children. As highly effective cognitive-behavioral programs were available for these adolescents (e.g., Bodden et al., 2008), this was not the most obvious start of mindfulness in a child and adolescent mental health care setting. But what about children suffering from externalizing problems, that is, problems of behavioral control, inattention, and impulsivity that are primarily manifested in outward behavior rather than in their internal thoughts and feelings? These children may have been classified as suffering from attention deficit and hyperactivity disorder (ADHD), autistic spectrum disorders, and oppositional defiant or conduct disorders. Few evidence-based approaches were available for them, and adolescents with these disorders, which are often comorbid in clinical settings, typically present with attention and impulsivity problems.

Although mindfulness training was not originally developed for these kinds of attention and impulsivity problems, there were reasons to believe that mindfulness practices could help. Children with externalizing disorders may have in common certain attention problems, such as maintaining attention over prolonged periods of time, paying attention to various aspects simultaneously, inhibiting their first response when needed, or a too narrow attention span. Children with externalizing disorders also have certain behaviors in common such as impulsivity, hyperactivity, or restlessness, which may result from the same underlying information processing problems. In mindfulness, attention skills such as focusing, becoming aware of the wandering mind, widening attention, and being aware of restlessness and action tendencies without doing them are trained, and therefore, mindfulness training may directly intervene in the attention and hyperactivity or impulsivity problem of these children.

While developing a program for these children, I felt that at least one of their parents should be included in a parallel mindfulness program for parents. The idea was that as these children still lived with their family, the mindfulness skills that they would learn in order to deal better with their attention, behavioral, and social problems would have to be embedded in a family context in which mindfulness is somehow installed, in the way a family eats dinner and spends time together, in family relations, and in dealing with family stress and conflicts. Moreover, some of the parents had similar attention and impulsivity issues as their child, and mindfulness could help them become less impulsive and more attentive in their contact with their child. Also, raising a child with one or more of these disorders is inherently stressful. Many parents had stressful years behind them where they were often called by the school because of the difficulties administrators encountered with their child, by other parents because of the misbehavior of their child, or even by the police. Their child would not meet their expectations and hopes they had for their child in terms of performance at school, having friends or the "right" friends, and being engaged in extra curricular activities. Or, the relationship they had built with this child would not meet their expectations for closeness, as their child would avoid contact with the parent; expectations of reciprocity, as their child had difficulties seeing the world from the perspective of the parent; or expectations of honesty, as the child had developed a pattern of lying or even stealing from the parent. Or, parents could not sleep at night, because their adolescent would come home very late or not at all, and they would worry about alcohol and drug abuse, or aggression they would meet on the street at night. Mindfulness could perhaps help parents deal with such stress and develop acceptance towards the, often severe, problems of their child, of which it was unclear whether they would be susceptible to change, given the chronic history and lack of success of previous treatment. The idea was that if we cannot change the problem, we can at least work on our own relation towards the problem, by taking care of ourselves as parents, and practice an open, mild, and nonjudgmental attitude towards the problem.

We called the parallel mindfulness training for parents Mindful Parenting. The term "mindful parenting" was first used by Myla and Jon Kabat-Zinn in their book. *Everyday Blessings: The Inner Work of Mindful Parenting*, from 1997. They described how intentionally bringing here-and-now nonjudgmental attention to parenting, children, and the family leads to deeper understanding of our children and ourselves. They suggested how Mindful Parenting can be healing and transformative for both children and parents.

Most of the parents participating in 2000 had never heard about mindfulness. Some were intrigued and motivated; others were just there because parental participation was a requirement for their child to participate in the training. Many parents were impressed by the effects of the practices on their parenting, family, and personal lives. For example, simply allowing themselves to feel how tired they were made a difference in their day. Some stated afterwards that they wished they had participated in a Mindful Parenting course when their child was younger, as they are now dealing with a sometimes very difficult adolescent in a very critical period, almost leaving home.

Annette Heffels, a marital and family therapist, was a participant observer in one of my early Mindful Parenting courses, in order to write about it for a popular magazine targeting mothers. She commented on the strong group cohesion and safety she felt in the group, early in the 8-week process. She noticed that parents could not do it wrong in the group, even if they were late or had not done their home practice; they were just as welcome and accepted, simply for being present. Her observations made me think about what Jon Kabat-Zinn calls "heart-fulness" or Jeffrey Young "reparenting": the feeling of being taken care of (by the group, the teacher, the meditations), and learning to take better care of yourself as a parent, may be essential for parents, who are carrying the heavy task of taking care of their children, sometimes in very difficult circumstances.

The combined effects of these first mindfulness groups for adolescents with externalizing disorders, and parallel Mindful Parenting for their parents, were that adolescents had improved in their externalizing and attention problems in important ways (Bögels, Hoogstad, van Dun, Schutter, & Restifo, 2008), but it remained unclear whether this was the result of their own mindfulness training, or the Mindfulness training for the parents, or both.

MINDFUL PARENTING AS A COURSE ON ITS OWN

When I started to work in Amsterdam in 2008, I had the chance to collaborate with Joke Hellemans, a clinical psychologist and experienced mindfulness teacher, trained by Jon Kabat-Zinn's group in the Center for Mindfulness of the University of Massachusetts medical school. We benefited greatly from Joke's expertise and depth of experience with, and embodiment of, MBSR and MBCT and their clinical use with adults suffering from stress (MBSR) and from depression (MBCT). Thus, she was able to contribute significantly to the curriculum of Mindful Parenting around the essential elements of these two approaches, namely, (1) their emphasis on the systematic formal and informal practice of mindfulness and (2) group discussion about the participants' life experiences with the practice.

Joke and I started our first Mindful Parenting course without parallel mindfulness training for their children. The advantage of this approach was that we could now include parents of children of all ages and all kinds of psychopathology and also parents whose children had no particular problems but who themselves were suffering from problems that interfered with their parenting. Parents interested in taking this course had encountered a wide variety of issues in their parenting. Some had difficulties related to their marriage, such as having gone through a divorce and their children not accepting their new partner. Others had parenting issues related to their own mental health, such as having suffered from postnatal depression and feeling guilty towards their child as a result. Some had parenting problems related to their background, such as having experienced trauma as a child and revisiting that while having children themselves. Still others had problems related to balancing parenting with other tasks, such as being ill from work since having children. And finally, others confronted parenting problems around mental health-related difficulties of their children, such as separation anxiety disorder, autistic spectrum disorder, and ADHD.

The duration of the sessions was now twice as long: 3 hours instead of the 1.5 hours of the Mindful Parenting course that was offered parallel to a child mindfulness course (since for children 1.5 hours was found to be the ideal duration for the mindfulness course; we kept the time the same for their parents for practical reasons of bringing and taking the children and also to make the Mindful Parenting intervention more acceptable for parents who simply participated because it was required). Around two-third of the new 3 hours course was based on the 8-session MBSR and MBCT program. Around one-third was Mindful Parenting, relying on our own previous protocols and experience in the shorter Mindful Parenting parallel to child mindfulness groups and on newly developed practices for which the book *Parenting from the Inside Out* of Dan Siegel and Mary Hartzell (2003) gave much inspiration. We were touched and impressed by the results. Parents described transformational changes in their own lives and in the ways they related to their children and partners. On questionnaire measures, they reported large improvements on their children's as well as their own psychopathology symptoms as well as on parenting and family functioning measures (Bögels et al., 2010).

Joke and I each ran many more Mindful Parenting groups, using the same program, in the academic mental health center for parents and children *UvA minds* in Amsterdam. Many child and family therapists, and mindfulness trainers, accompanied us in this process by sitting in as a participant observer during one of the courses and giving us feedback on what they observed and how the Mindful Parenting helped them in their own lives, balancing family and other obligations. In 2010, Kathleen and I ran a Mindful Parenting course together, for English language parents. From her background as a child and family therapist, her training as a mindfulness trainer, her research into family factors in child depression, and her interest in evolutionary psychology and compassion-focused approaches, we started to rewrite the program, integrating our thinking about mechanisms of change in Mindful Parenting as well as important theories and mindfulness-related interventions for preventing inter-generational transmission of psychopathology and negative parenting practices (e.g., Bögels & Brechman-Toussaint, 2008; Bögels et al., 2010; Restifo & Bögels, 2009).

COMPASSION, LOVING KINDNESS, AND MINDFUL PARENTING—KATHLEEN'S STORY

During the course of my training in mindfulness practice, I was influenced by exposure to loving kindness meditation, which I first came across in Sara Napthali's (2003) book Buddhism for Mothers. I recognized myself in Napthali's constant struggle to be a "good" mother, measuring herself up to some inchoate but absolute standard, and the inevitable fail-ure to live up to it. As a psychologist, I had worked for many years with people struggling with self-esteem issues, perfectionism, self-hatred, and suicidal thoughts or attempts. I had also struggled with my own perfec-tionism and high standards, which could leave me feeling inadequate in my work and in my role of being a mother. Here was a practice which had love and kindness at the center of it and which assumed that kindness, love, and compassion can be cultivated by anyone. In my training as a psychologist, I had learned to emphasize the deficits that people had rather than looking at their inborn potential as human beings. Loving kindness meditation offered a different possibility: by intentionally prac-ticing kind, compassionate, and loving wishes towards oneself and oth-ers, we can cultivate our innate capacity for these positive states, towards ourselves and towards others.

Shortly after this, I had my first guided experience with this prac-tice during a silent retreat with Martine and Stephan Batchelor. Martine Batchelor's (2001) simple and poetic phrasing touched me and became the foundation for my own loving kindness practice. A year later, when I co-led my first Mindful Parenting group with Susan, we were struck by how self-critical and depleted the mothers seemed. Despite their obvious strengths professionally and as parents, they seemed to all struggle with feelings of guilt, of failure, and of not succeeding as parents. At the same time, these were clearly devoted mothers who loved their children and who wanted to do their best with them. I wondered if loving kindness meditation would speak to them as well, especially since the metaphor that the Buddha invoked to describe the attitude of kindness was a mother's love for her only child. We introduced loving kindness practice, and many parents responded positively to it.

Soon after, I learned of Kristin Neff's work on self-compassion. A developmental psychologist as well as long-time mindfulness practitioner, Neff has translated self-compassion practice into psychological terms and has conducted research on it. Her idea of using self-compassion practice to help deal with self-esteem issues fit into our sense of what was missing in the parents we saw in our group: self-compassion for their difficulties and struggles as parents (Neff, 2011). At the same time, I became aware of Gilbert's (2009) work on compassion-focused therapy. His description of patients who suffered from feeling shame and self-judgment and who could understand intellectually that their thoughts were not facts, but who could not feel loving or kind towards themselves, matched what we were seeing. Gilbert's point that we can cultivate compassionate states with certain kinds of practices and imagery, and that these practices may activate the underlying neuroendocrine processes subserving feelings of contentment and affiliation, was exciting. I also read Christopher Germer's work on compassion and mindfulness, and Susan and I attended a workshop with him to learn some of the self-compassion techniques which he and Kristin Neff had developed, to see if we could integrate them in the Mindful Parenting course (Germer, 2009; Neff, 2011).

We began to wonder how we could incorporate these practices into the Mindful Parenting course from the beginning, so that it would become a red thread through the entire course, since we felt that parents would need to practice this over time. We struggled to understand the relationship between compassion and mindfulness. Through conversations with mindfulness trainers and psychologists—Nirbay Singh. Joke Hellemans, Mark Williams, Christopher Germer, Christina Feldman, John Teasdale, Myla Kabat-Zinn, Jon Kabat-Zinn, Rebecca Crane, and Franca Warmenhoven—we began to understand loving kindness as the basic underlying attitude of all mindfulness practice, something which cannot be separated from mindfulness practice. At the same time, we felt that teaching the specific practices of self-compassion and loving kindness might help parents cultivate this attitude.

SCHEMA MODES AND MINDFUL PARENTING

In our Mindful Parenting groups, and in our own parenting experiences, we noticed how a stressful situation between a parent and child could sometimes erupt into a very emotional interaction. The hallmarks of these interactions were quick, automatic, and often angry emotional reactions as well as quick escalation of the conflict between parent and child. Many parents describe these interactions as "losing it" with their child and afterwards feel remorse and shame about having lost control of themselves and having behaved in a destructive manner towards their child.

We began to think about what exactly was going on in these situations. Clearly, parents were becoming emotionally triggered by something in the interaction with their child; once triggered, they seemed to go into an almost altered state of consciousness from which there was no turning back. In this "altered state," they reacted quickly, automatically, and with strong emotions. This would often lead to the child responding in anger and hurt, which further escalated the strong negative emotions. We wondered (1) what is it about the parent–child relationship which seems so ripe for this kind of interaction, and (2) what is the parent's experience during these interactions and (3) how can we help parents interact more wisely in these situations?

We were very much helped by psychiatrist Dan Siegel and early childhood educator Mary Hartzell's description of "low-road" parenting in their book "Parenting from the Inside Out." This refers to fast, automatic reactions to perceived threat, which can be triggered in stressful interactions with our children which we discussed above. These reactions are mediated by the limbic system and amygdala, and bypass higher cortical involvement. Dan Siegel describes such a low-road moment between himself and his 12-year-old son, which began over a dispute about a video game his son wanted to purchase. His example of "losing it" matched what we were seeing clinically and what we had sometimes experienced in our own relationships with children and partners (Siegel & Hartzell, 2003). We saw that mindfulness practice, especially the 3-min breathing space, was helping parents become more aware of these reactions, and to sometimes pause before reacting, but often the emotions were too strong. We were struck by the repetitive quality of these parent–child interactions. It seemed that when parents "lost it" with their children, these repetitive patterns would ensue. We wondered whether these patterns were related to parents' own childhood experiences; that is, were parents reenacting some core relationship issues from their own relationship with their parents in their interactions with their child?

We developed an exercise to help parents bring mindful awareness to the interactions with their children, in which, in a curious and open way, they investigated whether there were repeating patterns and also whether these patterns reminded them of patterns in their own upbringing. In this way, parents could connect their "low-road" experiences with their children with unresolved or difficult patterns in their own childhood. Parents often found this helpful in a profound way. They could now see their own contribution to these difficult interactions which they had blamed on their child's difficult behavior or strong emotions. In this way, they were able to become more empathic toward their child and become more curious about, and compassionate with, their own reactions. They also began to see that their reactions, far from being random, were specific to their own background and development. Connecting these superficially out of control reactions to these very personal and early patterns helped them to be more accepting of themselves and their child.

We began to see that these repetitive patterns were very similar to what Beck, Freeman, and Davis (2004) and Young (1994) describe as early schemas: automatic or unconscious experiences of the self which include cognitive, emotional, and bodily representations. We were struck by how the schema description is similar to "mindstates" which have been described in the mindfulness and Buddhist literature. Like schema modes, mindstates refer to a complex interacting pattern of thoughts, feelings, and body sensations which are experienced simultaneously and as total state. Mindstates can reflect any emotional state—anger, happiness, depression, and peacefulness—and they shape our perception of our world as well as our reactions. What makes mindstates and schemas so powerful is that we experience them as reality. When we are in a particular mindstate or schema, we believe that we are perceiving the world, others, and ourselves accurately, and we are not able to see how much our perceptions, thoughts, feelings, body sensations, and actions are determined by the particular mindstate or schema. Buddha's instructions from 2,500 years ago to "know mindstates as mindstates"—that is, not to mistake them for reality and not to identify with them—are completely consistent with the MBCT approach of recognizing "thoughts as thoughts" and not facts. But we found that schemas captured, in a more experiential way, the intense, entangled mess of distorted thoughts, feelings, body sensations, and reactions which can feel like an altered state of consciousness. We also found that schemas made the link between the parent's current difficult interactions with their child and their own unresolved interactions with their parents. This link seemed crucial to help parents become aware of the pattern, understand its emotional force, recognize its negative effect in the present, and, eventually, be able to let go of it and bring mindful awareness and choice to difficult interactions with their child. We know from developmental research that dysfunctional parenting patterns can be "transmitted" across generations, and the same is true for parent–child attachment patterns (Egeland et al., as cited in Gelles and Lancaster, 1987; van IJzendoorn, 1995). From our own experience as parents, and from the experiences of the many parents going through the Mindful Parenting groups, we had anecdotal evidence supporting this: our own childhood experiences of being parented can be strongly evoked, in the context of an emotional or stressful interaction with our children.

To conclude, the development of this Mindful Parenting course has been a joint effort involving the input of many people. The program has evolved with the feedback of the parents and of mindfulness teachers who completed the Mindful Parenting training course. Our personal journeys in mindfulness training and retreats have also fed this process. We have worked on the program as professionals but also as parents. As professionals, we have relied on our background as family-, cognitive-behavior-, and schema-focused therapists and have tried out the practices in our clinical practice and while training other professionals. As parents, we have used the practices in our own family lives, being aware of our own "low-road" moments and our intergenerational parenting experiences.

ORGANIZATION OF THIS BOOK

In the next 13 chapters, we describe the Mindful Parenting program as we have developed, implemented, and tested it in a child and parent mental health clinic, *UvA minds*, in Amsterdam, the Netherlands. In Part 1, Chapters 1 through 3, we present the theoretical, clinical, and empirical background for the program. In Chapter 2, we widen our lens and explore parenting and parenting stress in the context of our evolutionary history. In Chapter 3, we present findings from two clinical trials of the Mindful Parenting program and pilot findings on our latest version of the program including the compassion and schema techniques described in this book.

In Part II, Chapters 4 through 13, we present the Mindful Parenting manual. We begin with an overview of the program in Chapter 4. We describe the goals of the program, the themes and practices of each session, and some suggestions based on our experiences leading these groups. We also describe the kinds of families and parents for whom the program was developed and our assessment procedure. Finally, we describe the process of cultivating one's own practice which we see as integral to becoming a Mindful Parenting teacher. In Chapters 5 through 13, we describe in detail the 9 sessions of the program (8 sessions plus a follow-up session 2 months after the completion of the group). Each chapter describes one session and includes a brief discussion of the theoretical or clinical background to the session, a detailed description of the practices and inquiry for that session, examples parents, and handouts for participants describing the home practice and other relevant themes. Finally, in Chapter 14, we allow the parents to speak for themselves about the longer-term impact that this course has had on their lives.

NOTE ABOUT PERSONAL EXAMPLES

Many examples are given to illustrate the practices. These examples are anonymous descriptions from participants of one of the many courses and workshops. We have changed the names and some characteristics of participants and their families in order to ensure their privacy. A few parents write prose and poems about their experiences with their name. We also give personal examples from our own lives, which start with "I," referring to Kathleen or Susan. When we use "we," we refer to all of us as Mindful Parenting teachers, as participants in a Mindful Parenting course, or as parents, or as authors.

CHAPTER 2

AN EVOLUTIONARY PERSPECTIVE ON PARENTING AND PARENTING STRESS

INTRODUCTION: WHY TAKE AN EVOLUTIONARY PERSPECTIVE ON PARENTING AND MINDFULNESS?

PARENTING—THE EFFORT required to bring one human child to maturity—can be one of the greatest joys in our lives. But for many parents, raising a child also brings along new stresses (Cohen, Kessler, & Gordon, 1997). For parents struggling with psychological problems such as depression or anxiety, or raising children with developmental or emotional difficulties, the stress of parenting is even higher (Deater-Deckard, 1998). The seeming ubiquity of parenting stress has led us to wonder whether there might be an evolutionary basis for parenting stress. To paraphrase evolutionary anthropologist Sarah Hrdy, do we have an "evolutionary right" to our parenting stress (Hrdy, 1999)?[1] In other words, can an evolutionary perspective on parenting help us to understand the stresses which modern parents face? And how can mindfulness help with this?

Parenting has clearly been shaped by natural selection (Hrdy, 1999). In our evolutionary history, parenting traits and behaviors which increased the chance of a child surviving to maturity were more likely to be passed on to the next generation. Much as we may wish to believe that our parenting style is a product of our conscious choice, our own upbringing history, or our culture, the bulk of what makes us tick as parents may lie in our shared evolutionary past. To quote psychologist Paul Gilbert, "We

1. Sarah Hrdy uses this expression to describe infant's evolutionary right to want to sleep near its parents, not to describe parental stress. We have borrowed her expression and applied it to parenting because we find parents respond well to the phrase.

are evolved creatures," and we might add, we are evolved *parents* (Gilbert, 2009).

What relevance does evolutionary theory have for the kinds of stresses that we face today as parents? Many parents judge themselves harshly for what they see as their failures to parent effectively or for their children's difficulties. But from an evolutionary perspective, many of the traits which hinder us now may have been the very traits which hinder us now may have been the very traits which enabled our forbearers to survive.

How can mindfulness help us with the inherited traits which may not be helpful in our current environment? In mindfulness, we learn to be present with our full experience—the positive and negative alike—and to acknowledge and accept it. When we acknowledge our reactions as parents and accept them for what they are, we can take a more kind and compassionate stance towards ourselves and our children. Paradoxically, when we accept our situation and see it clearly, we are more likely to be able to make changes.

In this chapter, we will discuss the evolutionary basis of parenting and parenting stress and the evolution of attachment, empathy, and compassion. We will discuss how this perspective is relevant to our experience as parents in the twenty-first century and how mindfulness can help us to respond more wisely to our inherited reactions.

SOURCES OF OUR PARENTING STRESS

Why is parenting stressful? From an evolutionary perspective, there are at least four sources of parenting stress: the enormous resources required to raise a human child to maturity, the difference in our modern family environment compared to the environment in which we evolved, our inherited affect regulation system, and our inherited attachment system.

RAISING A HUMAN CHILD TO MATURITY TAKES A LOT OF RESOURCES

Raising a human child requires an enormous expenditure of resources. No other species invests as much time and resources in the rearing of its young. For example, even compared to our closest primate relatives, the great apes, who care for their young for 4–7 years, our burden as human parents is much greater, extending to 18 years or more of caring and providing food (not to mention paying for college after that!) (Hrdy, 2009). Yet we rarely acknowledge the enormousness of this burden. Instead, we are often confronted with images of parenthood, and especially motherhood, which are idealized. This can leave many parents feeling guilty or inadequate when they fail to live up to these unrealistic standards.

In fact, throughout the course of our human history, motherhood and fatherhood have required a balancing of the resources a parent needs to take care of herself against the enormous resources required to raise her offspring. Sarah Hrdy points out that when resources are insufficient, "maternal instincts" such as the motivation, commitment, and ability to care for infants will also be diminished. For example, Hrdy notes that human pregnancy and child-rearing have evolved to ensure an optimal balance between the resources required to raise a child and the resources available to a mother. Among our hunter–gatherer ancestors, the number of offspring born by a mother was regulated through a delicate balance between the environmental conditions and her reproductive physiology. For example, the onset of menarche is triggered only when girls have developed a sufficient proportion of body. During the Pleistocene era, when modern humans evolved, only girls living in an environment of plentiful food who were being fed by their own mothers or other caretakers would have been able to reach menarche and bear children. In this way, natural selection ensured that young women who became pregnant would bear children in an environment which could help them provide for those children—an environment rich in both resources and caretakers. Breast-feeding provided a further form of birth control: during the 2–4-year period of breast-feeding which was typical during this period, a mother would not ovulate and usually would not be able to become pregnant. This prevented mothers from being burdened by caring for too many infants or young children at once. These natural checks on pregnancy have been lost in modern times. Having enough body fat to trigger the onset of menarche is no longer a mark of having enough resources to care for a child, and most women do not breast-feed long enough to benefit from the natural contraception it provides (Hrdy, 1999).

SHARED CARE: MOTHERS HAVE ALWAYS NEEDED HELP WITH CHILDCARE

Another source of stress for modern parents is that our current environment differs radically from the environment of our hunter–gatherer ancestors, in which over 90% of our evolution took place (Konner, 2010). In contrast to our modern idea of the nuclear family—parents and children living separately under one roof—in most of our evolutionary history, communal living was the norm. Evolutionary anthropologists have studied modern hunter–gatherer cultures in Africa and South America to learn more about how our ancestors are likely to have lived. From systematic observation of many of these cultures, they have concluded that humans evolved as *cooperative breeders* (Hrdy, 2009; Konner, 2010). In other words, mothers had help from others to care for their young.

In cooperative breeding species, offspring are cared for and given food not only by mothers but also by other individuals or *allomothers*, which can include fathers, grandparents, older siblings, aunts, and even unrelated members of the community. While cooperative breeding has been described in many other species, from bees to some canine and primate species—it is only recently that evolutionary theorists have recognized the importance of cooperative breeding for human evolution. The evidence from evolutionary research indicates that for most of our evolutionary history, mothers have had help from multiple caregivers to raise their children (Hrdy, 2009; Konner, 2010). Our Western expectation that mothers should care exclusively for infants and children without other help is simply not consistent with our evolutionary history and adaptation.

IMPLICATIONS FOR MODERN PARENTING

From an evolutionary perspective, the nuclear family is actually an aberration in the history of human beings rather than being the "natural" way things have always been. Sarah Hrdy dates the nuclear family back to the 1950s ideal of one parent working and one parent staying at home full-time, which was only possible due to the postwar economic boom. As she puts it, the nuclear family is just a "blip in time" when viewed from the longer perspective of evolutionary history (Hrdy, 2009). Ironically, the improved standard of living which we now enjoy in Western cultures comes at a high price for mothers: a job which formerly was shared by multiple, closely-related, trusted, and highly motivated caretakers, including grandmothers, aunts, and cousins, now falls largely on the shoulders of mothers (and in some cases fathers). Although most women in the West have access to unparalleled reproductive freedom, it is not uncommon for women to bear children at much closer intervals than our ancestors in the Pleistocene. When we consider that most mothers and fathers in industrialized societies work outside the home, and the lack of good-quality or affordable childcare, it is not surprising that many parents experience stress. Put simply, compared to our hunter–gatherer ancestors, our childcare burden is *higher* (our children are more closely spaced) and our childcare resources are *lower* (we have less support from other caretakers, we live in relative social isolation, and we have less time for caring for our children due to demands of work). While we may beat out our forbearers in a fashion competition, for quality parenting, our hunter–gatherer ancestors take the prize.

HOW CAN MINDFULNESS HELP?

The lesson from our evolutionary history is that we have always needed to balance the demands of parenting with taking care of ourselves, and that we can only care for our children when we have sufficient resources to care for ourselves *and* for them. Even when parents have sufficient financial resources to provide for their children, they may struggle to balance the demands of children, family, and work. When the physical and emotional demands of parenting exceed our limits, we may feel stressed, exhausted, inadequate, depressed, or self-critical. In modern Western culture, we put a high premium on doing as much as possible, and acknowledging our limits can be perceived as weakness. But in our evolutionary history, children were more likely to survive when parents had sufficient resources to raise them, including childcare help from others (Hrdy, 2009).

In the initial Mindful Parenting sessions, we invite parents to become aware of their parenting stress as they experience it in their bodies, thoughts, and feelings. We acknowledge that parenting is very demanding and that we evolved in environments which provided greater communal support for rearing children. This can help parents acknowledge and accept their own parenting stress with self-compassion. It also helps parents make room for their own needs, by asking *What do I need?* instead of *What's wrong with me?* We can begin to examine the balance of our lives and ask how we can take better care of ourselves and how we can get additional resources and help.

EVOLUTION OF SHARED CARE

How and why did we evolve to be cooperative breeders, and what are the implications for parenting, child development, and human nature? These are some of the questions Sarah Hrdy has asked in her study of the evolutionary basis of motherhood and parenting. Her answer to these questions begins with another question: how could human beings ever have evolved to have such slow-growing, big-brained offspring who are born entirely dependent on parental care and who remain dependent on parental care and provisioning for so many years? This question becomes especially difficult to answer when we consider the fact that the fathers' involvement in caring for their children, though much greater in humans than in most other primates, has been extremely variable throughout the course of our evolution, up until the present (Hrdy, 2009).

Hrdy's answer is that mothers have always needed to find extra help to raise their children. The only way mothers could have possibly raised their slow-growing, costly, and dependent children during the period in which anatomically modern humans evolved is if they were able to get help in rearing these young. Human children require huge caloric and caretaking resources from birth to maturity in order to survive. Even compared to our closest ape relatives, human children are dependent on parental care much longer. Yet despite the enormous caloric needs and length of dependency of human young, human mothers actually give birth more frequently than do ape mothers. (Modern hunter–gatherer mothers give birth roughly every 3–4 years, whereas great ape mothers give birth at intervals of approximately 6 years.) How could human mothers have evolved to be more successful at breeding than other great apes, given the higher costs of raising a child? Hrdy's answer is simple: they had good help. Cooperative breeding—extra hands to help out with childcare—may explain why our ancestors were able to outbreed their ape relatives and go on to populate the world (Hrdy, 2009).

WHO HELPED MOTHERS RAISE THEIR CHILDREN?

If our ancestors needed help rearing their costly and dependent young, who would have been available to help? One answer is fathers, and indeed human fathers are unusual compared to fathers of most other mammalian and primate species in the degree of parental care they provide. However, paternal involvement in childcare is extremely variable among all human populations studied, ranging from the extremes of no contact after fertilization, to high degrees of father involvement observed in a few hunter–gatherer societies or among Western stay-at-home dads (Hewlett, 2004; Hrdy, 2009; Konner, 2010). It's not that dads aren't important—they clearly are and have been from an evolutionary point of view. The puzzle is how our ancestors could have been so successful at reproducing, outbreeding our other primate relatives, and eventually populating diverse environments around the world, given that mothers could not possibly rear their offspring alone and that mothers could not necessarily count on fathers helping out.

A couple decades ago, a few evolutionary anthropologists began asking the question: who else could have helped mothers provide for their young during our long evolution? Their answer to that question is grandmothers. Anthropologist Kristen Hawkes and her colleagues systematically measured the amount of food brought back by each individual in a modern hunter–gatherer society. They discovered that grandmothers were bringing back substantial amounts of food such as root vegetables and nuts, much more than had previously been recognized (Hawkes, O'Connell, & Blurton Jones, 1989). In contrast, men often came back empty-handed from hunting expeditions, due to the difficulty of killing large game. While previous evolutionary theorists had emphasized fathers' hunting of meat as the most important source of food for children, Hawkes' research documented that the vegetables and nuts obtained by grandmothers were essential for sustaining the population on a day-to-day basis, in the absence of a big game win. With this study, Hawkes and her colleagues provided empirical evidence for the role of grandmothers in providing food and increasing the survival chance of their grandchildren.

The positive effect of grandmothers on child survival rates may help explain one puzzling aberration in our life history: human females are the only mammals who live out a significant portion of their lives after menopause. Hawkes hypothesized that mother-child food sharing among our ancestors may have led to the evolution of longer postmenopausal lifespans in human females. After weaning, human children are too small to be able to get their own food. Mothers' sharing of difficult-to-obtain foods like root vegetables would have been critical for child survival. (While it may seem obvious that mothers would share their food with their children, among the great apes, very little food sharing takes place between mothers and offspring after weaning.) A grandmother, by helping her daughter to obtain these foods and sharing them with grandchildren, would have increased her daughter's reproductive success, allowing her daughter to care for a newborn infant while the grandmother helped provide food for older but still dependent children. Over time, this would have led to selection for women living longer past menopause, as the effort of postmenopausal women would have increased the survival chance of their daughters, granddaughters, and nieces (Hawkes, O'Connell, Blurton Jones, Alvarez, & Charnov, 1998). There is evidence supporting this hypothesis from studies of modern hunter–gatherer cultures demonstrating that having a maternal grandmother around increases the likelihood of grandchild survival (Hrdy, 2009). While in current Western cultures we may emphasize the younger generation taking care of older people as an important ethical value, Hawkes points out that in our evolutionary history, it went the other way: postmenopausal women would have only survived if their presence increased the reproductive success of their daughters and the survival of granddaughters and nieces.

A final puzzle in our evolution as cooperative breeders is the question of why our ancestors would have trusted anyone else to care for their young. In the wild, an ape mother will almost never relinquish her baby to another ape even to hold, much less to "babysit." This is because of the very real risks of infanticide by a male from another troop or of being stolen by another female. Sarah Hrdy wonders what conditions might have enabled a primate mother to risk allowing someone else to care for her young. She hypothesizes that two factors may have been important for the evolution of mothers' entrusting their young to other caretakers. First, apes that were able to live close to their own mothers might have dared to let their own mother, a trusted figure, care for their young. Second, as our ancestors evolved to have increasing cognitive abilities, mothers would have been able to make risk-benefit calculations. For example, a mother could weigh the risk of leaving her baby alone compared to allowing a trusted relative to hold her. To the extent that this increased her reproductive success and the survival of her young, this trait—being willing to trust another with her baby—would have been selected for over the course of our evolution (Hrdy, 2009).

Indeed, in contrast to our ape relatives, human mothers share their babies very easily and eagerly (Hrdy, 2009). Think about what happens in many cultures today when a new baby comes into the family. Everyone comes to visit, and everyone wants to hold the baby, especially grandma and grandpa! I still remember the smile on my mother's face when she first held my newborn daughter. What a prize to hold a new baby in your arms! In some family gatherings, the new baby is held so much by others that the mother barely has a chance to hold her newborn herself, as the baby is passed from one eager relative to the next. Among modern hunter–gatherer groups, baby sharing can be even more extensive. For example, Hadza newborns are held by alloparents—grandmothers, great-aunts, older sibling, or fathers—85% of the time in the days following birth. Efe and Aka women pass newborns around to other female relatives, even allowing them to suckle in the period before the mother's own milk comes in. Efe newborns have been found to have on average 14 different caretakers in their first days (Hrdy, 2009). Among all hunter–gatherer peoples studied, babies are held, cared for, and provisioned by multiple caretakers from birth on. This provisioning would have been essential to help a mother provide food for her children during the many years of dependency, especially after weaning (Hrdy, 2009).

Sarah Hrdy understands human mothers' greater willingness to trust others to care for their newborns compared to other apes as a consequence of their awareness of their need for help from their community to raise their babies:

> Conscious awareness that they will need help rearing their babies renders human mothers more discriminating. Mothers also understand how beneficial it is for a baby to be introduced to a community of others. By sharing her baby, the mother sends a clear signal that both she and her offspring will be counting on help from the clan. By exposing alloparents to the sight, sound, and smell of her alluring little charge, the mother lays the groundwork for emotional ties binding her baby to potential caretakers and vice versa. . . . If human mothers exhibit greater postpartum tolerance of others, it must be because they are more confident of the benign intentions of those around them. Their trust is sufficient to override the compulsive hypervigilance universally found in new ape mothers.
>
> (Hrdy, *Mothers and Others*, pp. 78–79)

Being close to trusted family members—her own mother, sisters, aunts, and so on—may have given early human mothers the degree of trust and security needed to risk allowing others to care for her baby, helping to set the stage for the evolution of shared care (Hrdy, 2009).

SOCIAL SUPPORT AND MATERNAL AMBIVALENCE

One consequence of human mothers' need to assess and find adequate help to raise her young is that we have evolved to be very sensitive to social support. A mother raising her young in the Pleistocene, where infant mortality could be as high as 50%, would almost certainly have needed help from others in order for her children to survive. Human mothers have therefore evolved to be sensitive to social support. In our evolutionary history, a pregnant woman has needed to ask the question: *Who's going to help me raise this baby?* Assessing who is available—*and safe*—to help her take care of her baby is a skill which would have been highly adaptive for a mother (Hrdy, 2009).

However, as Hrdy points out, there is a serious downside to our sensitivity to support. If a human mother perceives that there is insufficient help for raising her infant, her commitment to her infant may be affected. Human mothers, unlike our great ape relatives, show maternal ambivalence. For example, while abandonment or infanticide by a great ape mother is virtually unheard of, it does occur among human mothers, albeit rarely. Hrdy understands this in the context of the importance of shared care in our evolutionary history. Human mothers, who could not possibly have raised their young without help from others, have evolved to be sensitive to the availability of support from others. When a human mother perceives that support is lacking or insufficient, her investment in her child may be diminished, and in some cases, she may abandon her child (Hrdy, 2009). This is usually a last resort and a very painful one for the mother. Nonetheless, it does occur in humans, whereas it is unknown among our ape relatives.

Unlike her ape counterpart, a human mother has the cognitive capacity to assess her situation and imagine the future. She knows that she cannot raise her infant without help. Her ambivalence arises out of needing to assess her infant's prospects, based on the amount of help she thinks she will get. For an ape mother, however, perception of support is simply not relevant. She does not depend on shared care, and furthermore, she would not hand her child over to another ape because the risks would be too high. The social support that a human mother perceives is available to her is therefore extremely important for her commitment and motivation to care for her infant (Hrdy, 2009).

IMPLICATIONS FOR MODERN PARENTS: SOCIAL SUPPORT AND MATERNAL AMBIVALENCE

What are the implications of this for modern mothers and fathers? As mothers, we have evolved to be sensitive to the availability of support in raising our children. On some level, we are constantly assessing who is available to help, whether our child will be safe and well cared for, and how we can line up more help when needed. Not surprisingly, both material and emotional support have been associated with positive maternal behavior (Konner, 2010). The amount of social support a mother feels has also been found to affect the quality of her attachment to her infant in studies of both Western and non-Western cultures (Belsky, 1999). Given our sensitivity to help, it is logical that when we perceive that we don't have enough help, we will feel stressed, anxious, and potentially ambivalent about our childcare burden or commitment. This in turn may be communicated to our child, thereby affecting our attachment relationship and other aspects of our parenting.

HOW CAN MINDFULNESS HELP?

In our Mindful Parenting groups, social support for parenting is an important theme. Many mothers feel they should be able to cope with the demands of parenting, regardless of how much help they have or how burdened they are with other responsibilities. For example, Linda, a mother with a new baby and two toddlers at home, felt disappointed in herself for not being able to enjoy her children more and for how exhausted she felt when she had to take care of them by herself. She had returned to a demanding job and felt that she should be able to handle that as well. It was difficult for her to accept just how demanding her childcare load could be at times. Her attitude was, "It's not so bad, I can handle it." Yet emotionally, she was exhausted and felt disappointed in herself. This kind of dichotomy—thinking, on the one hand, "I can handle it" but feeling emotionally overwhelmed, tearful, depressed, or guilty—comes up often in our groups. Intellectually, these mothers have absorbed the message that they should be able to handle it all—the kids, the career—and without complaining. But their bodies and emotions tell another story, which has to do with their sensitivity to the emotional and practical support that they need. Our assumption is that when we feel stressed, tired, anxious, or depressed or ambivalent, this is not a sign of pathology but rather a sign that we need to pay closer attention to our situation and our needs. Instead of asking, *What's wrong with me?* or *Why can't I handle this?* we encourage parents to ask themselves: *What do I need right now? What kind of support would help me?*

IMPLICATIONS OF SHARED CARE IN A MODERN WESTERN CONTEXT

What relevance does our history as cooperative breeders have for the struggles of modern parents, most of whom are living in relative isolation from extended family, and who have limited opportunities to share the burden of childcare? From an evolutionary perspective, mothers have always looked for help raising their children, but now that help is more difficult to come by. One consequence of Western family lifestyle is that parents shoulder more of the burden of childcare directly. Informal childcare by family members or as-if family members is hard to come by (although I am impressed by the number of friends who try to move close to their mothers, if possible, when they have children). For most of us raising children far away from close family in modern Western societies, paid or institutionalized care—babysitters, daycare, school teachers, and after-school programs—has replaced kinship-based alloparental care. One of the practical issues is ensuring the availability and quality of this care, which lies more in the hands of government or community agencies. In our evolutionary history, a mother tried to ensure the best care possible for her children by lining up fathers or other trusted close kin like grandmothers, aunts, or older siblings. She also could count on these family members being motivated to invest in caring for her children. Nowadays, parents often have less choice and control over who cares for their children. For example, while the sensitivity of daycare providers has been linked to infant attachment (e.g., NICHD Early Child Care Research Network, 2003), high quality daycare is not available for many parents who need it, particularly lower-income parents. Furthermore, unrelated caretakers may not be as motivated to invest in a child as they are in a relative. Mothers often express worry or guilt about their childcare choices, yet this is not a new problem! We have always needed to find good help for raising our kids.

One interesting phenomenon is the development of near-kin relationships. When parents find themselves far away from biological kin, they often attempt to re-create kinship-like relationships which serve many of the same functions as actual kin such as providing social support and care for children (Bailey & Wood, 1998). I was fascinated to read about this because, raising my children in New York City where I had no close relatives nearby, I indeed created my own near-kinship support system, although I wasn't aware of it at the time. Brooklyn was (and still is) a paradise for new parents. Apartments are tiny, and new parents flock outside to escape their tiny living rooms and to meet other adults in the playgrounds which are found every few blocks. What we lacked in living space—875 sq. ft in a third story walkup with no garden—was vastly compensated for by this community, ready and waiting, outside our door. Everywhere you went you would see groups of new mothers congregating on park benches and in coffee shops, with babies in tow or strapped to them in baby bjorns. Soon I had a cadre of new friends, all new mothers with infants born within weeks of my own. These mothers provided the emotional support—the pat on the back when you were feeling exhausted, incompetent, anxious, or insecure—and actual support, taking your baby for a few minutes while you ran to the bathroom, later on caring for her for a whole morning if necessary, and even "provisioning" your baby as well. It was like a warm bath for all of us mothers, and the fact that many of us were transplants to New York who didn't have family close by helped us to bond with each other as if we were family. Looking back at this, I am astonished to think how much of the new parent bonding fits in our long evolutionary history of shared care.

WHAT ABOUT FATHERS?

By now many of you, especially the fathers among you, may be asking, what about fathers? Michael Lamb has conducted decades of research on the impact of fathers on children's development and has documented the social, emotional, and educational benefits that fathers bring to children (Tamis-Lemonda, 2004). Yet the evolutionary perspective shows that fathers have not always been necessary for survival and that there is a great deal of variation in the involvement of fathers. For example, in some hunter–gatherer cultures, father involvement has not been associated with increased child survival (Marlowe, 2000). How can we make sense of this?

Reading the literature on father involvement, the key word which comes through is *variability*. Compared to most other mammals and primate species, human fathers' involvement in parenting is much greater (Konner, 1010). However, in our evolutionary history and in modern industrialized and non-industrialized cultures, fathers' involvement in their children's lives has been highly variable, from no involvement, to full-time "househusbands" or the highly involved fathers among the Aka foraging people (Hewlett. 2004). The lesson of our evolutionary history is that while the involvement of fathers has very often increased the survival chance of children, fathers have not always been around to help raise children. This variability has meant that a savvy mother has had to line up additional help for her young to ensure their survival. Mothers' flexibility in finding care for their young may be one of the most adaptive traits with regard to successful child-rearing. It's not that mothers don't want or need fathers to be involved. On the contrary, human mothers have found all sorts of ways to keep fathers involved in helping to raise children (Hrdy, 1999). But, when fathers have not been available, the flexibility and resourcefulness of human mothers have enabled them to find extra help from other trusted sources: grandmothers, older siblings, aunts, and even non-related members of the community (Hrdy, 2009). This point is still relevant today: no matter how good the intentions of all parties involved, relationships end, marriages break up, and there is no guarantee that every child will have an involved father—or any father— in the picture for his entire childhood.

What factors lead to fathers becoming more involved with their children? Barry Hewlett, an anthropologist who has studied father–infant relations among hunter–gatherer cultures, suggests that proximity breeds paternal caretaking and loving impulses. Hewlett lived among the Aka foragers, who have the highest degree of father involvement ever recorded in a culture. Hewlett observed that Aka fathers were often in close physical proximity of their infants and were more likely to show physical affection such as kissing or hugging infants, compared to Aka mothers. Furthermore, in contrast to the rough and tumble play which has been found to characterize father–child interactions in urban industrialized cultures, Aka fathers did not often play in a vigorous or highly stimulating way with their children. To explain the difference between Aka and Western fathers, Hewlett notes that Aka fathers, by virtue of their close contact with their children, knew them intimately and could more easily understand their communications (Hewlett, 2004). Knowing their children intimately, they interacted with them in more quiet ways and did not need to resort to vigorous physical play to interact with their children:

> . . . Aka fathers were not vigorous because they intimately knew their infants through their extensive care. Because Aka fathers knew their infants so well, they did not have to use vigorous play to initiate communication or interaction with their infants. They could initiate communication and show their love in other ways. Infants often initiated communication, and Aka fathers knew how to understand their infants' verbal and nonverbal (e.g., via touch) communication. Fathers (or mothers) who are not around their infants are less likely to be able to read and understand infant communication and therefore more likely to initiate communication, often with the use of physical stimulation and play.
>
> (Hewlett, 2004, p. 189)

Hewlett also notes that among the Aka, mothers, fathers, and children participate in net hunting. Through hunting, Aka fathers stay in close contact with their children, which may explain their intimate knowledge of them (Hewlett, 2004). Sarah Hrdy likewise emphasizes the importance of proximity and experience for eliciting paternal caretaking impulses. When fathers have the opportunity to be around their children and be directly involved in their care, they can develop very strong paternal caretaking feelings and attachments, and there is research showing that fathers show hormonal changes when in the presence of pregnant women and babies (Konner, 2010). Hrdy hypothesizes that paternal caretaking, while variable in our evolutionary history, goes back a very long time and was probably already present in the Pleistocene (Hrdy, 2009). The idea of proximity breeding intimacy for fathers brought back memories of my husband caring for our newborn daughter. He had a flexible job, and every Thursday he took full responsibility of her. During this day I had to get out of sight so that he could be the only parent, without my interference. Their time alone together was critical for their bonding, since I was not available for breast-feeding or comforting. Instead, my husband gave our baby a bottle, changed diapers, comforted her, put her down for naps, and did whatever else was necessary. On these Thursdays, he gravitated to other dads pushing babies in swings or simply hanging out in the playgrounds, separate from the groups of mothers. Pretty soon he had found one, then two, then three other dads with flexible schedules who also had infant daughters. They began to meet informally on Thursdays, often picking up a new member at the park. Before long, there were 8–10 regulars in the dad's group, who would meet en mass on Thursdays, take care of and play with the babies, and go out for breakfast at a local coffee shop, where they would receive solicitous attention from the (typically young female) waitress who would be tickled by the sight of eight guys with eight baby girls in tow in slings, baby bjorns, or strollers ("babe magnets with babies" as he liked to joke). What strikes me now about this time he had alone with our daughter was not only the proximity but also that he had sole responsibility for her during this day. He had to learn, just as I did, what all her communications meant, how to get her to sleep, when she was hungry, when to change her, and so on. And he also developed the confidence that he was just as capable of caring for her as I was.

RELEVANCE FOR MODERN FATHERS: WHAT ARE THE
CHALLENGES MODERN FATHERS FACE?

In some ways, expectations have never been so high for fathers. In postindustrial cultures, a father's success and his family's social status are measured in large part by his economic success. At the same time, fathers are expected to be more involved than ever, changing diapers, doing dishes, and providing sensitive care to children while still providing financially for their families (Tamis-Lemonda, 2004). These expectations may conflict with each other. Fathers may want to have more contact with their children, but the financial pressure of providing for their family often takes priority over having time to spend with their family.

A second challenge is that fathers come to parenting with extremely variable experiences with their own fathers, ranging from fathers who have never met their own father, to fathers who have had a close relationship with a nurturing father who was emotionally available, and many types of relationships in between. Some fathers say things like "My father did not know how to relate to me emotionally. He worked hard, paid the bills, but it was my mother I turned to when I needed someone. I don't know how to be the kind of father I want to be for my children."

MINDFUL FATHERING: HOW CAN MINDFULNESS HELP?

We often hear the poignant longing from fathers wishing they had been able to connect with their own fathers or wanting to be emotionally present for their children. This is the first step towards becoming the father they would like to be. By recognizing the emotional impact of their own experience, fathers can emotionally integrate their own experience into a coherent understanding of themselves. Fathers can also draw on relationships with others who may have been there for them emotionally—an uncle, teacher, stepfather, and so on. Fathers who have had a close relationship with their mother or other female figure can draw on this as well. One of the important findings from the research on fathers is that the qualities of a father and his relationship with his child are more important for children as maternal warmth and closeness (Tamis-Lemonda, 2004). Research on attachment also shows that having multiple secure attachments is optimal for a child's development, so a secure relationship with the father is beneficial (Van IJzendoorn, Sagi, & Lambermon, 1992).

Not only can fathers provide warmth and closeness as mothers do, they also may provide different parenting behaviors from mothers that may have an important function in raising children. Several researchers have proposed that fathers' more frequent rough and tumble play and their greater tendency to challenge their children and compete with them may help to "toughen them up" and prepare them for dealing with the outside world (Lamb, 2003; Paquette, 2004). Bögels and colleagues suggest that fathers' evolutionarily based greater expertise in dealing with certain challenges in the outside world and in taking risks may make them particularly important in helping their children overcome fears and develop confidence (Bögels & Perotti, 2011; Bögels & Phares, 2008; Möller, Majdandzic, de Vente, & Bögels, 2013).

What's our message to fathers? The message from research is clear —you can make a big difference to your children. But perhaps the strongest message is to simply ask, "What would you have wanted or needed from your dad?" or, "What did your dad give to you that was important?"

and, most importantly, "What do you want to give to your own children?" By connecting with their own experience, fathers can feel the importance and weight of their role in their children's lives.

EVOLUTION OF OUR AFFECT REGULATION SYSTEMS: THREAT, DRIVE, AND CONTENTMENT

Another reason that modern parenting can be stressful is that the brain and hormonal systems underlying much of our automatic and emotional reactions evolved long ago, when we lived in very different environments with very different types of threats. Anatomically modern humans have been around for roughly 10,000–100,000 years, yet the lives we lead, and the environments and threats to our survival have changed dramatically (Konner, 2010). One of the goals of mindfulness is to replace automatic reactivity in parenting situations with nonreactive awareness. But it's important to acknowledge that the biological systems which have evolved to subserve our emotional and behavioral reactions are set up for automatic reactivity, and these reactions can be triggered by situations quite different from what our forbearers were facing. It therefore takes consistent and intentional effort to learn to respond differently. It also means that we are not entirely to blame for our reactivity.

Paul Gilbert's model of three circles of affect regulation—threat, drive, and contentment/affiliation—can help us put parental reactivity in a larger context. Gilbert describes how our threat system evolved in tandem with our drive system and our contentment/affiliation system to regulate our emotional lives and behavior. Our drive system is essential for motivating us to seek rewards, resources, mates, and achievements, and it is associated with feelings of pleasure. But for many of us, this system is on overdrive. We are constantly doing, achieving, and striving, and when we are not, we may feel depleted or self-critical. Our threat system is also overactive but is triggered now more often in interpersonal or social situations than in situations of actual physical danger. Gilbert argues that our drive system also interacts with our threat system. For example, we may pursue achievements and goals in order to avoid feeling inferior or rejected, or we may feel that we "should" do certain things, to avoid feeling shame, guilt, or bad about ourselves. The third system, our contentment/affiliation system, has evolved from our attachment system. Unlike the charged, excited, pleasurable positive emotions of our drive system, this system is associated with feelings of calm, peacefulness, security, and safety (Gilbert, 2009). Oxytocin, the hormone which is released during breast-feeding, lovemaking, and during other bonding experiences, is associated with this system. Oxytocin plays a role in calming the autonomic nervous system after a stressful experience and helps us to establish close emotional bonds in times of stress (Carter, 1998). In our modern lifestyle, this system is often underactivated.

IMPLICATIONS FOR MODERN PARENTING

As Gilbert points out, these systems have evolved to help us survive, and we still need all three systems. However, when these systems get out of balance, we suffer. When our drive system is too strong, we are too much in doing mode; when our threat system is overactive, we react in fear and aversion. Our contentment/affiliation system which supports our need to bond with others, and which enables us to feel calm, content, and soothed, tends to be underemphasized in Western industrialized cultures (Gilbert. 2009). This can lead us to feel driven to achieve and by our automatic stress reactions. Yet a growing body of literature shows that secure attachments bring not only psychological benefits such as feelings of security and trust but also physiological and neurochemical benefits (Carter, 1998).

HOW CAN MINDFULNESS HELP?

The goal of mindfulness is not to eliminate any of these systems but to help restore the balance. With mindfulness, we learn to be aware of our experience, noticing when we are in doing mode or when we react with fear and aversion. We learn to accept these experiences as being part of our inherited human nature, instead of rejecting them or criticizing ourselves for these reactions. We can respond more compassionately towards ourselves, when we understand our reactions as a part of how we have evolved as humans. We can form the intention to respond differently to our automatic reactions, by pausing and simply allowing things to be the way they are.

With mindfulness practice, we shift into being mode instead of doing mode, reducing activation of our drive and threat systems. We can also actively strengthening our natural contentment system, in order to help reduce the negative effect of our drive and threat systems and to increase the positive emotions of calm and contentment. For example, spending time by simply being with our children with full attention rather than having to achieve something can help us activate our affiliation system and develop a stronger attachment with our children. Meditation practices which cultivate compassion may also activate our affiliation system and reduce our threat system, leading to greater balance. There is increasing scientific evidence demonstrating that mindfulness and compassion meditation lead to changes in brain activation which are associated with positive emotional states, supporting this hypothesis (Davidson & Begley, 2012).

REACTIVE PARENTING FROM AN EVOLUTIONARY PERSPECTIVE: OUR THREAT SYSTEM

In our experience as parents, and in our parenting groups, we have observed how we often have strong, even explosive emotional reactions more often with our children and partners. Why we would have evolved as a species to be more likely to "lose it," in exactly the situations where it can do the most harm—with our children or other loved ones? From an evolutionary perspective, *reactive* parenting may have evolved precisely because it short-circuited higher cortical functioning, thereby saving precious seconds which could prove crucial in life or death situations of our forbearers. In situations of potential danger, reacting without thinking may have been the strategy that won the day, leading over time to selection for this trait.

When we look at anxiety from an evolutionary point of view, it is easy to see how reactive, anxious, or overprotective parenting may have helped our ancestors in the Pleistocene survive. As Joseph LeDoux's research on the brain mechanisms underlying anxiety makes clear, we have evolved to be really good threat detectors. Put simply, in the environment of our ancestors, it paid to be a little paranoid. That is, individuals with brains that could quickly detect potential threats and react automatically were more likely to survive and leave offspring. LeDoux gives the example of a hiker who mistakes a stick on the path for a snake and who reacts automatically by jumping back in fear. This so-called low-road reaction—the fast, automatic reaction to perceived threat which is mediated by the limbic system and which bypasses higher cortical involvement—was clearly advantageous in our evolutionary past, when we lived among predators. Our modern-day hiker, after his initial shock, may sheepishly laugh off his mistake, but it's no coincidence that we have the tendency to react first, think later when in danger: this capacity gave our ancestors a survival advantage (LeDoux, 1996). Paul Gilbert uses the expression "Better safe than sorry" to describe how our brains are designed to make mistakes when it comes to assessments of threat (P. Gilbert, p.c., June 23, 2012). Keeping in mind just how vulnerable infants and children were to threats, we can see how a mother who was "overprotective" or "anxious" would have been more likely to leave behind surviving off-spring who would carry those traits.

IMPLICATIONS FOR MODERN PARENTING

Once again, the problem is that our environments have changed radically since that time, while our affect regulation system has not had time to evolve further. It's still set on "maximal threat detection" when, in fact, these kinds of physical threats are no longer our greatest threat to survival. As parents, our caretaking and protective traits towards our precious young are highly evolved. That means that our threat system can be easily triggered when we worry about our children. In situations of actual physical danger, this can still occasionally be useful. When my son used to run blindly into the street, my automatic reaction of running after him, yelling at him to stop, and grabbing him was clearly beneficial to his survival. But some of our worst parenting moments occur when we react automatically if we feel threatened or feel our children are threatened. When stressed, we can overreact emotionally, and when anxious, we can become overprotective of our children.

Nowadays, however, most of the triggers for feeling threatened involve social threats, as opposed to threats to physical survival. The perceived threat when our child is not invited to a birthday party, or when we are passed over for a promotion at work, are the more likely triggers to feeling threatened nowadays. I was interested to read Sarah Hrdy's description of how high-ranking baboon mothers pass their social status on to their daughters, who in turn enjoy greater reproductive success (Hrdy, 1999). It helped me to understand why sometimes I feel like I am back in junior high school when I'm picking up my children on the schoolyard. Not only do I find myself attending to who is "in" or "out" among the children, I also notice it among the other mothers. While nowadays we may view a mother's anxiety about her child's or her own social status as pathological, in our evolutionary past it may have been crucial for her children's survival.

HOW CAN MINDFULNESS HELP?

From an evolutionary perspective, there is nothing abnormal or pathological about parental anxiety or our automatic reactions (S. Hrdy, p.c., July 1, 2012). We don't need to pathologize a mother or father as being overprotective or overanxious; this is part of our species' inheritance as much as upright walking and speaking are. This perspective can help us to be more accepting of our larger human nature. Mindfulness practice offers the possibility that as we become more aware, we can slow down our automatic reactions, pay attention to what our body is telling us, and pause before allowing our automatic reactions to take their course. We can choose how we want to react or, for that matter, choose *not* to react.

EVOLUTIONARY PERSPECTIVES ON ATTACHMENT

Our attachment system has clear evolutionary advantages for survival and reproduction. John Bowlby defined attachment as "the propensity of human beings to make strong affectional bonds to particular others" (Bowlby, 1977, p. 201). Although attachment behaviors are seen in most mammals, attachment is particularly important for human survival, given the long length of dependence that human children have. In particular, a child's drive to seek proximity with his mother, especially when threatened, had clear survival advantages in our ancestors' environment. Attachment behaviors are triggered by threat or stress situations: when a mother or infant felt threatened, seeking proximity was often the best survival strategy. Bowlby understood attachment behaviors to be normal, evolutionarily adaptive reactions to separations from the mother or to threats of predation. An infant who cries when separated from its mother or is afraid of loud noises or the dark is not pathological, since separations and loud noises would have signaled danger from predators in our evolutionary past. When a child is upset, he naturally seeks proximity to his mother, whose presence comforts him. Having been comforted, he is able to go back out and explore the world (Bowlby, 1971, 1977). Infants who are able to do this after a brief separation from the mother or father are considered "securely attached," and these infants tend to have better social, emotional, and cognitive development (Bretherton, 1992). When a mother responds sensitively to the child's needs, for example, providing comfort and protection when a child is frightened, a child is reassured, and this builds up his experience of feeling safe in the relationship. He also learns that he can turn to his mother when afraid or distressed (Stams, Juffer, & van IJzendoorn, 2002).

Attachment processes also evolved because they helped ensure a mother's commitment of resources to her baby. As we have seen, maternal commitment among humans is not a given. The development of a mother's attachment to her infant is therefore important for ensuring her commitment to him (Hrdy, 2009). Even before a woman gives birth to her infant, her attachment system has been primed through the multiple hormonal and biochemical changes which support her investing in, caring for, and loving her child. When an infant is born, its behaviors also trigger the mother's attachment system. For example, nursing triggers the release of oxytocin, bringing feelings of relaxation and calm, reducing anxiety, and supporting bonding (Carter, 1998). Fathers also undergo similar hormonal changes in reaction to the birth of their infant, although the magnitude is not as great (Carter, 2006).

NEUROENDOCRINE BASIS OF ATTACHMENT

Our attachment system, and the neuroendocrine reactions which subserve it, helps us to fall in love with our infant, motivates us to care for her, and makes us feel happy, safe, and calm when we are bonding with our baby. Oxytocin, the neuropeptide associated with this system, is arguably Mother Nature's love potion, and it's free, 100% natural, and has no negative side effects (except lowered productivity, see below)! Release of oxytocin triggers labor contractions, reduces the stress of birth, and promotes feelings of calm and relaxation after birth. Oxytocin supports bonding between a mother and infant: it stimulates milk let down during breastfeeding and contributes to the feeling of calm that mothers experience after breastfeeding. Oxytocin also buffers the response to stressors, for example, by reducing autonomic nervous system reactivity associated with stress reactions, such as heart rate and blood pressure. Oxytocin also helps restore our feeling of calm, safety, and trust after we have experienced a stress, helping mothers and infants to bond after a stressful experience (Carter, 1998, 2006).

I still remember the slightly drugged, happy, and contented feeling I would have after breast-feeding my newborn daughter, which in the early days seemed to take up the majority of my time. As she would fall into a contented sleep on me, my brain would weakly try to convince myself to get up and do something useful: throw in a load of laundry, empty the dishwasher, clean up the mess in the house, or at least take a shower. But my mind seemed to be slowed and groggy and my body coaxed; why not just sit here for a while, staring at her, inhaling her smell, falling asleep with her? Looking back, I wish I could have enjoyed that precious state more, and turned down the volume in my mind which kept telling me everything I needed to be doing. In fact, I *was* doing everything I needed to be doing.

IMPLICATIONS FOR MODERN PARENTING

Our attachment system is responsible for many of the ways in which we connect and care for our children, and the underlying neuroendocrine reactions ensure that much of this occurs out of our awareness. We have this amazing built-in system which kicks in automatically when we bond with our baby or others, helping us to feel soothed, comforted, and calm, and enabling us to help our children feel soothed, comforted, and safe. All of us have this capacity, built in, and the beauty of it is that our attachment reactions often happen automatically, without our needing to think about it. When our child is suffering or needing something, we often respond immediately by comforting her—this is our attachment heritage in action.

HOW CAN MINDFULNESS HELP?

All we have to do to develop this system is to use it. Although this is a bit of an oversimplification, the basic point is supported by research. When we engage in activities such as being with our children, comforting a friend, acting compassionately towards another, or caring for someone, we activate this system. Touch is the most highly developed sensory modality at birth and is important for caregiving and bonding. Physical touch has been found to release oxytocin, reduce the stress hormone cortisol, and reduce activation of brain areas related to stress. When we engage in soothing activities, especially those involving soothing touch, such as holding our children, physically comforting them, or even physically comforting ourselves when we are upset, we activate this system, which helps us to feel calm and content (Gilbert, 2009; Goetz, Keltner, & Simon-Thomas, 2010; Neff, 2011).

When we practice compassion and loving-kindness meditation, we may also strengthen this system. For example, Richard Davidson and his colleagues have examined the effects of meditation practices on the brain and have found that mindfulness and loving-kindness meditation shifts the brain into a pattern associated with positive mood states (Davidson et al., 2003).

INTERGENERATIONAL TRANSMISSION OF ATTACHMENT

Unfortunately, there can also be a down side to our automatic attachment reactions. We tend to repeat the automatic attachment and parenting interactions we experienced with our own parents (van IJzendoorn, 1995). If we've had less than optimal parenting experiences, this can make it difficult for us to establish a secure attachment relationship with our child. For example, parents who were abused as children may have a higher risk for abusing their own children, although many parents who were abused do not abuse their own children (Egeland, Jacobvitz, & Sroufe, 1988). Think about your own experience as a parent: how often have you found yourself, in the heat of the moment with your child, saying or doing something exactly like your mother or father, despite the fact that you swore never to do that?

Marinus van IJzendoorn has examined how attachment patterns are transmitted from one generation to another. In a large meta-analysis (a study combining the findings of many separate studies), he found that a mother's understanding of her own attachment relationships during her life was the strongest predictor of whether her infant would be securely or insecurely attached to her, better than observed interactions between her and her infant. Think about this for a moment: what counts most for your infant's attachment to you is your internalized story about how you felt in your most significant attachment relationships, more than what you actually *do* as a parent. Van IJzendoorn calls this the "transmission gap," since we are unable to measure exactly how these mental representations of attachment lead to the observed attachment behavior in infants (van IJzendoorn, 1995). This transmission gap might be the reason why some parents don't respond as well to behavioral parent training courses, which focus on teaching parents basic parenting skills. For parents with insecure attachment backgrounds, "doing" all the right things might not be sufficient if they are experiencing other feelings about their own attachment relationships from the past. What we communicate nonverbally, on an emotional level, may be more important for our children than what we say or do, especially when it comes to attachment (Siegel & Hartzell, 2003). And, as we will explore below, human babies have evolved to be very sensitive to reading the intentions of their mothers and other caretakers, since their very survival has depended upon securing their commitment (Hrdy, 2009). Not surprisingly, human children may be more sensitive to the nonverbal communication about attachment rather than what parents actually say.

IMPLICATIONS OF ATTACHMENT RESEARCH FOR MODERN PARENTING: A SILVER LINING?

There is an important silver lining behind these findings about the transmission of attachment patterns from one generation to the next. These studies measure mothers' attachment *representations*—how mothers make sense of their attachment in a coherent and emotionally inte-grated way. This is regardless of whether a mother has had a secure or insecure attachment to her own parents. In fact, the research suggests that adults can "earn" attachment security, even if they had an insecure attachment to their own parent, by reflecting on their attachment experi-ences and understanding the emotional impact on relationships in the present.

It's also important to keep in mind that attachment relationships continue to develop and change throughout an individual's life. For example, developmental psychologist Alan Sroufe found that infants who had been insecure in infancy but were rated as secure in adolescence had a better outcome than those who were insecure at both time points or than those who switched from being secure in infancy to insecure at adolescence (Sroufe, Carlson, Levy, & Egeland, 1999). An experimental study of infants born in a Romanian orphanage makes an even more com-pelling case for the plasticity of attachment relationships. In this study, infants were randomly assigned to care as usual (remaining in orphanage) or placement in foster care. Children who were placed in foster care made significant gains in their attachment security compared to those who remained in the orphanage, despite the fact that before placement, more than 75% showed insecure attachment or no attachment behaviors (Smyke, Zeanah, Fox, Nelson, & Guthrie, 2010).

HOW CAN MINDFULNESS HELP?

These findings offer a beacon of hope for parents. Many of the par-ents we see in Mindful Parenting groups have not had the best experi-ences with their own parents. Some ask, "How can I be there for my child when I never had that myself?" The answer to this question, based on the research, is that it *is* possible to overcome even a very difficult or abusive childhood, if we are willing to do the emotional work of integrating these experiences and becoming aware of how they may arise in our pres-ent relationships with our children and other attachment partners. It is by no means easy, and not every parent will be willing to do the work or capable of making change. But, we are certainly not doomed to repeat the patterns of our parents, if we are motivated to become aware and make the intention to do things differently.

We address this in the Mindful Parenting course in two ways. First, we invite parents to become aware of repeating patterns of interaction with their children. Then, we ask them to explore whether these pat-terns, are similar to interactions from the past and the emotions attached to it as something which doesn't belong to the current situation with their child, and make a conscious choice how to respond. This recognizing and letting go of older patterns can help parents disengage from dysfunctional or even abusive parenting interactions.

A second way we address it is by exploring parent's attachment relationship with their child. We begin by inviting parents to observe their child mindfully and to practice mindful listening and speaking with their child. Simply giving this kind of full attention to a child helps to build the attachment relationship. We also use Dan Siegel and Mary Hartzell's (2003) idea of "rupture and repair" in attachment relationships to help parents deal with the conflicts that occur with children and adolescents. These conflicts may be experienced as a rupture in the attachment relationship. What is important is that we go back after a conflict and "repair" the relationship. This means going back to our child, after the emotions have cooled down, to revisit what happened. In particular, we ask our children to share their emotional reactions, and we empathize with their experience. In this way, we validate their emotional experience, which helps them to understand and accept their emotional states. This helps our children develop empathy and compassion for themselves and others. We also restore the emotional closeness and safety of our relationship with them so that we can remain a safe haven for our children to return to when they are upset.

EVOLUTION OF MULTIPLE ATTACHMENT RELATIONSHIPS

Earlier we discussed how human beings evolved as cooperative breeders, raising children with multiple caretakers. How can we understand parent–child attachment in light of this evolutionary history? One of the most important developments in attachment research is the recognition that children can have multiple attachment relationships to different caretakers and that multiple secure attachment relationships may in fact have advantages over a single secure attachment. For example, psychologists Marinus van IJzendoorn and Abraham Sagi conducted studies of children in the Netherlands and Israel who were raised either primarily by their mother or by their mother and another caretaker. They found that children's attachment relationships to different caretakers varied; for example, a child could be insecurely attached to one parent but securely attached to another parent or grandparent. Based on their evidence, they concluded that the overall quality of the child's attachment *network* is the most important predictor of his social and emotional development and that having three secure relationships was optimal (Van IJzendoorn et al., 1992).

IMPLICATIONS FOR MODERN PARENTING

The above findings do not mean that mother–infant attachment is unimportant. It just means that we have to widen our lens when we think about attachment, to include the larger circle of significant others involved in caring for a child: mother, father, stepparents, grandparents, aunts, older siblings, daycare providers, and even teachers. These findings also leave room for a variety of caretaking and attachment arrangements, calling to mind the flexibility in our evolutionary past. For example, studies have shown that a secure relationship with a father can buffer the negative effects of an insecure relationship with his mother (Chang, Halpern, & Kaufman, 2007). A child growing up in a single-mother home could have a secure relationship with his mother and grandmother, and a child in a stepfamily could have a secure relationship with mother, father, and stepfather. This flexibility in being able to form different kinds of caretaking networks for children evolved in our species due to the need for mothers to get additional help raising their young. Another lesson from our evolutionary history as cooperative breeders is that infants are eager to form attachments to other caretakers, especially when they are sensitive, caring, and consistent. The fact that infants readily form attachments to other caregivers, and the fact that other caregivers are so attracted to human infants, is a legacy from our evolutionary past that made it possible for our ancestors to survive and outbreed our other primate relatives. This capacity for human infants to form multiple attachments may ultimately give us the flexibility (I like to hope) to find solutions for caring for our children in the twenty-first century.

But being securely attached to multiple caretakers is not just a good substitute for attachment to one primary caretaker: it actually appears to bring certain cognitive and social benefits to children. For example, in the above study of Israeli kibbutzim, children securely attached to their nursery caretaker showed greater self-confidence and social skills later in kindergarten (Van IJzendoorn et al., 1992). Children who have secure relationships with multiple caretakers seem to develop a feeling of security in their relationships as well as cognitive advantages including being able to see things from multiple perspectives (Hrdy, 2009).

EVOLUTION OF EMPATHY, COOPERATION, AND COMPASSION: GIFTS FROM OUR ANCESTORS

Finally, evolutionary theory may have something to teach us about the development of the capacity for empathy, cooperation, and compassion, capacities central to parenting, mindfulness, and our very nature as humans. Evolutionary theorists and psychologists trace our unique human abilities for empathy and compassion back to the unusually close and long-lasting relationship between mother and child which is the source of our attachment system. Psychologist Jennifer Goetz and her colleagues argue that compassion arose in our evolutionary history as an affective state designed to reduce the suffering or needs of vulnerable offspring. Over time, increased survival of children raised by more compassionate mothers would have selected for this trait. But mother–child attachment is a hallmark of all mammalian species, particularly primates (Goetz et al., 2010). Why would empathy, compassion, and cooperation have developed to such a high degree in our species, and not in closely related great apes such as chimpanzees?

Michael Tomasello, a developmental primatologist, argues that human beings differ from other primates in their ability to "mind read" or share mental states. Unlike virtually all other higher primates, human beings (1) understand that other human beings have thoughts, motivations, and intentions and (2) try hard to understand what these thoughts, motivations, and intentions are. We actively try to read each others' minds, all the time. What's even more impressive, we act in ways to help other human beings, once we think we understand what they are intending. We share a common assumption of mutual cooperation and helpfulness: our motivation for understanding the intentions of others is to be cooperative with them, to help others achieve their goals, or to create shared goals together (Tomasello, 2008).

From a young age, children are motivated to understand what others think about them and others' intentions for them (Hrdy, 2009). Human children and adults are also very concerned about how others feel about them: Do you *really* love me? Do you *really* care for me?

Why did we evolve to be so motivated to understand how others feel about us and to be so good at it? Sarah Hrdy argues that these mind-reading abilities would have helped infants secure their mothers' commitment to raising them. At some point in our evolutionary history, the burden of raising human infants became too high for a mother to be able to do it on her own. Mothers had to have help to ensure their children's survival, and they began to allow others to care for their young. With this increased need for help came an increased cognitive awareness of the need for help. Unlike the apes who came before them, these mothers' commitment to their young was not a given—rather, it was dependent upon how much help they perceived was he available. Infants who could better read the intentions, motivations, and emotions of their mothers, and who could respond in an engaging way, would have had an advantage in securing their mother's attachment and commitment to them. In other words, since a human mother's commitment to her baby is not guaranteed, human babies have had to "work" to get mama's attention. Natural selection would have favored infants who could engage with their mother by gazing into her eyes, cooing, and smiling reciprocally. Human babies are capable of making eye contact within a few days, and this helps attract new mothers and fathers to gaze into their new baby's eyes for long bouts of mutual gazing and babbling which help develop attachment, language, and mind-reading abilities. Hrdy hypothesizes that human infants, unlike other apes, evolved these abilities to such a high degree because they helped win the attachment and commitment of their mother (Hrdy, 2009).

In addition, being raised by multiple, sensitive caretakers would have further developed the capacities for perspective taking, shared emotional states, and empathy. When another caretaker holds an infant, the infant gains a new perspective on the mother. Instead of being pressed up close to mother's body, the infant now views her from a distance. To survive, an infant needs to develop the capacity to read the intentions on its mother's face (Will mother take care of me? Is mother anxious? Am I in danger? Is this stranger safe or harmful? Can she take care of me or feed me?). We have seen how infants who were good at understanding the intentions of their mothers and other caretakers would have been favored by natural selection. Likewise, a mother who is physically separated from her infant will also be more motivated to try to read the intentions on her infant's face. Thus, the mutual sharing of experience, as well as communicating through facial display of emotional and motivational states, would have given our forbearers survival advantages. Hrdy argues that intersubjectivity—the capacity to share mental states as well as share mental goals—evolved to a such a high degree in our species, and *not* in our nearest ape relatives, because these abilities were crucial to an infant's survival once cooperative breeding appeared on the scene. Our ancestors' motivation and capacity to share emotional and mental states led to the evolution of the most pro-social, cooperative line of apes of all: *Homo sapiens* (Hrdy, 2009).

COMPASSION AND COOPERATION IN THE NYC SUBWAY

A recent trip to New York City illustrated for me just how motivated humans are to read the intentions of others in order to help them, even complete strangers in a large city. I had just flown in from Europe, and, travel weary, I jumped onto a subway car, before checking whether it was going in the right direction. As I stepped into the car, the doors began to shut on me. A young man wearing gold chains and a baseball cap held the door for me as I boarded the train. Realizing I didn't know whether I was heading in the right direction, I sought out a friendly looking woman to ask which way the train was going. She wasn't sure, but she pointed to the man across from her, suggesting I ask him. The man assured me that the train was going in my direction. As I thanked him, another man from across the aisle called to me, "Excuse me, Miss, but you should wait until the next station to get off, because if you get off here you'll have to pay twice." I had to smile to myself: in contrast to the stereotype of New Yorkers being unfriendly, in the space of about 3 min, my hapless behavior had motivated four separate individuals from all walks of life to spontaneously offer their assistance to me.

Only later did I think about how this illustrates Hrdy's and Tomasello's point about our highly evolved capacity for mind-reading and cooperation: contrary to our view of human beings as being primarily aggressive and out for ourselves, human beings are the only primate species to have evolved to understand that other human beings have minds, to be able to share in the experience of these minds, and to be motivated to help other humans achieve the goals which originate in these minds. These people on the subway were hardly heroes: they simply noticed a somewhat frazzled woman boarding the train with suitcases, inferred what I wanted to do from my behavior, and were motivated to help me to achieve these goals. We are so accustomed to this behavior that we take it for granted, not realizing what an evolutionary leap it represents.

FINAL THOUGHTS: EVOLUTION, COMPASSION, AND MINDFULNESS

In the course of our long evolution to becoming human beings, we have evolved to become more in tune, more empathic, and more compassionate than the rest of the primates we left behind. And in the course of our children's development, we can observe the unfolding of our species' potential for empathy, compassion, and intersubjectivity (Hrdy, 2009; Tomasello, 2008). From a young age, children show concern for others, are eager to share and help others, and are interested in sharing mental states (Zahn-Waxler, Radke-Yarrow, Wagner, & Chapman, 1992; Hrdy, 2009). These are unique abilities of our species. When children are raised with sensitive and responsive caretakers, these innate abilities for intersubjectivity, empathy, cooperation, and compassion develop. As parents, we have an important role in helping our children develop empathy and compassion, by being emotionally present with them and tuning in to their emotional states (Siegel & Hartzell, 2003).

Traditional mindfulness practice emphasizes not only mindfulness as an individual skill but the goal of mindfulness practice: to become more compassionate human beings and for our actions as humans to reflect compassion. This does not mean that we are only compassionate, but, as meditation teacher Thich Nhat Hanh says so eloquently that the seeds of compassion exist in all of us, along with the seeds of aggression and fear (T. Nhat Hanh, p.c., July 2010). In our genes, our bodies, our emotional reactions, and our automatic action patterns, we carry the weight of our evolutionary past. We cannot help but be stirred to feel and act compassionately; it is our evolutionary heritage, in the same way that we sometimes cannot help to be stirred to feel aggression or fear. We are part of the flow, and we could say that we have an evolutionary right to all of these reactions. Mindfulness doesn't change any of this; it simply gives us the possibility of choosing our course of action, intentionally, and with awareness.

CHAPTER 3

EFFECTS OF THE MINDFUL PARENTING COURSE

Running Mindful Parenting groups, we as teachers have been impressed by the depth and breadth of the effects of the course on most participants, as we have illustrated with case examples in Session 8 and the follow-up session. However, we should be aware of the rose-tinted glasses that we as therapists wear when we evaluate subjectively the effects of what we do: research has shown that therapists tend to strongly overestimate their effects (Margraf, p.c., April 2012). An objective assessment of the effects of a course by all participants, including the ones who have not completed the course (the so-called treatment dropouts), or have not completed all measurement moments (the so-called measurement dropouts), is therefore important to estimate the true effects of Mindful Parenting, also in order to compare it to other interventions focusing on parenting, such as Parent Management Training, and to other interventions focusing on decreasing problem behavior in children.

Below, we describe the results of three empirical studies on the Mindful Parenting course. In the first study, we report results of the program on child and parental psychopathology, parenting stress and parenting styles, co-parenting, and marital satisfaction of the first 10 groups we ran. In the second study, we evaluated whether the Mindful Parenting program increased general mindfulness as well as mindfulness in the parenting context and parental experiential avoidance and parental stress. The second study included participants from the next 10 groups that were run not only in our own center but also in other mental health care centers, in which the trainers were trained in Mindful Parenting by us, to unsure that they would carry out the program in similar ways. The third study evaluated our latest version of the Mindful Parenting program including self-compassion, loving-kindness, and schema mode practice, as was presented in this book, and concerned only one group of 14 parents.

In all three studies, participants were measured before, immediately after, and around the follow-up session. The Mindful Parenting course lasted 2 months in all three studies, 8 weekly sessions of 3 h, and a follow-up session 2 months after Session 8. The follow-up measurement results indicate to what extent the effects of the course are maintained in the absence of the group. In the first study, we also included a wait-list assessment, in order to be able to control the results of the Mindful Parenting course for the effect of assessment (sometimes assessment itself may lead to improvement) and time (sometimes spontaneous recovery occurs).

STUDY 1: EFFECTS OF THE FIRST 10 GROUPS

In this first study of Bögels, Hellemans, van Deursen, Römer, and van der Meulen (2013), we sought to evaluate the acceptability as well as the possible effects of the Mindful Parenting course. Parents attend Mindful Parenting courses for very different reasons, and Mindful Parenting can have very different outcomes on different parents (see Chapter 4 for a discussion of this). Therefore, we measured possible effects on a wide range of measures: child psychopathology symptoms (Achenbach & Rescorla, 2001; Verhulst, van der Ende, & Koot, 1996) and parental psychopathology symptoms (Achenbach & Rescorla, 2003; Ferdinand, Verhulst, & Wiznitzer, 1995; Wiznitzer et al., 1992); parental stress (Abidin, 1983; Dutch translation De Brock, Vermulst, Gerris, & Abidin, 1992) and parenting behavior (Bögels & van Melick, 2004; Verhoeven, Bögels, & van der Bruggen, 2011); co-parenting (McHale, 1997; Dutch validation Karreman, van Tuijl, van Aken, & Dekovic, 2008), that is, the tendency of parents to support or undermine each other in the presence of their child; marital conflict (the scale "Spouse/Partner" of the parental psychopathology measure (Ferdinand, Verhulst, & Wiznitzer, 1995)); and marital satisfaction (Gerris et al., 1993).

Participants in the study were 86 parents (89% mothers), mostly white, and their educational level was on average high. They took the Mindful Parenting course in 10 different groups. In 64 (81%) families, parents experienced problems with at least one of the children. These children were labeled the target children, 40% were girls, and their mean age was 10.7 (4.6). The children were diagnosed with ADHD (47%), autistic spectrum disorder (21%), anxiety disorder or depression (12%), ODD or conduct disorder (4%) learning disorder (3%), and schizophrenia (1%). A parent–child relational problem (DSM-IV V-code 61.20) was classified in 58% of the families. In the other families (19%), parents' own mental health problems, which interfered or had interfered with their parenting, were the reason they attended the course.

Some families had to wait before the Mindful Parenting group would start and conducted wait-list assessments. Immediately before treatment all parents were assessed and immediately after the Mindful Parenting course of 8 weeks again. A follow-up assessment took place 8 weeks after the end of the course. In total one family (1%) dropped out of treatment, which means the participating parent missed four or more sessions. Effect sizes of change (Cohen's *d*) were calculated and were considered small when less than 0.4, medium from 0.4 to 0.8, and large when greater than 0.8 (Cohen, 1988).

What did we find? Wait list did not have any positive effect, except for a decrease in parental externalizing symptoms. After Mindful Parenting, parents reported significant reductions in target children's internalizing problems (e.g., depression and anxiety) and externalizing problems (e.g., behavior problems, aggression); effect sizes of change were medium. At pretest, 59% of the children had subclinical or clinical levels of internalizing and 63% of externalizing symptoms, whereas at follow-up, these were 39% and 43%, respectively. Also, significant reductions in parents' own internalizing and further reduction in externalizing problems occurred, of medium effect sizes. With respect to parenting, parents reported significantly reduced parental stress, of medium effect size, and significant improvements in their parenting of small to medium effect sizes. That is, they reported that they encouraged the autonomy of their child more and were less overprotective and rejecting towards their child. On the rearing dimension acceptance, a borderline significant improvement only occurred at follow-up. Also, improvements were observed in co-parenting, of small to medium effect sizes. Changes were maintained at follow-up or further improvement occurred. No changes on marital variables were found.

Participants filled in an adapted version of the program evaluation of the stress reduction program, developed at the Center for Mindfulness of the University of Massachusetts medical school, to evaluate how they appreciated the Mindful Parenting program (see handout 12.3 for a slightly adapted version of the scale concerning the new program). The vast majority (over 90%) felt the training gave them something of remaining value, that it changed their lives and parenting, and that they became more aware of parenting issues. Also the vast majority (95%) intended to remain aware in daily life, and 88% intended to keep meditating. Most parents had practiced less than advised: 1–4 times a week. Parents gave the course a grade of 8.1 (on a 1–10 scale, which is the standard school grade scale in the Netherlands).

From this study, it was concluded that the Mindful Parenting course is feasible, as only one (1%) of the participants did not finish the course. Moreover, the Mindful Parenting course was shown to be effective on a wide range of measures—child and parental psychopathology, parenting stress, parenting styles—somewhat effective on co-parenting, but not effective on marital functioning. Although improvements on child psychopathology were only of small to medium effect size, it should be noted that this is an important effect taking into account the following two aspects. First, as children suffered from a wide range of problems (a so-called heterogeneous group), measures of more specific target complaints that are more sensitive to change could not be applied. Therefore, the smaller changes on the broadband measures may well be clinically significant. Second, the course was short (only 8 sessions). It is interesting that changes were as pronounced on parental psychopathology as on target child psychopathology, particularly because the vast majority of parents were referred because of a mental disorder of the child rather than of their own. This improvement in parental psychopathology is however consistent with the focus of the Mindful Parenting intervention, that is, becoming aware, in a nonjudgmental way, of (parenting) stress and anxiety, (parenting) sadness, (parenting) anger rather than acting upon these emotions, practicing focused and nonbiased attention, cultivating nonreactivity, and taking care of oneself. Such practice can be expected to effect internalizing psychopathology symptoms, such as anxiety, depression, somatic symptoms, and social withdrawal, as well as externalizing psychopathology symptoms, such as delinquent and aggressive behavior of parents.

The improvements in (self-reported) parenting are also remarkable, given that the focus of the course was not about changing certain parenting styles or behaviors as in Parent Management Training, such as giving praise or time-out. The reduced parenting stress is important as parenting stress is found to negatively affect parenting (Crnic, Gaze, & Hoffman, 2005). Finally, the improvements in co-parenting are remarkable given that only a few couples participated. This is an important finding, as the negative effects of conflict in the presence of the child, and unsupportive co-parenting, on child psychopathology are well documented (Cummings, 1994; Majdandzic, Vente, Feinman, Aktar, & Bögels, 2012). The finding that marital functioning does not improve gives a clear indication of what Mindful Parenting does and does not do, on average, for family functioning. Note that although we do encourage parents to attend the course with their partner, the majority of parents take the course without their partner. This may explain the lack of improvement on marital functioning: parents may need to take the course with their partner in order for the course to have an effect on marital functioning. See Chapter 4 for a discussion of the advantages and disadvantages of running a Mindful Parenting group with couples only.

STUDY 2: EFFECTS OF THE NEXT 10 GROUPS

Now that we learned about the effects of Mindful Parenting on child and parental psychopathology, parenting, and co-parenting, we wanted to know whether Mindful Parenting indeed made parents more mindful, in general and in their parenting, and whether parents would become less avoidant of their children's strong emotions and accept those emotions more, which are thought to be underlying mechanisms of change in Mindful Parenting. We also wanted to evaluate Mindful Parenting now in a wider range of child mental health centers, given by a wider range of trainers.

In the second study by Meppelink, de Bruin, and Bögels (in prep.), 74 parents (91% mothers) of 72 target children (mean age target children = 8.9; SD = 3.3) participated, in 10 different groups. Five mothers (6.8%) dropped out of the course before the end of the course. Parents were all referred because of their child's psychiatric symptoms to one of three community infant, child, and adolescent mental health care clinics collaborating in this project, of which *UvA minds* was one. Primary psychiatric DSM-IV classifications of the children were autistic spectrum disorder (29%); ADHD (23%); anxiety (3%), oppositional defiant (1%) or adjustment disorders (1%), and V-code parent–child interaction problems (24%). Some children (4%) were characterized as "other," and for a few children (5%), the diagnosis was unknown. For the other children (11%), no DSM-IV classification was made but psychiatric symptoms were present.

Parents who attended the course completed a pretest, posttest, and at 8-week follow-up set of questionnaires: the short Five Facets Mindfulness Questionnaire (Baer, Smith, Hopkins, Krietemeyer, & Toney, 2006; Baer et al., 2008), which we first validated for the Dutch population (de Bruin, Topper, Muskens, Bögels, & Kamphuis, 2012); the Interpersonal Mindfulness in Parenting scale (Duncan, 2007), which we also validated for the Dutch population (de Bruin et al., 2013); the Parental Experiential Avoidance Scale, which assesses parents' tendency to avoid taking action in the context of emotional experiences of their children and their unwillingness to experience the emotional experiences of their children (Cheron, Eichenreich, & Pincus. 2009), which we adapted to fit for children with internalizing and externalizing problem behavior; parental stress (Abidin, 1983); and finally parental reactivity (Arnold, O'Leary, Wolff, & Acker, 1993; Dutch valilation Prinzie, Onghena, & Hellinckx, 2007). Results were analyzed with multilevel analysis, according to an intent-to-treat analysis, implying that the 5 mothers who intended to follow the course but did not complete the course were included as well.

Results indicated no effect of the center in which the course took place. There was a significant increase in parents' reported mindful parenting after Mindful Parenting training as compared to before, and a somewhat further increase in mindful parenting at follow-up. These findings are in line with the randomized pilot trial of Coatsworth, Duncan, Greenberg, and Nix (2010) of a mindfulness enhancing parenting program versus the regular parenting program and a delayed intervention group (65 families). Effect sizes on reported increase in mindful parenting in Coatsworth et al.'s study were, as in our study, medium to large. Looking in more detail into changes in mindful parenting (note that the Dutch six subscales are somewhat different from the ones proposed by the developer of the scale Larissa Duncan), parents indicate significant improvements at posttest and follow-up compared to pretest, on listening with full attention to their child, on emotional non-reactivity as parents, on emotional awareness and compassion for self, and on nonjudgmental acceptance of parental functioning. A significant change on compassion for child and on emotional awareness of child was found only at follow-up.

Moreover, parents reported a significant increase in general mindfulness after Mindful Parenting training and a significant further increase at follow-up. They indicated that they were better able to not let things get out of hand in a stressful situation, to be less explosive and step back, and to think and feel more instead if instantly reacting. Parents also reported significantly reduced parental experiential avoidance at posttest, and some further reduction of experiential avoidance at follow-up, indicating that they avoided experiencing the emotions of their children less and had become less avoidant of taking action when their children had emotional experiences. Finally, they reported reduced parental stress, which became only significant at follow-up.

As this study took place in three different mental health care centers, results suggest that the positive effects of Mindful Parenting as obtained in the center where the course was developed can be achieved in other centers as well.

STUDY 3: EFFECTS OF THE LAST GROUP, USING
THE PRESENT MINDFUL PARENTING PROGRAM

The final version of the Mindful Parenting program, as described in
this book, has been tested in a new group of 14 parents, referred to our
child and youth community mental health care center *UvA minds*. There
were 3 fathers and 12 mothers: one was a (female) couple. The target
children were nine boys and five girls, their age ranged between 4 and 14.
The problems of the target children concerned autism or autistic spectrum disorder (2), ADHD (3), separation anxiety disorder (1), post-
traumatic stress disorder (PTSD) (1), an infant disorder (1), or V-code
parent–child relationship problem (3), or a diagnosis of the parent was
the referring problem, generalized anxiety disorder (1).

Parents completed questionnaires about their child's and their own
psychiatric problems, their parenting stress, their parental reactivity,
their mindful parenting, their general mindfulness, their parental experiential avoidance, and finally their overactive parenting. They also completed the program evaluation about the training at posttest, as was done
in Study 1, but the form was somewhat adapted to the new format of the
program.

Results (see Table 3.1) showed significant and substantial improvements in mindful parenting, general mindfulness, and parental experiential avoidance, all with large effect sizes. Parents also improved on their

Table 3.1 Effects of the new format Mindful Parenting course, as described in this book,
on measures of mindfulness, measures of parenting, and measures of child and parental
psychopathology, in one group of 14 participants; measures at pretest posttest, and
follow-up after 2 months; and the effect sizes of change from pretest to follow-up
(*=significant change compared to pretest, # is borderline significant change compared
to pretest) (Note that mean scores are mean item scores)

	Pretest	Posttest	*fu*	Pre-fu
	M (SD)	M (SD)	M (SD)	Effect size
Mindful parenting	3.0 (.48)	3.5 (.28)*	3.6 (.35)*	1.3
Mindfulness	3.0 (0.77)	3.7 (0.79)*	3.8 (0.38)*	1.0
Parental experiential avoidance	3.8 (0.89)	3.2 (0.28)*	3.0 (0.35)*	1.0
Parental reactivity	3.7 (0.87)	3.0 (0.54)*	2.9 (0.88)*	0.6
Parental stress	2.8 (1.1)	2.5 (0.73)	2.2 (1.1)*	0.6
Child internalizing symptoms	0.46 (0.15)	0.38 (0.27)	0.30 (0.21)*	0.8
Child externalizing symptoms	0.35 (0.27)	0.32 (0.24)	0.28 (0.26)*	0.4
Parent internalizing symptoms	0.55 (0.36)	0.47 (0.34)	0.39 (0.31)*	0.5
Parent externalizing symptoms	0.37 (0.24)	0.36 (0.12)	0.26 (0.25)*	0.7

parental stress and perceived over-reactive parenting, with medium effect sizes. Parents also reported improvement with respect to their child's internalizing psychopathology, which became only apparent at follow-up, with a large effect size, as well as a medium effect size improvement on their child's externalizing problems. With respect to parents' own psychopathology, a significant decrease in their own internalizing and externalizing problems became apparent, again only at follow-up, of medium effect size (Table 3.1).

Parents were extremely positive on the evaluation form concerning the training. All parents (100%) found Mindful Parenting was of value; reporting that they changed their lifestyle, their interaction with child or family, or their parenting; that the way they relate to their emotions, cognitions, and action tendencies in parenting had changed; that they intend to continue meditation; and that they intend to continue practicing mindfulness in parenting. Of the 14 parents, 13 found the training sufficient for continuing their life as a parent. They reported that they practiced on average five times a week.

They gave the training a 9.1 on a 1–10 scale. They rated the importance of different elements of the training on a 1–10 scale as follows. Of the formal meditations, 3-min breathing space had the highest rating (9.4), followed by the sitting meditations (8.4), body scan (7.9), yoga (5.9), and walking meditation (5.6). These findings do not necessarily mean that the lower-rated practices are unimportant; for some participants they clearly were (i.e., 7 of the 14 participants gave a rating between 7 and 9 for the value of yoga, and 5 participants gave a value of 7–8 for walking meditation), and one of the goals with yoga and walking meditation is also to bring variety in the range of possibilities to practice meditation. Note also that less time was dedicated in the program to yoga and walking meditation compared to the other meditations, so the rating of the participants may also reflect the relative importance that we gave it.

Of the themes, they found awareness in daily (parenting) life (8.5), awareness of patterns and schemes in parenting (8.4), and self-compassion and metta (8.1) all highly important. Of note, one participant deviated by giving a 1 on the value of compassion and metta, suggesting that this is not everyone's cup of tea. For a discussion of "backlash" effects of loving-kindness meditation see Chapter 4 and Session 7. In terms of work forms, they valued the group discussions and psycho-education (8.4), the diary record forms (7.4), and the reading of handouts (7.1).

It is difficult to compare the effects of the third study, using the new Mindful Parenting program, to the previous two studies, as the third study consisted of only one group, and thus we cannot rule out that a particular selection of participants or particular group processes may have influenced the results. In and of itself, the results of the new group are very good in terms of the program evaluation showing that parents were extremely happy with the course; the overall grade of 9.1 they gave for the course is very high. Furthermore, the results are very good in terms of large effect sizes of change in parental stress, parental reactivity, mindful parenting, mindfulness, and parental experiential avoidance. Finally, the positive effects on child and parent psychopathology that only became apparent 2 months after the course had finished are promising. Such delayed effects of intervention on central outcome measures have been called in the prevention literature "sleeper effects." These effects suggest that once the seeds of mindful parenting are planted, in time this will positively affect the mental health of children and parents.

CONCLUSIONS AND FUTURE RESEARCH ON MINDFUL PARENTING

The three studies described here all show that Mindful Parenting is well accepted in community mental health childcare, which is indicated by the extremely low dropout and the very positive program evaluation. Also, the studies show that Mindful Parenting has clinically significant and substantial effects on a wide range of measures concerning parenting, mindfulness, and child as well as parental psychopathology. The newer program, as is presented in this book, appears even more effective than the older one, but we have to be very careful with such comparisons as we evaluated the new program only in one pilot group, so that the particular selection of parents, children, teachers, or aspects of this particular group, such as the group cohesion, may have influenced the results.

The most important next step is to randomly assign referred parents to Mindful Parenting versus a proven effective parenting training, such as Parent Management Training, in order to compare the effects of the two approaches. Furthermore, it would be interesting to examine whether some parents might benefit more from Mindful Parenting, whereas others might benefit more from Parent Management Training. Another, perhaps more creative way to look at this question, would be to investigate which parents self-select or are selected for Mindful Parenting and which parents for Parent Management Training. In addition, a combined approach of a Mindful Parenting program plus a Parent Management program could be tested; particularly order effects are interesting. That is, is it better to first take a course of Mindful Parenting and, second, Parent Management or the other way around? Multiple informants (e.g., child, teacher, nonparticipating parent) and objective assessments (e.g., observed parenting behavior) are recommended in order to evaluate whether the subjectively reported effects also translate into objective changes. Longer-term follow-ups are needed to examine the hypothesis that Mindful Parenting leads to transformational life changes, as some of the parents who have completed a Mindful Parenting course describe (see Session 8 and Chapter 14 for some descriptions). Such transformational life changes may be more visible over time.

PART II

MINDFUL PARENTING: A GUIDE TO THE 8-WEEK PROGRAM

CHAPTER 4

OVERVIEW OF THE MINDFUL PARENTING PROGRAM

In this chapter, we present an overview of the Mindful Parenting program and discuss the main themes of each session. We also address some of the practical issues involved in setting up a Mindful Parenting course: who the course is intended for and in what kinds of settings, what kind of training is necessary for the teacher, how to get started, and some of the potential difficulties you might encounter.

AIMS OF THE PROGRAM

In Mindful Parenting, parents learn to apply the skills of mindfulness to themselves and to their experience of parenting their children. Most parents come to the course wanting help with parenting and their children: they hope to reduce their stress, improve their relationship with their child, parent more effectively or less impulsively, or help their child be more calm or well behaved. We try to hold the paradox of acknowledging these legitimate and worthwhile goals while remaining open to whatever experience parents have, balancing being with what there is with parents' desire to change things.

Yet we know from our research and from feedback from parents who have completed the course that many parents and children do change as a result of this course. And we feel that the program can help bring about these changes, as our research evidence demonstrates. To describe the aims of the program, we present below some of the ways this program has helped parents who have completed the course. The first set of aims comes from what we have seen as teachers and what parents have told us at the end of the course. The second set of aims comes from our research. Of course, for each parent, the process and outcome will be different.

Mindful Parenting may help parents in the following ways:

- Respond less reactively to parenting stress.
- Take better care of themselves.
- Develop more empathy and compassion for themselves and for their child.
- Tolerate difficult emotions in themselves and their child.
- Become more accepting of themselves and their child.
- Recognize patterns from their own upbringing as they arise in the here and now relationship with their child.
- Resolve conflict better with their child.
- Develop a stronger bond with their child.
- Fully experience both the joys and difficulties of parenting.
- Relate differently to parental suffering: while not all problems will change, parents' attitude towards these problems may.

The results of three clinical trials of the program (see Chapter 3) indicates that Mindful Parenting helps in the following ways:

- Reduces parents' behavior and emotional problems
- Reduces child behavior and emotional problems
- Reduces parenting stress and parental reactivity to stress
- Improves parenting and co-parenting
- Increases general mindfulness
- Increases mindfulness with children
- Reduces parental experiential avoidance

OVERVIEW OF THE THEMES AND PRACTICES
OF MINDFUL PARENTING

Mindful Parenting is based on an adaptation of MBSR and MBCT. We introduce all of the formal meditation practices such as the body scan; mindfulness of the breath, body, sounds and thoughts, and emotions; choiceless awareness; mindful seeing; mindful walking; and yoga, in roughly the same progression. We also introduce mindfulness of everyday activities from the beginning but with a focus on day-to-day parenting and family activities. In addition, we weave short self-compassion practices throughout the 8 weeks, culminating in the teaching of formal loving-kindness meditation in week 7. We also help parents recognize patterns arising in their relationship with their child that may originate from their own childhood, using experiential techniques adapted from schema therapy. We include exercises to help parents become aware of their own personal limits, in order to help them set limits with their child. Finally, we include exercises to help parents reconnect emotionally with their child after a difficult conflict. The core Mindful Parenting themes and practices are summarized in Box 4.1.

SUMMARY OF THE THEMES OF EACH SESSION

Session 1: Automatic Parenting. The central theme of the first session is becoming aware of parenting on automatic pilot, during daily interactions with children, and under stress. We explore parents' reactions to a typical parenting stress situation and connect these to our fight–flight–freeze stress reaction. In this way, we give the rationale for one of the main goals of the course: learning to pause before we react, particularly when under stress, to give time to respond intentionally. We invite parents to experience what happens when we parent more intentionally and mindfully. Just as eating a raisin mindfully as if you have never eaten a raisin before may open you to the full and rich experience, being mindful of your child and with yourself as a parent may open you to the full and rich experience of this child at this very moment and what it's like to be a parent of this child.

Session 2: Beginner's Mind Parenting. Parents share their experience observing their child with beginner's mind and often discover positive qualities which they had overlooked due to focusing on their child's difficulties. Alternatively, some parents discover just how difficult it is to view their child with beginner's mind, as they become aware of their judgments and preconceptions of their child. We discuss how we can become biased towards seeing the negative in our child, especially when our children have been given a diagnosis or when we have given them a label, and how we tend to see view our children in the context of that diagnosis or label. A second theme is the attitude of kindness which we invite parents to embody in their experience as parents, especially when they are struggling or under stress. We explore how we often have difficulty being kind to ourselves, whereas we naturally feel kindness and sympathy towards another parent who is struggling.

Session 3: Reconnecting with Our Body as a Parent. The central theme of this session is becoming aware of our body sensations when we are parenting, experiencing pleasurable sensations, or experiencing parenting stress. We explore how we often ignore our bodies' signals and our

Box 4.1. Themes and Practices of Each Session

Session title	Themes	In-session formal practice	In-session mindful parenting exercises	Home practice
1. Automatic pilot parenting	Rationale (nonreactive parenting) Automatic pilot Doing versus being mode	Bodyscan Raisin	Morning stress exercise	Bodyscan Child as raisin Mindful routine activity Mindful 1st bite
2. Beginner's mind parenting	Seeing child with beginner's mind Attitude of kindness Obstacles to practice Expectations and interpretation	Bodyscan Sitting meditation: breath Seeing meditation	Morning stress from perspective of a friend Gorilla video Gratitude practice	Bodyscan Sitting meditation: breath Mindful routine activity with your child Savoring pleasant moments calendar
3. Reconnecting with our body as a parent	Body sensations Awareness of pleasant events Watching the body during parenting stress Recognizing limits Self-compassion when we're stressed	Yoga (lying) Sitting meditation: breath and body 3-min breathing space	Exploring bodily reactions to parenting stress Imagination parenting stress: self-compassion	Yoga (lying) Sitting meditation: breath and body 3-min breathing Mindful activity with child Stressful moments calendar
4. Responding versus reacting to parenting stress	Awareness and acceptance of parenting stress Grasping and pushing away How thoughts exacerbate stress Responding rather than reacting to stress	Sitting meditation: breath, body, sounds and thoughts Yoga (standing) 3-min breathing	Fight-flight-freeze-dance Imagination parenting stress + 3-min breathing + doors	Yoga (standing) Sitting meditation: breath, body, sounds and thoughts 3-min breathing under stress .b Parenting stress calendar with 3-min breathing Autobiography

5. Parenting patterns and schemas	Recognizing patterns from own childhood Being with strong emotions Awareness of angry and vulnerable child modes and punitive and demanding parent modes	Sitting meditation: breath, body, sounds and thoughts, emotions Walking meditation inside	Pattern recognition exercise Holding strong emotions with kindness	Sitting meditation: breath, body, sounds and thoughts, and emotions Walking meditation 3-min breathing when your child is behaving . . . Parental stress calendar + schema mode recognition
6. Conflict and parenting	Perspective taking, joint attention Rupture and repair Turning in to your child's emotional states	Sitting meditation: choiceless awareness Walking meditation outside	Imagination: parent–child conflict + perspective, rupture and repair	Own 40-min practice Rupture and repair practice Breathing space when you . . . Mindfulness day
7. Love and limits	Compassion and loving-kindness Befriending yourself and your (inner) child Awareness of limits Mindful limit setting	Loving-kindness Self-compassion	Imagination: limits Role-play: limits What do I need?	Own 40-min practice Bring in symbolic object Write narrative Mindful limit setting Loving-kindness
8. A mindful path through parenting	Review of personal growth via symbolic objects or narrative Looking to the future Intentions for practice How can I care for myself (and my child)?	Bodyscan Loving-kindness	Sharing process through symbolic objects or narrative Gratitude practice	Own practice
Follow-up session: each time, beginning anew	Experiences, obstacles and renewed intentions for practicing mindful parenting	Bodyscan Stone meditation	Mountain meditation Wishing well	Own practice

own physical boundaries and limits, especially when parenting. Returning to the body, again and again, and taking care of the body, is the foundational skill that we practice.

Session 4: Responding Rather than Reacting to Parenting Stress.   The first step in responding to parenting stress is to become aware of it, in the body, and to accept it rather than push it away. We explore the variety of automatic reactions that occur when our fight–flight–freeze stress response is triggered. We also explore how our thoughts can exacerbate our stress reactions. Mindful awareness and a breathing space can help us to step out of our automatic reactions when stressed, to pause and respond more intentionally.

Session 5: Parenting Patterns and Schemas.   How do our childhood experiences affect how we parent our own children? Parents investigate reactive parenting patterns with their child and whether these are similar to patterns in their relationship with their own parents. Parents learn to recognize their own angry or vulnerable child modes and their punitive and demanding parent states which may arise during difficult interactions with their child. We practice bringing self-compassion and acceptance to our inner child when we experience these difficult emotional states.

Session 6: Conflict and Parenting.   In this session, we explore parent–child conflicts, which we reframe as opportunities for growth and closeness with our child. Mindfulness can help us create more space, so that we can take into account both our perspective and the perspective of our child. Parents have previously practiced self-compassion for their own emotional states; now we ask parents to expand their awareness to include a sense of compassion for their child's emotional experience. We invite parents to practice holding their emotional experience and their child's simultaneously. We practice coming back to our child after a difficult conflict from this new place, in order to emotionally repair the relationship.

Session 7: Love and Limits.   This session has two main themes. First, we extend our compassion practice by introducing formal loving-kindness practice, as a means to cultivate our inherent capacity for kindness and love. The main message is that we all have the capacity for love and kindness and that no matter what the difficulties have been, we have what it takes to love and care for our children. We can cultivate this even further with the intentional practice of loving-kindness meditation. Secondly, we explore limit setting as a form of "ruthless compassion," since by setting limits, we are actually showing our child love. We have practiced being in touch with our own limits as we feel them in our body. Now we apply this to limit setting: becoming aware of when our own personal boundaries and limits have been crossed by our child and responding from this awareness. Setting limits is viewed as a way of taking care of ourselves while providing the structure that our child needs. We also explore obstacles to setting limits, for example, related to our own experience with limits in our childhood or to the particular difficulties our child has.

Session 8: A Mindful Path Through Parenting. We reflect on what this experience has been like for us, what have we have invested, what we have learned, and what if anything has changed. Parents have struggled to find the time to practice, have dealt with frustration and lack of progress, and have sat with difficult emotions. Some have also had moments of insight and made changes in their lives or their perspective on their life and children. This process has also affected the children. To facilitate this reflection, we invite parents to bring in an object, drawing, poem, song, or short narrative that symbolizes their own personal journey and to share this with the group.

Follow-Up Session: Each Time, Beginning Anew . . . How have parents taken care of themselves and continued with the process of mindful parenting in the last 8 weeks in the absence of the group? What difficulties have they confronted? The main theme is that we can renew our intentions to bring mindfulness into parenting each time again. Just as we can always come back to the breath when we become distracted, we can always come back to the present moment experience with our child. What formal and informal meditation do parents want to continue from this point on, in order to nourish themselves, their parenting, and their children?

HOME PRACTICE

The practice in between sessions, or "home practice," is where parents experience and practice many of the new skills that they are learning. Every week we devote the first part of the session to discussing how the home practice has gone. We encourage parents to make notes in their workbooks and to bring them to each session to help recall their experiences and to help us discuss the home practice concretely. We usually discuss how the home practice went in pairs and then open up the discussion to the larger group. Parents often struggle with finding the time to practice during the week, so exploring this is important. There is often overt resistance to doing the practice, due to lack of time or difficulty with the practices, and it is important for the teacher to meet this with openness. The home practice includes both formal, longer meditations practices, as well as shorter practices that can occur throughout the day, such as mindfulness of daily routines or the 3-min breathing space. We try to embody an accepting stance of whatever the parent brings in. For example, many parents report at the end of the course that the 3-min breathing space is the most useful practice for them (see Chapter 3), so if this is all they have been able to do during the week, that is fine. At the same time, we invite parents to see if they can make space for the formal meditations as well, so that they can get a taste for how this may affect them. At the end of each session, we reserve time to review the home practice for the following week so that everyone understands them. As we discuss in the section on teacher qualifications, it is important for teachers to have experience with the home practice assignments themselves. It is essential that you incorporate these practices into your own life before giving them to others.

For the formal meditation and yoga practices, audio-recordings are available from different sources, for example, from the authors of MBSR and MBCT. Teachers may also choose to make their own recordings.

NEWER ELEMENTS TO THE PROGRAM

In the latest version of Mindful Parenting, we have incorporated compassion practices as well as experiential practices taken from schema therapy. In the next section, we describe these in some detail.

COMPASSION PRACTICES IN MINDFUL PARENTING

In our latest version of the Mindful Parenting program, we incorporate practices to cultivate self-compassion and compassion throughout the 8-week course. As in all MBSR and MBCT programs, we try to embody openhearted kindness, friendliness, and acceptance in our stance towards participants in our group and towards ourselves.

In addition, in Session 1, we invite parents to become aware of their reactions to an imagined stressful parenting situation. Parents often react to this situation with self-critical or judging thoughts, so the first step in developing self-compassion is becoming aware of our lack of self-compassion in these situations. We end Session 1 with a short meditation from Sylvia Boorstein, "May I meet this moment fully; may I meet it with kindness," which captures so simply the attitude of kindness inherent in all mindfulness practice (S. Boorstein, p.c., October 22, 2011).

In Session 2, we ask parents to imagine how they would respond to a friend in the same parenting stress situation introduced in Session 1.

Most parents respond with compassion to their friend, in contrast to their punitive and judging reaction to themselves the previous week. Parents recognize the difference between their self-critical approach to themselves compared to their compassionate approach towards a friend and often express surprise when they realize that they could choose to approach themselves with compassion.

In Session 3, we invite parents to imagine a recent stressful interaction with their child or partner and to first explore their automatic reactions, which often include self-critical thoughts. Then, we ask them to try bringing self-compassion to themselves in the ways Kristin Neff and Christopher Germer suggest, for example, by placing their hands over our heart or other self-compassionate touching, speaking kindly and compassionately to themselves, and recognizing that other parents have also struggled (C. Germer, p.c., November 2011).

In Session 4, we teach the 3-min breathing space to use during stressful parenting interactions, and, in addition, we invite parents to bring self-compassion in at the end, simply by placing one hand over the other on their heart and directing a sense of kindness to themselves.

In Session 5, we invite parents to look at patterns in their own childhood that may arise in their current relationship with their child and to recognize when child or adult schema modes are activated (described in the section below). We invite them to bring self-compassion to their vulnerable or angry child, as a way to soften their punitive parent voice.

Having spent time cultivating self-compassion in these sessions, we move to compassion and empathy for our children and partners in Session 6 where we explore the theme of rupture and repair in close relationships. We ask parents to call to mind a recent conflict with their child and to become aware of their body sensations, feelings and thoughts, and action tendencies. We invite them to bring a sense of compassion, kindness, or forgiveness to themselves, as they have learned in the previous sessions. Then, we ask them to shift their awareness to their child and imagine how he or she is feeling, with kindness, empathy, and compassion. Many parents are surprised at how easily they can empathize with their child, simply by bringing their awareness to his or her experience and suffering. We feel that the emphasis on first bringing compassion to themselves helps develop this capacity.

In Session 7, we introduce formal loving-kindness practice. Since we have already been practicing mindful embodiment of kindness, as well as self-compassion for the previous 7 weeks, we present loving-kindness practice as a continuation of what we have already been practicing. We emphasize the importance of intention over feeling in the practice: we intend to bring an attitude of kindness to ourselves and others, but we may or may not feel that, and that's okay. We also warn participants that some people prone to rumination or depression may experience what Christopher Germer calls a "back draft" of negative feelings towards themselves, and we offer different ways to work with this gently (Germer, 2009; Neff, 2011). For example, they can simply be aware of the feelings and thoughts, or they can play with first bringing kindness to their child or another beloved figure, or bringing kindness to an image of themselves as a vulnerable child.

In Session 8, we do not introduce any new material, since it is a session to reflect on participants' experience and how they want to use what they have learned in the future. However, we have noticed that themes of self-nurturing and self-compassion often arise. For example, one mother brought in a quilt her mother had made for her and talked about the chain of caring, from her mother, to her, to her boys, and how the group had helped her to recognize the need to care for herself as well.

Since we only recently added these compassion practices and have only evaluated them in one group, our anecdotal and experimental evidence is still limited (see Chapter 3 for details). However, our overall impression, based on the experience of the teachers and parents, is that the practices are very valuable for parents. It is interesting to note that mindfulness practice *without* formal loving-kindness practice has been found to increase self-compassion in a recent study by Willem Kuyken and his colleagues. We don't yet know whether adding formal practices to cultivate compassion will further enhance this effect. But a recent study by Neff and Germer (2012) suggests that it might: participants who completed their Mindful Self-Compassion (MSC) program showed a significant increase in self-compassion, mindfulness, and well being compared to those on the wait list. An ongoing study comparing MBSR to MSC should help to answer this question (C. Germer & K. Neff, p.c., September 2012). So stayed tuned for further developments.

A NOTE ABOUT LOVING-KINDNESS MEDITATION

We would also like to say a few words about issues to keep in mind when teaching loving-kindness meditation (but see especially Chapter 11, Session 7, in which we go into this in more detail). A number of meditation teachers and clinicians working with depressed individuals or people prone to rumination have raised the concern that these individuals can sometimes react quite negatively to loving-kindness meditation, become more ruminative, depressed, or even suicidal in reaction to feeling not worthy of love and kindness themselves. Loving-kindness practice seems to elicit feelings of loss and grief related to early experiences in the attachment relationship. Therapists like Paul Gilbert and Christopher Germer working with compassion-based approaches emphasize that this is part of the healing process. When we can hold feelings of pain, shame, or loss with compassion, we can begin to heal them. This is consistent with schema therapy approaches as well. In order to be able to integrate painful experiences, we need to re-experience them to some degree and bring a compassionate stance of the therapist or ourselves to the healing process. Mindful Parenting is not therapy, but we have seen that the compassion practices, together with the support of the group and the teacher, seem to have a healing effect on some participants.

We have also experienced some parents struggling with loving-kindness practice, especially the part of the practice where they send friendly wishes to themselves. In Chapter 11, when we discuss loving-kindness meditation, we offer suggestions about how to work with these kinds of experiences. It's helpful to keep in mind people will have different reactions to the loving-kindness practice (and to all the practices). For this reason, we recommend that you only teach loving-kindness meditation if you have practiced it yourself. This way you will be more intimately familiar with your own reactions which will help you to guide others.

There is also a recent research study from the lab of Barnhofer, Chittka, Nightingale, Visser, and Crane (2010) comparing the effects of mindfulness versus loving-kindness meditation on EEG patterns. In this study, novices to meditation were taught either mindfulness or loving-kindness meditation. After the training, experimenters measured changes in their EEG patterns. Previous research has shown that mindfulness meditation alters the pattern of brain waves, increasing left temporal activation, which is associated with positive emotional states. In this study, *both* forms of meditation led to an increase in the left-side activation associated with more positive mood states. However, when they separated participants into ruminators and non-ruminators, they found something really interesting. Among the ruminators, only mindfulness meditation led to the shift to left-side brain activation (indicating increased positive affective state), whereas if they learned loving-kindness meditation, they did not show the left-side shift. Among the non-ruminators, they found the exact opposite pattern: non-ruminators who learned the loving-kindness meditation showed the left-side shift (indicating increase in positive affective states), where as non-ruminators who learned the mindfulness meditation did not show the left-side shift. This was a very small study of only 15 participants, so we have to be very cautious interpreting it. However, if the findings prove to be robust, it adds some empirical evidence to the anecdotal accounts of depressed or ruminative individuals having a more negative reaction to loving-kindness meditation practice. One take-home message is that different people will respond differently to all of the various practices. This doesn't mean that you shouldn't include the loving-kindness practices, but it's important to be aware of these potential reactions and that you feel comfortable working with them.

SCHEMA MODES AND MINDFUL PARENTING

In our latest version of the Mindful Parenting course, we have incorporated language from Jeffrey Young's Schema-Focused Therapy (Young, Klosko, & Weishaar, 2003). A schema is an internalized representation of how we experienced our relationship with our parents. Schema *modes* refer to states of thinking, feeling, and acting which reflect activation in the present moment of these early childhood schemas. When we are emotionally triggered by something—for example, a conflict with our child—one of our schemas may be activated, and we shift into a schema mode and react automatically. The hallmark of schema modes is strong negative emotion. When we feel flooded by intense negative emotion, cognitions body tension, and strong impulses to act, there's a good chance that we have shifted into a schema mode. Schema modes are action oriented rather than verbal or conscious recollections. Often we do not even realize when we have been triggered into a schema mode. Mindful awareness can help us to recognize when this happens.

When we are in a schema mode, we experience ourselves as either being in the child role or the parent role of the schema. In the most common child modes—angry or vulnerable child—angry or vulnerable child—our thought, feelings, body sensations, and actions are experienced in a childlike way, and the strong emotions and negative thoughts are not modulated by our healthier, integrated adult side. Since our childhood schemas also include representations of our parents, we can also shift into a parent mode. The most common parent modes are punitive parent, where we beat up on ourselves, or demanding parent, where we expect world of ourselves. Of course, we also have our healthy side—our healthy adult mode, which reflects our more balanced, emotionally aware and integrated state, in which we can recognize our emotional reactions for what they are and respond to the situation based on our full understanding as an adult.

The schema modes—angry or vulnerable child and punitive or

demanding parent—seemed to capture something which was happening when parents would report that they had "lost it" with their child. Parents told us that the language of angry child, vulnerable child, and punitive parent helped them become aware when they had become emotionally triggered by a negative interaction with their child. It also helped them to recognize that some of their strong emotions did not actually belong to the present interaction but belonged to something they had experienced in the past.

For example, a mother described an explosive interaction with her teenage daughter, which began when she told her to clean up her room (healthy adult mode). Her daughter responded defiantly, refusing to clean up her room. The mother became enraged and started yelling at her (angry child mode). Becoming more enraged, the mother screamed that she was ungrateful, never did what she was told, and was grounded for the next 2 weeks (punitive parent mode). Her daughter, now also provoked, screamed "I hate you! You're the worst mother ever!" The mother felt hurt and rejected by this (vulnerable child mode). When the daughter burst into tears and ran up to her room, the mother felt guilty about how she overreacted and berated herself for having lost it with her child (punitive parent mode). All parents get angry with their children at times and that does not necessarily indicate a schema mode. But in this instance, the mother became so carried away with anger that she lost her healthy adult perspective in which she might have recognized that her daughter was just being a teenager who didn't feel like cleaning her room or was just expressing anger. What is also striking about schema modes is that in a short but emotionally heated interaction, we can shift from mode to mode without realizing it, which can escalate the conflict. When we become aware of this happening in the moment, we have the chance to interrupt this kind of destructive escalation with our child.

DO WE NEED THE SCHEMA CONCEPT IN MINDFUL PARENTING?

The schema mode language seems to help parents become aware when their childhood experiences become triggered in their present-moment interactions with their children, particularly when under stress. For example, the language of an "angry or vulnerable child" helps parents connect with a part of themselves which they may have tried to deny or ignore. The language of "punitive or demanding parent" helps them recognize when they are being overly punitive or judgmental towards themselves or their child. As parents get to know which situations may trigger them, they can anticipate them and be aware, rather than simply reacting automatically.

The metaphor of angry or vulnerable child also adds the emotional and interpersonal richness which is important for the healing process. When we connect a strong emotion in the present with feelings from the past, our emotions can deepen, connecting us with the childhood roots of our suffering. We can bring empathy and compassion to this child part of ourselves who still suffers. When we can be compassionate with this child part of ourselves, we can also be more compassionate towards our own children's suffering, especially the suffering we may inadvertently cause them when we overreact.

Finally, noting schema modes can help parents decenter from the negative interactions with their child which they have been caught up in, in much the same way that noting thoughts as thoughts helps depressed people to decenter from negative stories about themselves. When we recognize our own schema modes *as* modes, we can begin to let go of them (Segal, Williams, & Teasdale, 2002).

QUALIFICATIONS OF THE TEACHER

THE IMPORTANCE OF YOUR OWN MINDFULNESS PRACTICE

What kind of training do we need to lead a Mindful Parenting course? Let's begin with the most important starting point: our own personal journey with mindfulness. If you are reading this book, you are probably involved in a mental health profession, in education of children or adolescents, in parenting and child development, or you may be a mindfulness teacher—or you may be a student of these areas. Whatever our professional background, the common thread needed to use mindfulness in our professional context is an in-depth personal experience with the practice of mindfulness meditation. Although many books and articles have been written about mindfulness, the only way to gain a true understanding is through one's own experience. In fact, this is what makes mindfulness so powerful: what we ask of our participants is to try out the practices and see for themselves what happens. For this reason, it is important that, as teachers of mindfulness, whatever our other professional training, we have our own experience in mindfulness to draw on. This is different than training in other professions. No one would argue that a dentist should undergo root canal before conducting one on a patient. And while psychotherapists may benefit from their own personal psychotherapy, we don't assume that a cognitive therapist has been in cognitive therapy. So the personal commitment that we ask from ourselves as mindfulness teachers is qualitatively and profoundly different.

What does that mean on a practical level, and where do we begin? If you are a student, perhaps you feel, "I don't have enough experience to be a mindfulness teacher! I'm much too young, and I'm not wise like my teachers." Indeed, when we compare ourselves to our teachers, we feel quite humble. How do we begin to teach others when our experience seems so limited? But the point is that we all have to begin from where we are now, whatever our experience. Embodying a mindful attitude means bringing the intention and commitment to our own mindfulness practice, whether we are just starting out or whether we have a long-standing engagement with the practice, and to be present with our own experience from moment to moment.

My own experience with mindfulness began about 14 years ago. When I first did the raisin exercise as part of training in Dialectical Behavior Therapy for suicidal adolescents (Miller, Rathus, Linehan, & Swenson, 2007). I remember feeling critical and wondering what this had to do with helping suicidal teens. A couple of years later, I attended a workshop on mindfulness for psychologists. Once again, I noticed myself feeling skeptical of the whole thing. But, despite my critical mind, a little bit of mindfulness practice started seeping into my psychotherapy practice, as I began asking patients to become aware of their bodies, thoughts, and feelings in the present moment, and I saw how my patients began to experience their emotions more strongly. A little bit of curiosity opened up in me. It was several years later before I was ready to approach mindfulness again. I was attending a conference, and I signed up for a workshop by Mark Williams on mindfulness-based cognitive therapy for depression. There was still the criticism, the need to dismiss this as something ridiculous, but for the first time I allowed myself to be more open to the experience. And something about the practices touched me enough to make me feel that this could be something helpful for me. A few months later, when I was under some personal and professional stress, I decided to take an 8-week mindfulness course. At the time, I was motivated by my own personal stress, as well as my own professional curiosity about whether this was something that might help my patients. My father had been sick with cancer for several years and seemed to be getting worse, and my mother was diagnosed with lung cancer. I was under pressure at work and didn't feel I was performing well enough. At home, I was struggling to be a good mother but found myself so distracted by my work stress and my worries about my parents that I didn't feel I was doing a good job there. Everywhere I looked. I felt I was failing.

The funny thing about mindfulness is that it is so deceptively simple that you feel you're doing nothing and, at the same time, you can have moments of clarity that years of working in therapy haven't produced. So for me, within the first couple of sessions of mindfulness, I noticed how I was often in a struggle with someone, in my head at least—my father, my boss, my husband, my mother, my kids. And I realized that, I didn't want to be in such a struggle anymore, it was too exhausting. It was striking, since I had been in therapy before, but had never seen this so simply and clearly. I can't say that I instantly became happier or even less stressed. But something powerful changed, and perhaps the most objective indicator of that was that my husband, who had never shown much interest in mindfulness, decided to take the course as well, largely because of the change he had seen in me. So mindfulness came a bit more into our family.

So when embarking on your mindfulness journey as part of your professional training, it's good to keep this dialectic in mind: you have a professional goal, but you also have a personal experience with mindfulness. Graduating from professional programs requires that we finish proscribed courses in a proscribed amount of time, after which we walk up on a stage, get a diploma, and then go for a nice lunch with family and friends. And that works okay for the first part of your goal—your professional training. But for the second part, it's not that simple. For one thing, despite your professional intentions, you don't know what your own personal reaction is going to be to mindfulness practice, and you can't push this or make it go faster or different than it is. In my case, it took several years before I was really open to the practice, much less ready to make a commitment to it. Other people take to mindfulness practice immediately. Everyone's path is different, and that's okay, and in fact, it adds to diversity of experience that we all bring to this endeavor.

So what do you need, concretely, before you embark on this program? First, to have an honest look at how you feel about mindfulness and the place it has in your own life. Second, we recommend based on our own experience and the experience of many others before us that you have had your own mindfulness practice for some time. Your own personal commitment to the process is essential to being authentic, open, and to be able to hold the process for your participants. On a practical level, this means committing yourself to developing a regular mindfulness practice, starting from taking a structured mindfulness course such as MBSR or MBCT or participating in regular meditation within a more traditional meditation context. We also suggest that you have experience in guided silent meditation retreats, in order to deepen your practice.

Once you have established your own personal practice, you can continue your training by enrolling in formal mindfulness training programs, which are now widely available. Mindful Parenting teacher training programs or workshops are beginning to be offered in some mindfulness teacher training centers. Guidelines for teacher training in mindfulness have been developed (e.g., see the work of Crane et al. (2012)), but one's own personal practice is the most important foundation.

THE STANCE OF THE MINDFULNESS TEACHER

The stance we embody as mindfulness teachers may be different than how many of us have been originally trained in mental health fields, especially when working with parents and children. For example, as a child and family psychologist, I had led groups before and conducted family sessions but always as the "professional"—the psychologist with the presumed expertise. When I taught my first Mindful Parenting course, I was co-leading the group, but I was also present as another mother. The distance between therapist and patient was reduced to the meeting of one human with another. It was a relief to simply be in the group as another mother who also struggled with difficulties, as opposed to a professional who had all the answers. I also felt how different it was to simply be with parents in their struggles, without trying to help them "fix" their problems or their child. It was also interesting to hear parents describe their experiences with psychologists and other mental health professionals. So much of their contact with professionals was focused on diagnosing problems, and this left many parents feeling inadequate, blamed, or like they had failed. The attitudinal foundation of mindfulness—non-judgment, allowing things to be as they are, and kindness—was something new for them.

This does not mean we have to give up everything we've learned in our training as psychologist, teacher, or child development worker. But it's important to be aware that our relationship to the parents and children may be radically different in this context. We relate firstly as other human beings who also struggle to bring mindful awareness and compassion to ourselves and our task as parent, partner, friend, or colleague. We connect with others as someone who has also suffered, and who is aware of our suffering, and therefore able to be present and empathic with their suffering. This is why having our own mindfulness practice is so important. When we comment or ask questions of participants in order to help them clarify their experience, we do so not only from our professional expertise but also from our personal experience, with a spirit of co-journeying. This allows us to be genuinely in the room with others in a way that is usually not possible in traditional psychotherapy. We do not have all the answers, but we can help by joining together in investigation and sharing our own struggles with the practice and our own suffering as human beings.

We can also disclose more of our own personal experience, as a way of helping others to understand their experience. This can be tricky, because when we disclose something about ourselves, it's important that we do so in a skillful way which will help the group process or the individuals and not simply because we enjoy telling a good story about ourselves! We try to be mindful when we share an example from our own personal experience—*Am I doing this because I feel like talking, or do I think this will help the others?* In general, we have found that talking about our own struggles with our children and partners is enormously helpful and relieving for parents. Somehow they imagine that because we are mindfulness teachers or therapists that our relationships with our children and partners are perfect! Nothing could be further from the truth, and acknowledging our own struggles helps embody our sharing of universal suffering and helps parents feel more accepting of their own difficulties.

When I started leading Mindful Parenting groups, I had my own parenting stress, raising four children out of two different relationships, including one stepchild, which I could use as my personal test of how Mindful Parenting can help in dealing with the stress of parenting in general and dealing with stepparent and stepchild situations and with ex-partners. Sometimes I felt comfortable disclosing my own experiences as an example. But most importantly, being mindfully present with my own parenting stress and suffering helped me to be present with the parenting stress of other parents in the group. As a more recent example, one mother consulted me after the group because she kept crying during the meditations. She told me that she felt like a failure, not having a stable job and career while raising two young children, and compared herself to me being a director of a clinic, a professor at the university, and also raising a family. I replied with "But you have a partner with whom you raise your two children, while my second relationship with children has recently collapsed." I could easily identify with her feeling of being a failure, as I felt a failure on the relationship domain. She dried her tears, thanked me for the conversation, and continued the Mindful Parenting course. Two years later, I met her at a conference, where she was giving a professional training, and she appeared happy and confident, telling me how she still used her mindfulness practice.

We usually bring up personal examples briefly, so as not to burden the group with too many details about our own personal lives. And in the same way that we encourage parents to speak about their moment-to-moment experience, we also try to share in an experiential way, rather than telling a long story about ourselves or our children. For example, if we are discussing the stress we feel getting our children to school on time, I might mention, "Yes, this morning my daughter gave me an excellent opportunity to practice being mindfully aware of my body sensations when she overslept! I really began to panic, and I took a 3-min breathing space . . ." Or when we ask parents to think about the most difficult behavior of their child to use as their own personal meditation bell, I would share how this helped me deal with my frustration when my daughter would come out of bed at night, just when she was finally enjoying "my time." Hearing my daughter's footsteps, I would begin doing the 3-min breathing space before responding.

Of course, you have to find your own comfort level with disclosing personal experiences. It is possible to be fully present with another person without disclosing anything about yourself.

We have emphasized being present with parents as human beings and parents ourselves. Does this mean that you have to be a parent to guide Mindful Parenting courses? No. What is most essential is being authentically available and present in the group and having a basis of your own mindfulness practice. All of us bring different experiences to our role as teacher, but our essential humanness is what is universal, and in that sense, we are all more alike than different. One of our most experienced mindfulness trainers, Joke Hellemans, has led Mindful Parenting courses for years. Although she herself does not have children, her experience of caring for her mentally handicapped sister helps her to connect emotionally with the experience of caring for a child. And her groundedness in the practice, and authenticity, makes her a remarkable mindfulness trainer.

BRINGING A MINDFUL STANCE INTO THE EVERYDAY NITTY-GRITTY OF CHILD REARING

How do we help parents, and ourselves, actually bring mindful awareness into the moments where we need them the most—in the daily grind of our routine with children and partners? Many of us can experience the benefits that mindfulness offers during our practice in a course, or on retreat, or while sitting on our meditation cushion. But when we return to our usual situation with our families and work life, the pull of habit and routine inexorably lure us back into our old, often mind*less* ways. Nowhere is this more true than in parenting children! Whatever sense of awareness, calmness, understanding, peace, or intention we may have realized during our practice, it can be instantly dissolved in the face of a situation with our child, spouse, or ex-spouse which brings us into an emotional state in which we react unmindfully.

I remember one experience returning home after a retreat which brought this painfully home to me. After attending a weeklong silent retreat, which left me feeling invigorated and ready to reenter my life, this time more mindfully as a parent and wife, I recall being dropped off by the taxi and slowly walking up the garden path leading to our back door. In those few moments, I caught sight of everything in the garden which needed to be done, and my view through the kitchen door reminded me of how we needed to, finally, renovate our kitchen. By the time I had turned the key in the kitchen door, and stepped inside, I was already feeling demoralized, hopeless, and tired, and I felt as if I could literally feel all the positive energy of the week slowly seeping out of me, like a balloon with a hole in it deflating. I began to think about my relationship with my husband, and some conflicts we were going through, and I began to think about the stress of raising our children and our disagreements at times about how to deal with them. Standing in the kitchen, coat still on, luggage in hand, I felt like turning around and running back to the retreat center, perhaps to become a nun, which seemed more and more appealing.

So we are faced with the paradox that it's easier to be mindful when we are alone than when we are in interaction with others, even though our intention is to improve our ability to interact with others through mindfulness. Or, as Christina Feldman (2001) notes, "Mindfulness is easy. Remembering to be mindful is the challenge." Add to that the fact that our interactions with children and other intimates are rarely emotionally neutral. Even when we remember to be mindful in our everyday lives, when we are emotionally triggered, it becomes much more difficult to remain mindful, no matter how good our intentions were.

In Mindful Parenting, we invite parents to address this challenge full on. After all, what could be more real, stressful, enraging, exasperating, exhilarating, or available 24/7 than the tasks of parenting? "Parenting as practice" is a way to embrace the never-ending nature of parenthood and turn what is difficult about parenting into our most productive practice. Jon Kabat-Zinn uses the metaphor of your baby as your Zen master: every howl, every unsoothable moment, every demand needing to be filled is simply a gift from our best teacher ever, helping us learn how to grow as parent (Kabat-Zinn & Kabat-Zinn, 1997).

During the course, we ask parents to choose a routine activity which involves taking care of the children or household to do mindfully such as washing dishes, emptying the dishwasher, giving a child a bath, reading to a child, cooking, or putting a child to bed. Often these are tasks we rush through, wanting to get them over with as quickly as possible, so that we can finally do what we really want to do. But in fact, these mundane, routine, repetitive activities are simply the stuff of childhood itself. It is how we are with our children in these ordinary moments that they will remember. We try to separate moments into "quality time" moments versus boring or ordinary moments, but if we try to rush through them, we risk rushing through and missing precious moments with our child. The moments are not precious because our child is making us feeling happy, proud, or delighted to be a parent. They are precious because they are the only chance we have to experience and interact with our child *in that moment,* which will never be available to us again. How many of us have practically sleepwalked our children through the bedtime routine, eager to finally have some time to ourselves to relax or to take care of other pressing demands? Or rushed our children through the morning routine, with the only goal being getting to school and work on time? Nowhere is it more poignantly and painfully true than with children that the journey, not the destination, is what's important. After all, if the "destination" for children is reaching adulthood and leaving home, do we really need to race towards that?

Another way to bring mindfulness into our daily lives with children and partners is simply to remind ourselves at routine intervals to be mindful. So we recommend that parents choose their own "meditation bells": when the clock chimes, when the phone rings, when you start up your computer, when you get an e-mail or a text, when you are making a transition from one place to another, for example, picking up your child from school (T. Nhat Hanh, p.c., July 2010; N. Singh, p.c., March 31, 2010). All of these can become your own personal signals to stop and come into the present moment by following a few breaths with awareness. We also invite parents to pair up and send each other one text message at a random time each day; the parent receiving the text uses it as a reminder to take a few mindful breaths at that moment (Burnett, 2009).

In addition to these "meditation bells," we suggest using the following as parents' own personal meditation bells: my baby crying, my 4-

year-old throwing a temper tantrum, my child refusing to clean her room, my teen bursting out in anger or sadness, my partner coming home late, etc. In fact, we suggest that parents choose the most irritating or upsetting behavior of their child's and using that as their own personal meditation bell. My personal favorite was my daughter's screaming when something didn't go her way or if she were upset about something. In the past, I would immediately try to "help" her, and we would invariably end up in a fight. When I chose this as my personal meditation bell, the effect was surprising. The first time she began screaming, I started breathing: I followed my breath. In. And out. She looked at me, astonished. Where was the mother who would rush in and try to fix things, who she could get angry at for trying to control her? I was there, quietly watching my breath, not doing anything. The screaming stopped.

WHAT ABOUT PARENTS TEACHING MINDFULNESS TO THEIR CHILDREN?

Parents often ask us this question. In general, we don't suggest that parents teach their children mindfulness. Jon Kabat-Zinn (1944) suggests that the best way to bring wisdom or meditation to your children is by embodying yourself what you want to teach them. Paradoxically, the more we talk about meditation or want them to practice, the more they may resist. It is your truth, your path, not theirs.

I have to admit I have a dubious record when it comes to teaching my own children mindfulness. Perhaps the lowest moment was one night when my daughter was having trouble sleeping. A parent in a Mindful Parenting group that morning had told me, excitedly, how she had used mindfulness of the breath to help her 7-year-old fall asleep. Feeling like I should be able to do the same thing (*after all, I'm the mindfulness teachers!*). I suggested to my daughter that we could breathe together, and I began. This did not have the desired effect. Our mindfulness practice ended rather abruptly when my daughter said "If you don't stop that mindfulness crap now, I'm going to start screaming!" Very, very mindfully, we stopped the mindful breathing.

Really it was a gift that my daughter gave me. She helped me throw out the idea that a mindfulness teacher—a teacher of Mindful *Parenting* no less—should float through the house being calm, blissful and occasionally uttering mindful words while guiding her peaceful children in mindfulness practices throughout the day. Once I was able to give up this fantasy, it actually freed me up to be able to introduce the occasional mindful practice with my kids in a way that they could enjoy. For example, they loved picking out a mindfulness bowl at the gift shop in Plum Village (what kid doesn't love a gift shop, even a Buddhist one?). I borrowed a practice from the Mindful Schools program which we now use pretty regularly at dinnertime. Generally speaking, dinner at our house can be a rather frantic affair. It's always too late, because somehow my husband and I can't get it together to get dinner on the table earlier, so there's kind of a mad rush right at the end—*Television off! (But it's a new episode of my favorite show!) Computers off (But I have to reach one more level!) Set the table! (But my sister didn't set it this morning!) Wash your hands! (I did that this morning!)* So many things have to coincide simultaneous with food being ready that it's a small miracle that we over achieve it. In any case, what was happening was that I would dump all the food on the table, then run to the bathroom which I had needed to do for the past hour. By the time I got back to the table, the food would be gone! So I introduced the following practice, to help slow us all down so we could enjoy the meal together: one of the kids rings the bell. We all listen mindfully until we can't hear it any more. When you can't hear it anymore, raise your hand. It turns out my kids like this practice, especially being the last one to raise their hand. When it's a really good dinner, I can't say that we don't rush through the bell, but at least the bell is there.

Interestingly, my daughter now sometimes asks me at nighttime to do mindful breathing with her. My husband and I have always given her a "motion"—a little back massage—at nighttime. Sometimes I am impatient with the "motion." thinking, *Isn't she too old for this? Shouldn't she be able to fall asleep without it?* And, *I'm so tired, I can't do another thing for another person.* So I started to bring some mindfulness to my own impatience with this relatively small request of hers. My daughter likes to chat about her day while I'm giving her this massage, and sometimes she'll suddenly stop and say "Wait, now I'm *really* going to relax and enjoy this." I suggested to her that she pay attention to the sensations on her back and shoulders so she could fully enjoy her massage, which she did. Later she asked me if I could do a few mindful breaths with her to help her relax before going to sleep, and we do this now and again, when she asks.

So if we are feeling tempted to do mindfulness with our children, we can ask: who is the mindfulness for, really? If it's for our own egos, to feel good about ourselves as mindful parents, our kids are not going to be very receptive. But if they ask for it, or if we offer it and they can use it, then it's another story. On the other hand, we don't necessarily have to teach our children mindfulness practices; we can just focus on being mindful ourselves. When we can be with our own impatience, frustration, anger, sadness, joy, or whatever we are feeling, then eventually we will find a way to deal with the situation. So in the Mindful Parenting program, we don't teach parents to do mindfulness practices with their kids (although parents will sometimes spontaneously try things out with their kids). Instead, we keep the focus on bringing mindful awareness to all of these moments with our children and partners.

WHO IS THE MINDFUL PARENTING COURSE FOR?

The Mindful Parenting course grew in response to the needs of parents who were coming with their children to an outpatient child and adolescent mental health clinic. Many of the children and adolescents were receiving treatment for problems such as ADHD, autistic spectrum disorders, oppositional defiant or conduct disorder, anxiety, or depression. Some families were experiencing serious conflicts in the parent–child relationship. Most parents experienced a high degree of stress due to the challenges of parenting a child with difficulties. Many of the parents also struggled with their own difficulties related to depression, anxiety, autistic spectrum traits, or attention or impulsivity problems, often not diagnosed or treated. Many of the parents experienced stress from a host of other issues which impacted on their parenting and family life: balancing work and parenting, marital difficulties, being a single parent, co-parenting children after a divorce, raising an adoptive child, losing a child, lack of social support, caring for elderly parents, or other stressful life circumstances. Some parents had traumatic experiences growing up, and the emotional impact of these experiences resurfaced when they became parents. Despite the wide variety of issues that families struggle with, what most of these parents have in common is a period of heightened stress due to the high demands of parenting, which impacts on their parenting and their relationship with children and partners.

PREPARING THE PARTICIPANTS:
INITIAL MEETING WITH THE FAMILY

When parents express an interest in taking part in a Mindful Parenting course, the Mindful Parenting teachers invite the family for an initial conversation, preferably with both parents and the child or children for which the parents seek help in parenting. The interview consists of a first part with all members present, a second part with the parents separate from the children, and we end together (see Handout 4.1). If two teachers lead the group and they do the intake together, the teachers can split up for the second part, one talking with the parents, and one with the children.

We first introduce ourselves and tell a bit about our own professional background. We explain the concept of mindfulness and how we have found the Mindful Parenting course to be helpful for other parents. For example, we describe how many parents report that after taking the course they feel less stressed, are better able to deal with stress, are less reactive to their children, and feel more accepting of their children and of themselves as parents. Many parents also say they feel closer to their children and notice improvements in their own emotional state and in their children's behavior after the course.

If we already know something about the parents and children from previous assessments, we include this in our sketch of how the course may be helpful for them. For example, if a parent is struggling with depression, we may ask: when you feel depressed, does it feel more difficult for you to feel really present and connected with your child? If so, the Mindful Parenting course may help you to be able to deal better with feeling sad and depressed and may help you to be more present with your child. Or if we know that the parents have a child with ADHD, we may say: Mindful Parenting may help you to remain calm in the midst of your busy family life.

We ask whether family members have had any experience with meditation or yoga. We lead a brief sitting meditation with the breath for all family members to give the family a first taste of what we will be doing during the course.

Next, we want to get to know the other family members, and we invite each one to tell us something about their individual lives (school, work, friend, leisure time activities) as well as their experiences within their family: for example, we ask, what do they do together as a family, what is the family atmosphere like, and who do they turn to within the family when they have a problem?

After getting to know the family members a bit, we ask about problems which the children or parents may be experiencing, including any feedback from previous therapists about the nature of the problems or a specific diagnosis. We also ask parents to fill out several questionnaires about their children's difficulties, their own parenting stress, and marital satisfaction and conflict. In Chapter 3, we describe these questionnaires in more detail. We use this information to give participants feedback about their improvement, as well as for our ongoing research on the effects of the program.

We also ask a number of questions about family life. For example, we ask each of the parents about which areas of their parenting and family life they feel satisfied with and which areas they would like to improve. We also want to know how children feel about the way they are parented, for example, what do they like, what would they want their parent to do differently? What changes would they like to see in their relationship with their parents and in the family life? We also ask parents about what they like and would want to change in the marital relationship or their relationship with an ex-partner, or the father or mother of the children. We leave it to the judgment of the clinician whether to discuss this with the children present or not. Parents can often benefit from hearing their children's perspective on their marital relationship, and may forget to use their children as a source of feedback on how the family is doing. For example, one adolescent described how she felt excluded when her mother's new boyfriend was visiting, leading her to withdraw to her room. The mother was surprised, because she had assumed that her daughter didn't like her new boyfriend.

In the second part of the interview, we meet separately with the parent or parents, and ask them to talk about their own experience growing up in their family of origin: how they were parented, their relationship to their own mother and father, and so on. We also ask about possible traumas such as sexual or physical abuse, or emotional abuse or neglect, including asking whether the parent has received any help with this. If a parent has experienced abuse or neglect, we talk with them about how that may effect their experience in the course and whether they feel comfortable with that. Talking about the family of origin is often a personal and emotional moment in the conversation.

We ask about each parent's motivation to take the course. What does he or she expect to learn or to work on? We also discuss the importance of making the commitment to come regularly and do the at home practice of about an hour a day in order to gain the most benefit from the course. We discuss whether this is feasible for them.

We explain that during the Mindful Parenting course, the teacher will have the role of teaching and guiding the group in the meditations and will not be talking in this way, as a therapist, as we are doing now. We also make it very clear that parents will not get advice about how to parent their child. Rather we draw on inner wisdom that will be accessed when parents become more aware and attentive and better able to deal with parenting stress. These points are important to clarify so that parents know what to expect in the group. We also explain that after the group has ended, we will meet with them once more individually, to review their experience and to see if they want or need further treatment.

We also meet separately with the child or children during the initial meeting, to find out more about any difficulties and to talk further with the children about their perspective on the parenting and family problems. We invite the children to call or mail us, in case they have any further questions or feedback now or during the period in which their parents are taking the Mindful Parenting course.

We recommend asking parents if there is a professional working with the parent or child, in case serious problems arise during the Mindful Parenting course, for example, a parent who suffers from clinical depression or bipolar disorder, a child with serious problems who is not in therapy, or serious parent–child or marital problems. In general, given the intensity of the Mindful Parenting course, it may be good to consider taking a break from other treatments in which the family may be involved, during the 8 week of the course plus the 8-week follow-up period.

We end the initial meeting all together, giving a summary of what we have learned, and asking for any additional questions or remarks. Finally, we show the family the room in which the course takes place, to familiarize parents with the setting ahead of time.

SIZE AND COMPOSITION OF THE GROUP

Mindful Parenting groups generally consist of 8–16 parents who come alone or in couples. We invite parents to take the course with their partner: however, some parents indicate a desire to take the course on their own. We prefer to work with mixed groups of mothers and fathers together. We have no experience yet with Mindful Parenting groups that consist only of couples, but parents who take the course with their partner tell us about the additional positive effects on their partner and co-parenting relationship. As one-third of the parents that follow a Mindful Parenting course are divorced or single, it is important to take that into account in considering planning a Mindful Parenting group for couples only.

In general, very few participants have dropped out of the course, but we realize that in some settings, there may be more dropout. When someone misses a group, we mail the handouts and home practice and call the person to check in, to see if there was a particular reason why he or she missed the group, and ask if there are any questions about the home practice. The general attitude we want to transmit is care but, of course, participants are free to decide to stop the course if it is not what they expected or if it comes at the wrong moment in their lives. We try to embody an approach that balances supporting participants in making the commitment to the group, and accepting their limits, including if they decide to leave the group before it finishes. As Mark Williams once related to us, "It's how you respond when someone is walking out the door that in the end may be the most important."

PREPARING FOR THE GROUP SESSION

We need to be fully present and grounded ourselves when leading a group. In our busy lives as teachers and therapists, this is the first challenge. We find it helpful to plan enough time for preparing the room, in order to mindfully arrange the right number of mats, cushions, and chairs in the room; copying the handouts: preparing the whiteboard or flipchart: reading the notes from the previous session: looking ahead to this session: and sitting for a meditation. Most importantly, we ask ourselves before the group: *What do I need?*

HOLDING THE GROUP LEARNING PROCESS

In the first session, we want to establish the group norms and culture and to instill a feeling of safety in the group. We begin to do this from the first moments of the group. How we greet the participants sets a tone immediately. An attitude which is friendly and open, and warm begins immediately to communicate a mindful stance. The stance here is different than the stance of a typical group therapy teacher, who might present himself with more professional distance, as a way of making clear "I am the therapist, you are the patients." The stance of the mindfulness teacher is closer to "I am your teacher, but I am also another human being struggling to make my way through this world as best I can or another parent struggling with stress, expectations, and life balance issues." The stance needs to be an authentically humble stance: while as teacher we have knowledge and experience to share, as human beings or parents, we struggle with the same universal difficulties, although the content or degree of difficulty may vary.

We also give explicit instructions in the first session about confidentiality. Since personal issues often arise, sometimes unexpectedly, participants are asked not to discuss what other participants talk about outside of the group. We make arrangements with the group members about how to handle coming in late and missing groups. We always arrange for a place (mat and cushion) for participants that are late, so that they feel welcomed even if late. We explain to the group that no one needs to wait at the door when late and that latecomers offer an excellent practice for the rest in dealing with obstacles during the meditation. At the same time, we suggest that participants come on the early side, leaving space for the transition from whatever they have been doing. We invite participants to bring in cookies or a snack to eat mindfully during a 15-min coffee and tea break which we have in the middle of each session.

We try to model a stance of allowing things to be. This does not mean allowing anything to happen in the group or allowing participants to go on and on when it is not productive for the group. It simply means an open, curious, nonjudgmental stance towards the participants' communications of their experience.

At the same time, we need to structure the group in order to be able to cover the material and to give all members a chance to participate in sharing experiences. We also need to teach members what kinds of communications about experience are most helpful in a group. This is especially important when teaching Mindful Parenting in a mental health setting, where participants may have very different expectations about what they are going to talk about in the group. We tell parents in the first group, and in the initial family meeting which precedes the first group, that the purpose of the group is not to discuss their children's behavior problems or background history or to discuss specific parenting techniques. This is very important to clarify explicitly, since parents may have different expectations. Instead, the focus of the sessions will be learning mindfulness practices, applying them in our everyday lives as parents, and bringing this awareness into the group when we share our experiences. During the 15-min break period, and before and after the group session, however, parents are free to discuss other experiences with each other, including sharing helpful parenting resources or strategies.

Even after giving these instructions in the first group, however, some participants may describe their personal situation in great detail, in a manner more appropriate for a therapy group. When that happens, we can compassionately redirect them by asking them to share their present moment experience, for example, by saying "Can you tell us more about what you experienced—in your body, thoughts, and feelings—during the interaction with your daughter?" By focusing on present moment experiences rather than stories, we also make it safe for participants who do not want to share personal details to be able to reflect on their experiences in the group.

Another common experience is that sometimes participants will talk in an abstract or intellectual way about their ideas about a particular exercise, rather than describing their experience. When that happens, we can simply say, "It's most helpful when you tell us about the actual experience that you just had." In this way, participants learn to focus on their experience in the moment. Sometimes participants will comment on statements by the other group members, in some cases even taking the role of group teacher. Again, we can redirect this kind of comment, for example, by saying, "That's an interesting observation, but can you share with the group how *you* experienced the exercise?" Another common issue is that some group members will talk more than others. We try to pay attention to the balance in the group, for example, by encouraging more reticent participants to speak up and by limiting more talkative members if necessary. On the other hand, we stress that being present and listening is also a way of contributing to the group and that participants should feel free not to talk in the large group.

GUIDING THE MEDITATION PRACTICES AND YOGA

The formal meditation practices in the Mindful Parenting course are the same or similar to the practices in MBCT and MBSR. The handouts of these practices that we give out to support participants in their formal meditation practice are copied from the book *The mindful way through depression* by Williams, Teasdale, Segal, and Kabat-Zinn (2007). These texts are a guideline for teachers as well, but the full practices can be found on audio-recordings, made by the developers of MBSR and MBCT and in languages other than English by mindfulness teachers that have translated these practices and have made available their recordings. The yoga practices concern a series of easy lying and sitting/standing yoga practices, described in the book *Full catastrophe living* by Jon Kabat-Zinn (1990) and in Mindfulness-Based Cognitive Therapy for Depression by Segal et al. (2012). Again, audio-recordings are available from the developers of MBSR and MBCT of these yoga practices in several different languages.

RELATIONSHIP OF MINDFUL PARENTING TO BUDDHISM

The meditation practices which we teach in Mindful Parenting come from Mindfulness-Based Stress Reduction, developed by Jon Kabat-Zinn in 1979 and from the Mindfulness-Based Cognitive Therapy course, based on MBSR and developed by Zindel Segal, John Teasdale, and Mark Williams. One of the most extraordinary accomplishments of Jon Kabat-Zinn was his ability to translate meditation practices rooted in the Buddhist tradition into secular practices which could be accepted in mainstream medical and psychological settings. Particularly in America, where separation of church and state is built into the constitution, and where so many different religious traditions coexist, it was important to embed these practices in a secular program which would be acceptable to people from all kinds of backgrounds.

In the same way, the Mindful Parenting course is a secular approach which is not tied to any particular religious tradition. However, there are times when we want to acknowledge where these practices originate. And as clinicians and teachers, we find the poetry of some of the original Buddhist language inspirational. We also recognize that while Buddhism is practiced as a formal religion, the original teachings of the Buddha were not established as a religion. We therefore differentiate between Buddhist psychology—that is, the profound and universal psychological discoveries which date back to the Buddha—and Buddhism as a formal religion. To give full personal disclosure: while neither of us considers ourselves "Buddhists," we both have benefited greatly from Buddhist teachings, for example, through retreats, practices, or books we have been exposed to, and many of these influences have found their way into the Mindful Parenting course.

At the same time, we are sensitive to the fact that for many people, the word "Buddhism" brings up the idea of a religion and may also bring up other associations ("different, weird, spiritual") which may make them hesitant to come to a course. Since the program is secular, and since we want to make it available to as many parents as possible, we want to emphasize the importance of tailoring the language that you use for your population and the culture in your area. For example, in the handouts, we leave out specific Buddhist references (although we may have quotes from a variety of writers, including Buddhist scholars). In the guide to sessions, we sometimes refer to Buddhist psychology principles to illustrate points or deepen the understanding of various practices, but we deliver these practices in a secular context. We recommend that each teacher use their discretion about the language most appropriate for their group. For example, it is important to be sensitive about the use of some phrases: words like "meditation," "loving-kindness," and "Buddhist psychology" make evoke reactions from some people, and you are free to adjust the language to make it more accessible and acceptable to your group. The bottom line is that we don't want people to feel this is a course on Buddhism (which it is not) or to reject the program because the language makes them feel it is spiritual or religious. At the same time, we want you to have the freedom to use your own experience to guide and inspire your group and to be creative in finding different ways to present the material. We hope that we have been able to strike a balance between doing this ourselves; sharing what is most personal and inspiring for us from our own practice and as teachers and leaving you the freedom to choose the language and practices which will work best for your particular setting and participants.

STRUCTURE OF THIS MANUAL

Finally, a few words about the format of the rest of the book. Each chapter describes a session, which generally lasts about 3 hours, including a 15-min break in the middle. In the first part of each chapter, we introduce some of the broad theoretical or clinical background for the main issues of the sessions. We particularly focus on giving background to the newer elements in the program, which may be different from MBSR or MBCT. In the second section of each chapter, "Guidelines for the Session," we give step-by-step instructions for each session, including the basic meditation practices from MBSR and MBCT, as well as the additional Mindful Parenting practices. The texts for these practices are put in boxes. We also give examples from groups or our own practice, attention to common or difficult issues which arise, and some suggestions about how to conduct the inquiry process. Practices are always followed by a period of inquiry, in which participants have a chance to reflect on their experiences. Each session chapter ends with handouts for participants to take home, starting with the home practice instructions for after each session.

We should point out that the background section of each of the session chapters does not exactly match the "Guidelines" section since we have tended to highlight only the main themes or the themes which are new or different from MBSR and MBCT. While it certainly helps if you are familiar with these two programs, we have tried to make this book "stand alone," so that you can use this as your guide to the Mindful Parenting program.

COOKBOOK AND FLEXIBILITY

The risk of any mindfulness course manual is that it is might be used as a cookbook and that professionals will do the practices as they are written, without the full spirit of mindfulness. How do we combine an open, curious, here and now presence with our group, ourselves, and the unfolding experiences (or beginners mind), with the preset agenda for the session and our goals and expectations for that session? It is a paradox we have to hold. Sometimes, beginning teachers may be inclined to stick more rigidly to the agenda, at the expense of more open attention for what is going up in the present moment. With more experience, teachers usually become more able to flexibly combine the attention for the here and now experience in the session with the agenda.

This program has been in development for the past several years; as such, it is a work in progress. By the time these words are in print, the program will probably have changed again! In general, though, we can differentiate between the original program and the newer program, which includes the self-compassion, loving-kindness, and schema mode practices. The research results are primarily based upon the original program; the newer program has thus far only been formally evaluated in one group of parents, although our anecdotal evidence is promising (see Chapter 3). You can choose to use either the empirically tested original program or the newer program or elements of the newer program.

Finally, we would like to acknowledge that we realize that you will use this program creatively, adding and deleting elements as you see fit, depending upon your participants, your own mindfulness practice and background, and the particular setting you are giving this training in. This is of course fine and in fact will hopefully lead to newer developments in Mindful Parenting and beyond, which we look forward to hearing about.

And so with that, we wish you well on your path through Mindful Parenting!

HANDOUT 4.1 Intake Form

Composition of the family (names, ages):

Current functioning of each of the family members present, work, school, friends, leisure time activities, social contacts?

Problems of child(ren), including diagnoses?

Problems of parent(s), including diagnoses?

What areas of parenting and family life are going well according to family members?

What areas of parenting and family life family members want to improve?

What aspects of the partner relationship between both parents and/or with ex-partner do family members appreciate? What improvements would they want?

HANDOUT 4.1 Intake Form (continued)

With parents alone:
Description of each parent's family of origin, how were they parented, and what did they appreciate and what not?

Information about each parent's own developmental history, including any traumatic experiences?

What help do family members receive or have received for the current problems, and how did they experience this? Is there a professional available in case of acute problems during the Mindful Parenting course?

What do parents want to learn in the Mindful Parenting course?

With child(ren) alone:
Child(ren)'s further perspective on family functioning, parenting, their own problem behaviors?

CHAPTER 5

SESSION 1:
AUTOMATIC PARENTING

*It's 8:20. The children have to be at school at 8:30. You' already received a warning
from the principal that your daughter has been late too often. Your daughter is taking her time, doing her hair and changing her clothes again. "Come on, hurry up or
we'll be late" you say, several times, but she does not come down from her room. You
walk into your child's room, urging her to come, but she throws herself on the floor
screaming: "I'm not going to school!"*

WHAT WENT through your mind when you read this? If you're
like many parents, you can imagine only too well the sense
of stress accompanying this scene. Maybe you can imagine the feelings of
helplessness, anxiety, anger, and stress; maybe you can even imagine the
feeling of tension rising in your chest, your impatience, the thoughts that
might run through your mind, and what you might say and do.

For many parents, this kind of stress may be a daily occurrence. But
the funny thing is that while being late to school is not actually life threatening in any way, it can evoke in us strong sensations, feelings, and
thoughts, *as if something really terrible is about to happen.* We have evolved
as humans and as parents, to have quick, largely automatic reactions to
stress situations; however, these reactions are often out of proportion
with the actual degree of risk in the situation. This is one of the major
themes of Session 1 and the entire course: how we react to everyday
parenting stress and how that affects us and our children. When we do
this exercise with parents, we go immediately into the tempest of automatic parenting—those moments when we "lose it," which we all experience at one point or another.

But stressful situations are not the only ones in which we use automatic parenting. We may often find ourselves doing all sorts of routine
daily activities automatically: brushing our teeth, taking a shower, and

driving to work. We need very little active attention to complete these tasks, and, as a result, our mind goes elsewhere, thinking about work or future plans or ruminating about past events. In the same way, many aspects of parenting become automatic: we dress and feed our children, bring them to school, ask them how their day was, without being fully there. It's one of the amazing things about how our minds have evolved that we are able to be busy with one task, (e.g., giving our child breakfast), while in our minds, we are busy with a completely different task (e.g., imagining how our presentation at work will go today or thinking about what we will make for dinner tonight).

It is tempting to split ourselves in this way, since it feels efficient. After all, why not plan a bit of our day while feeding the kids? And this ability to complete tasks automatically clearly evolved because it has the advantage of being fast and efficient. But it comes at a price. How often have you had the experience of asking your child how his day was, only to realize a moment later that you missed something he said and are asking him again? "Mom, are you listening to me? I just told you I didn't have the math test after all." When we are physically present with our children but emotionally somewhere else, it affects our relationship with them: our ability to truly understand and empathize and to respond to them fully and sensitively. And automatic, mind*less* parenting has another cost: we miss out on fully experiencing the moment with our child. It's like a tiny gap in our consciousness—we literally don't fully process the emotions or even the words shared. When too much of our time with our children is experienced on automatic pilot, we run the risk of missing our child's growing up, perhaps only waking up periodically when we notice "He's growing up so fast! It's going too quickly!"

BEING MODE VERSUS DOING MODE

As parents, we are doing things all the time. We may make to-do lists on paper, or simply carry the to-do lists around in our heads. Many of us feel so overwhelmed by what we need to do that we are constantly pushing ourselves ahead: while we're working on one task, we're thinking about the next three ahead. Jon Kabat-Zinn (1990) introduced the term "doing mode" to describe our problem-solving, goal-oriented mind that helps us to get things done or reach our goals. Our doing mind is excellent at solving problems, planning strategies, and getting us from A to B. But when most of our time is spent in doing mode, it can be exhausting. No sooner do we finish one task then another appears in its place. We may feel driven, and if we don't finish the goals we have set, we feel incomplete or frustrated. In doing mode, the goal is what's important, and we don't necessarily pay much attention to the process of getting there.

Mindfulness offers the possibility of another way: "being mode." When we pay attention to our moment-to-moment experience, we are in being mode, we are experiencing what is happening as it happens, rather than jumping ahead to anticipate the goal or what we will do next. In being mode, we can more fully experience whatever is happening in the present moment. Jon Kabat-Zinn (1990) described meditation as non-doing—simply being present, without being attached to any outcome: " . . . in the meditation domain, the best way to achieve your goals is to back off from striving for results and instead to start focusing carefully on seeing and accepting things as they are, moment by moment."

The funny thing is that we can also *do* the things we need to do but do them in *being mode* rather than doing mode. Here's an example some parents might recognize. It's 8:00 pm, dinner has just finished. Your son's bedtime is 8:30, but he needs to take a shower. Meanwhile, the dishes are still piled up and need to be washed, the trash has to be taken out, and you need to throw a load of laundry in the washer. And at 9:00 your favorite show comes up, which you look forward to all week. You think to yourself, *Okay, if I hurry up, I can get this all done in time to settle onto the couch by 9 and enjoy 1 hour of peace and quiet for myself.* You go into doing mode: you send your son up to the shower; while he's showering, you tackle the dishes, thinking how as soon as you're done you'll put the trash out, then run up to the bathroom and make sure your son washed his hair. Then quick, out of the shower, towel him dry, quick story, into bed, and you'll rush down, throw the load of laundry in, then turn on the TV and collapse on the couch. Have you ever noticed what happens to your parenting when you try to do this? You might catch yourself reading the story quickly to your son, not really paying attention to the words or how your son's reacting. While saying goodnight, you go through all the right motions and tuck him in, but you're thinking about whether you'll make it downstairs in time for your show. In that moment, you can shift to simply being with your son. Instead of planning, thinking ahead, and focusing on the goal, you can simply be aware of what you are doing with him. It actually doesn't have to take a second longer. It's just being present with what is happening. It's paying attention to the process instead of the end result. When you shift to being with your son, you may notice his eyes, or what his body is doing, or you may notice that your breath slows a bit. You are still *doing* something but in *being* mode. You could do any of these tasks—the dishes, taking out the trash, the laundry—in being mode. But when we *do* things with our child in being mode, we get an extra benefit—the chance to be really present in our child's life in that moment.

The central theme of the first session is becoming aware of automatic parenting under stress and during daily interactions with children. The point is not to completely eliminate automatic parenting, which is impossible, but, to help parents become more aware of times when they are parenting on automatic pilot and to experience what happens when they begin to parent more intentionally and mindfully. When parents experience what it is like to be more present and mindful in their interaction with their children, they often feel what they have been missing— they fall awake, even for just one moment. And in that moment, they may see things they had not imagined possible, in their child, themselves, or in their relationship. Furthermore, when parents are able to be mindful of themselves and their parenting when under stress, and be more accepting of their own reactions and their children's, they can begin to examine whether the automatic way of reacting is helpful or not and whether they want to choose a different path.

WHAT HAPPENS WHEN WE TEACH MINDFULNESS IN THE FAMILY CONTEXT?

When we teach mindfulness through the prism of the parenting and family experience, something quite powerful happens. There is a kind of vulnerability and emotionality that is evoked from the very fact that people are discussing the one thing which is perhaps nearest and dearest to their hearts—their feelings about their children, with all the contradictions and intensity; their feeling about themselves as a parent, with whatever self-judgments that may contain; and their feeling about how they were raised themselves with their own parents. As a result of this focus, from the beginning, we engage parents at the level of several deeply emotional schemas: self as parent, self as child, self in relation to own parents. We use mindfulness to help parents turn a spotlight on their current family, including their family relations, parent–child relations, and marital relations and to connect this to patterns from their own family of origin. We invite them to broaden their view of themselves and to see that there are infinite possibilities of choice, no matter what experiences they may have had, if they can look closely at their own experiences with their children and in their family of origin.

We find that a focus on helping their children is very motivating for parents. Most parents will do just about anything if they feel it will help their child. Few parents attending our groups start out with an interest in mindfulness. They have come to the group because they have been told it will help their child. We have found that when parents believe that learning mindfulness will help their child, they are motivated to make the commitment to the group and to the practice. When they begin to experience directly the benefits of mindfulness, they become motivated to do the practice for themselves as well as their children.

GUIDELINES FOR SESSION 1

Box 5.1. Agenda Session 1

1. Meditation on intentions: hopes and longings for the course (10 min)
2. Introducing oneself (first in pairs, then in entire group) (20 min)
3. Practical issues, group rules (10 min)
4. Raisin exercise + inquiry (35 min)
5. Rationale for mindful Parenting: morning stress exercise (15 min)
6. Break: coffee, tea, and cookies in lounge; time to exchange information and experiences and to practice mindful eating and drinking (first bite/sip) (15 min)
7. Body scan + inquiry (1 hour)
8. Home practice (10 min)
9. Closing meditation—Mindfully reentering your world as parent (5 min)

1. GETTING STARTED: FIRST MEDITATION

The first session begins with the group leader welcoming the participants and inviting them to sit on either chairs or cushions arranged in a circle. It is helpful to begin immediately with a brief meditation, prior to the introduction and orientation to the group. In this way, we highlight the experiential nature of the course by beginning with an experience rather than an explanation of mindfulness. The first meditation has two additional purposes. It helps participants make the transition from the "doing mode" into the "being mode." Participants may have been busy with their morning or evening routine or rushing to get to the group. This is a chance to become acquainted with slowing down, paying attention, and coming into being mode. We then invite them to attend to their motivation for this course, by asking them to recall when they decided to take the course. What hopes do they have for this course? What longings? The purpose of this is to help parents connect with their motivation and bring a sense of intentionality and commitment to their work over the coming 8 weeks (See Box 5.2 for detailed instructions).

Box 5.2. Getting Started: Meditation on Intentions
                 (Text adapted from Joke Hellemans)

The teacher invites the group to sit for a short meditation, and invites the participants to either close their eyes or focus on a point on the ground before them. The teacher rings a meditation bell.

"Sit comfortably and close your eyes. Take a moment to connect with yourself in this moment, after the hurry or effort to get here this morning, after everything you had to do in order to get here on time: getting the children ready, leaving the house traveling, finding this building, the waiting room, this room. . . . And now, feeling the contact of your feet on the ground, the contact of your legs on the cushion or chair. Noticing any body sensations or thoughts or emotions. Taking a moment to land in this moment, here and now . . .

What brings you here? Just letting your reactions bubble up. If you like, seeing if you can connect with the moment when you decided to take this course. What challenges did you face? What did you want to change? And now, shifting your awareness back to the present moment, sitting here. . . . What are your expectations? What are your hopes? Your longings? Sitting for a moment with whatever comes up. . . . In a moment you will hear the bell again and you can open your eyes."

---

2. INTRODUCING OURSELVES

Following this brief meditation, participants are invited to break into pairs and introduce themselves by sharing their name, names of other parents and partners involved in the care of children, and names and ages of children. They then share why they have come to this group, what kinds of difficulties they are experiencing raising their children, with their partner or ex-partner if divorced, or in themselves. They discuss previous experience with mindfulness, any help with their children or parenting they have received, and what their expectations are for this course. The teacher briefly describes the practice of mindful speaking and listening, skills which we will practice in the group and eventually practice at home with children and partners. In mindful speaking, attention is focused on communicating clearly and honestly; at the same time, staying aware of one's bodily reactions, thoughts, and feelings that bubble up. In mindful listening, the listener brings full attention to the speaker, in order to understand her communication and receive it nonreactively, with empathy and compassion (see Box 5.3 on mindful speaking and listening). This format is used throughout the course, in order to practice mindful communication and also to allow more opportunities for sharing in larger groups.

We then invite participants to come together again in the full group, to share their experiences. Participants are invited to speak when they feel ready to speak. The teacher asks them to say their name, the names and ages of their children, and the name of other parents involved in the care of the children, and other partners, and writes this on a flipchart, as a way to "bring in" the other family members to the group and acknowledge each person's family situation. After saying their name and those of their children and other parents, participants are free to say more or to be silent, since learning takes place through listening as much as through speaking. The teacher does not write any other information on the flipchart, in order to avoid focusing on problems and diagnoses. The next week, the flipchart is taken to the group again to help parents get to know each other.

Box 5.3. Mindful Speaking and Listening

Mindful Speaking
When we speak mindfully, we bring our full attention to the act of communicating with another person. What do we want to say? How can we say that clearly and honestly? We bring our awareness to our thoughts, feelings, and body sensations which are activated as we speak. We use this awareness to help us glean more insight into ourselves. We also bring awareness to the listener. How does

our speaking affect her? We notice his/her facial expression or body language or her verbal reactions. Paying attention to the listener's reaction does not mean we have to inhibit what we say or change it to please the listener, but just that we are aware of the effect of our speaking.

Mindful Listening
When we listen mindfully, we bring our full awareness to the speaker. We do this by first orienting towards her and bringing our attention to her. What is she communicating to us, with words, facial expression, or body language? We bring our intention to listen openly, without passing judgment, criticizing, labeling, or assuming that we understand the situation completely. We bring a sense of empathy to the speaker, trying to understand her experience from her perspective. In other words, we listen with the mind of a beginner. At the same time, we are aware of how we react to the speaker's communication. We may notice certain feelings, thoughts, or body sensations. Despite our intention, we may find ourselves feeling judgmental, irritated, or bored, or we may feel we understand exactly how she feels. We become aware of these reactions but we deliberately do not share them, in order to give the speaker full space to express herself. This can feel awkward at first, because we are used to smiling, nodding, or responding in some other socially appropriate way. But in fact, to be *fully present* for another individual—to listen intentionally and mindfully, without reacting—is a precious gift we can give someone else.

VOICES OF THE PARENTS

Lily comes to the group wanting help for her 4-year-old son, who had just begun school. The school feels he is not adjusting properly, and the more the school raises concerns, the more anxious Lily feels. Then she tells about her husband's drinking problem, beginning to cry and apologizing for crying. "He hasn't had a drink in the last 4 weeks, but I don't know how long it will last."

Natalie comes to the group to get help in raising her 7-year-old son. Her husband has grown children from his first marriage, and this has put strain on their relationship. She notices that her husband is calmer with their son, and doesn't seem to get into the battles that she does, which makes her feel she must be doing something wrong.

Laura is a young mother raising her 4-year-old son alone. She struggles with feeling insecure as a parent, and with memories of her traumatic youth with a drug-addicted mother which come back to her as she raises her son.

Maria is raising two young children while caring for her aging father-in-law who lives with the family, and working. Her husband works abroad and only comes home on the weekends. As she talks about the stress she feels managing everything, she begins to cry, surprising herself. She apologizes for crying, explaining that normally she just handles everything and doesn't get emotional.

Maria's story is not uncommon. Sometimes we are so busy managing the stress of our day-to-day lives that we don't realize how we are feeling or the toll on our bodies. When we sit in stillness together for the first time, we may be surprised by what we feel and experience, especially if we have been fighting to keep certain feelings at bay.

Fred is an energetic and talkative father whose jokes keep the group laughing. He has taken a leave from work due to stress. At home, he is raising four children ages 4, 6, 10, and 11 with his wife. Although he loves his family life, sometimes his home feels like Grand Central Station, with his kids and their friends coming in and out, and he wants to learn to deal with it better.

Natasha has a 15-year-old daughter who is in therapy for depression, but she has mostly come because she wants help dealing with her ex-husband, who is a drug addict. She finds herself losing her temper and blowing up at him, and she wants to be less emotionally reactive to him.

Anna feels physically and emotionally exhausted, and she has suffered from depression. She recently lost her husband to cancer, and is still mourning him and learning to parent alone. She is also undergoing menopause, and she doesn't feel she can connect with one of her daughters.

Ellen has an adopted a teenage daughter who attended mindfulness group for teens with ADHD. Her daughter dropped out of the group, but said to her mom, "Hey mom, I think you need this more than I do!" Smiling, Ellen said she had to agree with her daughter.

Peter took his first mindfulness course 5 years ago, while recovering from depression. Since then he has become a parent and his meditation practice has fallen off. He wants to find a way to continue his practice, despite his commitment as father. He describes his son as a "handful," and feels his temperament is difficult.

Sophie and Alan have joined the group as a couple. They have a teenage son with autism, and a daughter who is doing well. Recently their son became violent at home, and had to be hospitalized. Their daughter complains that she doesn't get enough attention. Sophie and Alan are exhausted, and they worry that their marriage will fall apart from the stress. They hope that mindfulness will help them deal better with their family stress and help them to feel closer as a couple.

Helga, a single parent raising two boys after a divorce, described her 11-year-old as "difficult," and contrasted him to her 9-year-old "easy" son. She worries about him constantly, but realizes that the worrying doesn't help him.

Caroline worries about her 4-year-old son, born premature, and recently diagnosed with autism. She contrasted him with her "perfect" 7-year-old daughter who helps her so much.

These stories illustrate the variety of reasons which motivate parents to come to a Mindful Parenting group. Parents may be struggling to deal with a child with autistic spectrum disorder, ADHD, anxiety disorder, or behavior or developmental problems, and they may be struggling with their own emotional issues, such as ADHD (often undiagnosed), depression, trauma, marital conflict or violence, and alcohol and drug abuse. Many parents are also struggling to come to terms with emotional issues leftover from their own upbringing—issues which they felt were resolved but which have reemerged with emotional force in the context of raising their own child. Many parents come from "atypical" family situations: divorce, single-parent families, blended families with stepparents and stepchildren, or adoptive families. In fact, these families have become the norm now, but the stress accompanying these situations is worth noting and may lead parents to seek more support. Finally, many parents struggle to balance the demands of work and family responsibilities.

In listening to these stories, we sometimes feel the pressure these mothers and fathers feel to have normal or even perfect children and the pressure they feel to be good or even perfect parents. As therapists and parents ourselves, we wondered: Where do we get this idea that our children have to be perfect, and that we as parents have to be perfect? Sometimes parents put that pressure on themselves. But we also recognized that it also comes from schools, psychologists, and other agencies which are there to help parents. Often helping professionals focus on the child's negative behavior, leaving parents feeling criticized and defensive. Ironically, parents may increase pressure on their children to "behave normally," in response to the pressure they feel from these institutions. When parents feel this kind of stress, they are less able to be accepting of themselves and their children, and they may become less emotionally connected to their children. Paradoxically, this can lead to a worsening of children's behavior. The basic stance of mindfulness—accepting our children and ourselves as we are now in this moment—is radically different from the messages we often get as parents, especially parents of children who are different or diagnosed with a disorder. Whatever our children's difficulties, limitations, or problems, they are okay the way they are, they have what they need to grow, and we have what we need to provide for them and guide them. If parents are able to feel this stance in the first session, then we have accomplished the most important goal of Session 1. A collective sigh can sometimes be felt, a letting go of the tension of trying to live up to these expectations, and we can feel the spaciousness beginning to increase in the room.

3. PRACTICAL ISSUES

We take a few moments to discuss the general group rules, such as confidentiality, starting on time and ending on time, turning cell phones off, and missing sessions. We emphasize that this is a time fully for oneself. We explain that the focus of the sessions will be on participants' experience of the mindfulness and mindful parenting practices, rather than on problem solving for specific child behavior problems. We encourage parents to come early, to drink a cup of tea or coffee before the group begins and invite them to make a schedule for bringing cookies each week for the break. Finally, we open the group for any questions about practical issues.

4. STEPPING OUT OF AUTOMATIC PILOT: EATING A RAISIN MINDFULLY

We introduce the concept of beginner's mind, or stepping out of our automatic pilot, experientially, by asking participants to eat a raisin mindfully (see Box 5.3). This exercise introduces parents to the possibility of experiencing something ordinary and routine in a new way and allows them to experience how this stance can literally change their perception of that experience. This is the same skill which we will ask them to apply to their experience of their children, but we begin first with a more neutral example.

INQUIRY RAISIN EXERCISE

What did you notice about eating a raisin this way? Did you notice something about how it looked, felt, smelled, or tasted that you hadn't noticed before? How do you normally eat raisins? How did eating it this way make the experience different?

The teacher focuses in particular on the different sensations evoked: how does the raisin look (e.g., color, texture, ridges), how does it feel (rough, bumpy), how does it smell, how does it taste? Also, we can notice how our body reacts—what happens when we bring it up to our lips? What does our mouth do automatically? When we bite the raisin, what happens in our mouth, our gut, etc.? Did anyone notice any thoughts or feelings arising during this exercise? We give attention to the constant chatter in our minds which accompanies our experience. Participants may mention feelings of wonder and enjoyment, thoughts such as "I've never really tasted a raisin before!" as well as judgments ("This is really idiotic," "This is disgusting," "I hope the rest of the session is better than this," "I hate raisins"), and other thoughts ("I'm getting hungry for lunch"). The important point is that all reactions, positive, negative, or neutral, are interesting to explore.

Box 5.4. Eating One Raisin: A First Taste of Mindfulness
(Copied with permission from Williams et al., 2007, box pp. 55–56)

1. Holding
First, take a raisin and hold it in the palm of your hand or between our finger and thumb.
Focusing on it, imagine that you've just dropped in from Mars and have never seen object like this before in your life.

2. Seeing
Take time to really see it; gaze at the raisin with care and full attention.
Let your eyes explore every part of it, examining the highlights where the light shines, the darker hollows, the folds and ridges, and any asymmetries or unique features.

3. Touching
Turn the raisin over between your fingers, exploring its texture, maybe with your eyes closed if that enhances your sense of touch.

4. Smelling

Holding the raisin beneath your nose, with each inhalation drink in any smell, aroma, or fragrance that may arise, noticing as you do this anything interesting that may be happening in your mouth or stomach.

5. Placing

Now slowly bring the raisin up to your lips, noticing how your hand and arm know exactly how and where to position it. Gently place the object in the mouth, without chewing, noticing how it gets into the mouth in the first place. Spend a few moments exploring the sensations of having it in your mouth, exploring it with your tongue.

6. Tasting

When you are ready, prepare to chew the raisin, noticing how and where it needs to be for chewing. Then, very consciously, take one or two bites into it and notice what happens in the aftermath, experiencing any waves of taste that emanate from it as you continue chewing. Without swallowing yet, notice the bare sensations of taste and texture in your mouth and how these may change over time, moment by moment, as well as any changes in the object itself.

7. Swallowing

When you feel ready to swallow the raisin, see if you can first detect the intention to swallow as it comes up, so that even this experienced consciously before you actually swallow the raisin.

8. Following

Finally, see if you can feel what is left of the raisin moving down into your stomach, and sense how the body as a whole is feeling after completing this exercise unmindful eating.

VOICES OF THE PARENTS

Parents who are doing this exercise for the first time often describe this as a very powerful experience, which helps them to see how they can open to the new in themselves, their lives, and their children.

Gretchen responded in wonder: "I never ate a raisin that way before—really noticing it, tasting it—its smell, its texture, the feel of it in my mouth. If I could only experience the rest of my life in this way . . ."

Helga described her sense of wonder and appreciation of how her body knew just what to do, and her sense of being able to closely attend to her mouth sensations: "I really noticed how well my tongue supported my teeth—moving the raisin to one side or the other so the teeth could chew—they worked together to do the job. I felt like I was in my mouth, observing, like watching a play going on."

Marie observed that while she was feeling the raisin with her eyes closed, it felt so rich—she felt the ridges, valleys, and different textures of it, but when she opened her eyes she saw "just a raisin" and didn't see much on the surface.

It is also important to acknowledge responses which are less intense or less pleasant, which may reflect when our mind is in a critical or judgmental stance.

Lindsey noticed she was spaced out a lot of the time, and found herself thinking, "First I was so happy to be here, now I'm wondering if I belong. I am so distracted."

Fred experience impatience while eating the raisin: "It's much too slow that way—better to eat it quickly, so you don't lose interest."

Ann chose to mindfully bite the raisin, and then swallowed it quickly, without awareness.

These experiences are also helpful in bringing awareness to the automatic way we often deal with the experience of eating and also states such as frustration, impatience, boredom, distractibility, and judgment. With each meditation or experiential exercise, we try to model that there are no "right" or "wrong" responses and that we can learn as much when we experience our own automatic responses, even as we are opening to new experiences.

Because of the routine nature of many parenting tasks and the repetitive nature of parent–child interactions, it is easy for us to become stuck in a view of our child which is fixed and rigid and to miss out on the opportunity to see our child in a dynamic way. Since a child is constantly developing, our relationship with him is also constantly in flux and changing. Beginner's mind is a means of helping parents open to the fullness of their experience of their child, with all of the senses, and to be able to perceive the ever-changing nature of our child and our relationship with him. In the home practice this week, we ask parents to do a simple exercise to apply beginner's mind to their children.

5. MORNING STRESS EXERCISE (RATIONALE FOR THE MINDFUL PARENTING COURSE)

We ask everyone to sit comfortably, close their eyes, and imagine the following situation as if it were happening to them:

It's 8:20. The children have to be at school at 8:30. You've already gotten a warning from the principal that your daughter has been late too often. Your daughter is taking her time, doing her hair and changing her clothes again. "Come on now, hurry up or we'll be late" you say, several times, but she does not come down from her room. You walk into your child's room, urging her to come, but she throws herself on the floor screaming: "I'm not going to school!"

We then ask, "Imagine this situation as vividly as you can, as if it's happening to you now, and notice what you feel in your body, what emotions come up, what thoughts run through your mind, and what do you feel like doing?" Then we ask them to open their eyes.

INQUIRY AND VOICES OF THE PARENTS

On a whiteboard or flipchart, we write the following:

Body Sensations	Emotions	Thoughts	Action Tendencies

Usually there is much laughter as the parents recognize the stress of this common situation. We first ask about body sensations. Throughout the course, we emphasize going back to our body sensations as a way to connect immediately with the here and now and to open our attention beyond negative thoughts and emotions or impulsive action tendencies. The body serves as a safe haven, which helps parents anchor their experience in the here and now, without resorting to automatic judgments. When we ask a parent to really explore their physical sensations in detail, it has the effect of bringing their attention directly to themselves in that moment and away from the automatic flight of negative thoughts and feelings and the temptation to act on those feelings. The thoughts and feelings may still be present and are encouraged to be embraced under this larger, more spacious umbrella of experience, but the attention is focused on the body. Many parents can identify immediately where in their body they feel tension or stress—in the stomach, like knots or butterflies; in their neck and shoulders; and in their chest, for example. Parents can usually use fairly neutral language to describe their body sensations—"It feels like my neck and shoulder just tense up and tighten," "I feel like I have a 1,000 butterflies swarming in my belly," "I feel the air move up to my chest and get stuck there," "I notice my heart beating" This focus helps expand parents' awareness of their present experience, which fills the space of their awareness, allowing less room for negative thoughts and feelings to take up all the attention.

When we ask about feelings, we often hear about anger, feeling helpless, feeling out of control, feeling embarrassed. Participants also include statements which they experience as feelings but which in fact are more accurately described as thoughts (with a strong affective tinge). This allows us to begin a discussion of differentiating thoughts and feelings. For example, one mother offered "I cannot take this anymore!" as a feeling. We pointed out that this was in fact literally a thought: *I cannot take this anymore*, colored by strong emotion—anger and frustration. This differentiation is important in order to prevent the automatic coupling of feelings and thoughts that can lead to negative or fixed judgments. This mother's protest also hinted at a lack of acceptance of the current reality, as though telling a child "I cannot take this" will actually change his behavior. The situation is what it is, and although we don't have to like it or condone it, wishing it to be different in that moment is a denial of what there is and usually doesn't get us very far!

Then, we ask for thoughts, which parents readily offer: "Oh my god, late again!" "This cannot be!" "I cannot accept this!" "I'm leaving without her!" "What will other parents think?" "How come I'm the only one who's always late like this?" "Why do I always have to bring her to school?" "She's just doing this to aggravate me!"

Next, we ask parents what they would be inclined to do, their first impulses—their action tendencies. We usually get a lot of smiles of recognition—parents know what they tend to do or want to do in these situations. "Make her go to school in her pajamas!" suggested one smiling dad. "Yell at her!" comes up frequently. "Leave without her!" "Go back to bed and crawl under the covers." Interestingly, parents rarely suggest physical reactions, such as pushing, shoving, or hitting. However, if we stress that it is about action tendencies, your first impulses, and not what you would actually do, or when we disclose, "Sometimes I feel like giving my child a good wallop!" we see a lot of nods and rueful smiles, and most participants acknowledge that they have sometimes had the urge to hit their child or that they have actually responded physically. This can be a sensitive issue for some parents. For many parents nowadays, physically disciplining a child does not fit into their values as parent; however, some have found themselves hitting or pushing their children despite their intentions. It's important to encourage openness to discuss all forms of action tendencies, to acknowledge that sometimes as parents, we do things we don't intend and to model a nonjudgmental and gentle attitude towards ourselves when this happens.

This is not to say that we condone physical aggression towards children. The point of the exercise is to begin to train parents in the skill of going back to their body sensations in moments of high stress with their children, in order to connect with their experience in that moment and to deliberately create a pause between their experience and taking action. In this pause, the parent has the opportunity to forego action, until he is fully aware of his bodily reaction, and the accompanying feelings and thoughts.

For example, John talked about what happens to him when his son refuses to do what he's told. "It's rough—I go from 0 to 100 in a second. Sometimes he gets me so mad I feel like hitting him. My old man used to beat me, so I know I don't want to do that. But man, it is really hard sometimes." The teacher asked John how he recognizes his anger—where he feels it in his body. "My heart starts pounding, I have trouble breathing sometimes, sometimes I'm even clenching my fists without realizing it." John already had good awareness of his bodily sensations, and he knew what his action tendencies were—to strike out. It helped him to realize that he could focus on his body sensations and not take any action in the moment.

AUTOMATIC SURVIVAL RESPONSE:
FIGHT–FLIGHT–FREEZE REACTION

After filling in these four columns, we explain that the first column—physical sensations—are the bodily manifestations of stress. The reactions in the fourth column can be divided into flight, fight, and freeze reactions. These reactions are needed for survival in situations of real danger, such as if our child runs into the street when a truck is approaching. Screaming and grabbing the child forcefully are automatic survival responses that are actually needed in that situation. But being late to school is hardly life threatening! Unfortunately, when we are stressed, our bodies react with the same automatic survival response as if we were in actual danger. This survival reaction is evolutionary hardwired, automatic, fast, and not under our conscious control. Our fight–flight–freeze response involves activation of the *short route* in the brain, which involves pathways from the brainstem to the limbic area and which bypasses the prefrontal cortex which is important for judgment, control, and paying attention. A fast survival response such as fighting is functional in situation of real danger but is ineffectual and potentially destructive for our relationship with our child in cases where there is no actual danger (LeDoux, 1996; Sapolsky, 1994; Siegel & Hartzell, 2003).

How can we avoid reacting with our automatic survival patterns in stress situations which are not actually dangerous? By recognizing the physical signs of stress in our body (column 1), we can learn to identify such moments of stress. By taking a breath, and becoming aware of our body, we can slow down and step out of our automatic survival response. We can then use *the longer route* in the brain that involves our prefrontal cortex, which is important for judgment, paying attention, organization, planning, seeing things from multiple perspectives, and compassion.

When we step out of our automatic reactions, and pause, we are able to choose more wisely between several different actions. One choice is no action at all, which can sometimes be the most powerful action. Children can become so used to our reacting automatically to their behaviors in stressful situations that when we don't react in the automatic way, they are surprised. That surprise can shake them out of *their* own automatic reaction, opening a space for them to react in a new way to the situation.

Meditation helps us to recognize our body's signals of stress, as we learn to pay attention to our breath and body. This helps us to become less reactive in our parenting. We first learn to meditate for 45 min, but in the end, we can meditate in 3 min or even 3 seconds, which can be enough to interrupt reactive parenting (see Handout 5.2 for the rationale handout).

6. BREAK

During the break, we provide tea, coffee, and cookies. We invite parents to drink the first sip mindfully and to eat the first bite of the cookie mindfully, with full attention, just as we did with the raisin, aware of our tendency to eat and drink automatically, out of habit. For the following 7 sessions, parents arrange among themselves to bring cookies or another snack for the break. This is also a time for parents to share experiences and practical information and to bond with each other.

THE BODY SCAN

We use the body scan as the first formal meditation in Mindful Parenting in order to emphasize the importance of the body in developing mindfulness and as a means to connect with ourselves and with our experience with our children. Going back to our body sensations is a simple and fast way to bring our attention into the present moment.

We use a body scan based upon the MBSR and MBCT version (e.g., see Box 5.5 and Handout 5.4), but there are many versions of the body scan available which can also be used, as long as it is based upon mindfulness and is not a relaxation exercise.

Box 5.5. Body scan

Introduction to the Body Scan
In our culture in general, we have learned to cut the head off the body. We live so much in our heads, in our thoughts, and in our worries that we lose the wisdom of our bodies. Often times, we don't even realize what is going on in our bodies, how much stress or pain our body feels, until it gives out on us. When caring for children, we may be even more inclined to disregard our bodies, to push them aside as if they get in the way of our doing what we have to do. Our body's needs—food, sleep, rest and even going to the bathroom—are often put aside until after we care for the needs of our children. The same may happen when we are absorbed by the demands of our work. Ultimately this strategy backfires on us. If we don't take care of our bodies, who will? And how can we take care of our children without first taking care of ourselves? Becoming aware and connecting to our body is a powerful way of stepping out of our automatic pilot, our doing mode.
See Handout 5.4 for a summary of the body scan text.

COMMENT

In a Mindful Parenting group, the body scan is often met with eager anticipation—finally, a chance to lie down and rest! There is usually some joking about falling asleep. Lack of sleep is clearly an issue for new parents, but it is surprising how many parents of older children also feel they don't get enough sleep, and often this is an indication of a parent's difficulty balancing the demands of parenting, work, intimate relationship, and private time. It may also be an indication of a parent's difficulty establishing boundaries with children, such that their children are going to bed too late, leaving less time for other aspects of the parent's life. Other parents may view sleep as an escape from the stress and demands of their lives.

It is helpful to point out that the goal of the body scan is to become aware of everything that is going on in the body, rather than to relax. Paradoxically, when we try to relax, it can increase tension. In fact, many people do experience a feeling of relaxation after the body scan, but sometimes participants become aware of uncomfortable or painful sensations, such as tension or muscle pain. We also emphasize that there is no right or wrong way to experience the body scan. Feeling distracted, unfocused, or drowsy is a common experience; being distracted by mundane thoughts about the day's plans and thoughts about recent experiences, fantasies and daydreams, and emotional states is common. The goal of the body scan is simply to become aware of sensations arising in the body. We bring a curious ("Hmm, what do I feel in my left foot now?"), open ("Whatever is there, let me see if I can feel it"), and accepting ("Whatever I feel in my body is okay; even feeling nothing is okay; it is what it is.") stance to this investigation. Accepting isn't about liking or not liking the sensations but simply allowing them to be there instead of denying or fighting them. The awareness of the body also includes awareness of any thoughts, feelings, or other sensations which arise as well. We invite participants to notice when their attention has moved away from the body to thoughts or feelings or other sensations, to notice what is now in their mind, and then to gently return the focus to the part of the body they were attending to. As in MBSR and MBCT, we emphasize that this is simply the normal activity of the mind, the so-called monkey mind in which it seems our thoughts and perceptions are swinging from one thing to another, like monkeys swinging from branch to branch (Williams, Teasdale, Segal, & Kabat-Zinn, 2007). We call these "distractions," but in fact this is the normal state of our mind, which roves around seeking stimulating thoughts, feelings, and sensations. The stance toward distractions, thoughts, and feelings is that they can be lightly held in awareness. This is a form of attention which lies somewhere between following the chain of associations automatically, as our minds often do, and the tendency to push away distractions harshly. We note the distraction, we let our attention touch it lightly, we note what is there—sounds, judgments, thoughts, feelings—we try to hold all of this in awareness, allowing it to be, and then we gently let go of it by redirecting our attention back to the body.

INQUIRY

Following the body scan, we invite participants to share their experience by asking an open-ended question such as "What did you experience?" or "Who would like to share what they experienced?"

The inquiry process is one of the most important and most difficult for the beginning mindfulness teacher to learn. Following each mindfulness exercise, the teacher invites participants to describe their experience and may choose to follow-up with questions about this experience. The purpose of this kind of Socratic questioning is to help participants clarify their own experience and to model for the group the kind of awareness we are trying to develop, by holding a mirror up to one participant's experience. The teacher shapes that experience by asking questions which elicit responses about the here and now experience of body sensations, thoughts, and feelings. In addition, the teacher uses the inquiry to highlight certain themes, which she wants to convey in each session. These two purposes highlight the two different styles of inquiry: the in-depth, individual-focused inquiry and the more superficial level inquiry, emphasizing universal and group themes. The art of the inquiry is being flexible in using both approaches. However, when using either approach, the teacher remains attuned to the group level, so that the inquiry is beneficial to all group members. Even when exploring in finer details aspects of a participant's experience, the teacher uses the inquiry not only to help one participant clarify his experience but also to model for the group how they can look at their own experience. Other times, a teacher may respond to a participant by broadening it to the group or universal themes.

VOICES OF THE PARENTS

Gretchen described her "monkey mind" during her the body scan. The teacher choose to highlight this universal theme rather than asking for more details of Gretchen's experience by saying, "Yes, isn't it amazing how our minds just to leap from one topic to the next, even when we are trying to focus on the breath. That's just how our minds work, and the interesting thing is to see if we can observe that in action. Did anyone else notice their monkey mind in action during the body scan?" This kind of comment opens up the floor for the rest of the participants, and keeps the discussion from going into detail for any one participant. On the other hand, the teacher may choose to go in-depth with a participant by asking a series of questions to highlight one person's experience about an important topic.

Anna described: "I felt nauseous. I tried to go back to the body scan, but I couldn't focus any more. I couldn't wait for it to be over." The teacher asked permission to ask more questions about this experience:

T: Do you remember when you felt nauseous for the first time?
A: When we had to focus on our breath in the belly.
T: What did you feel, and where in your body did you feel it?
A: My mouth was dry and my throat was tense.
T: What happened next?
A: I tried to ignore it but I couldn't.. I tried to swallow but my mouth was too dry.
T: And what happened then?
A: I felt irritated because I could not control it, and embarrassed because I thought everybody could hear me swallow, and thought: How long will this practice still last? I wondered whether this course was a good choice.
T: (turning to the whole group) Isn't that interesting, how we start with a bodily sensation, then we add some thoughts, until we have concluded that this course was a bad idea! This is what our thinking mind does. There is a bodily sensation that is slightly uncomfortable, then negative thoughts are added that makes it more and more uncomfortable, and then our action mind wants to fix it, in this case by ending the course when other things have not worked. And we all struggle with something annoying during the mediation, whether it's nausea, pain, cold, noises, hunger, restlessness, falling asleep, or thoughts. . . . And this is exactly what meditation is: noticing what distracts us, and letting go, focusing again on the point of awareness, getting distracted again, going back . . . again and again. Training the muscle of awareness. (Turning back to the mother) So you were doing just what you needed to do.

Laura expressed the fear that she would fall asleep during the body scan. A single mother with a history of trauma, she felt that sleep was her only comfort and escape from her anxieties and stress, and described herself as a sleep addict. During the body scan in session one, she fell asleep after the ankle, and felt concerned about it. The teacher modeled a mindful and compassionate stance of accepting our experience and the wisdom of our bodies: "Sometimes we don't realize how tired we are until we lie down and let our body do what it needs to do. Although the intention is to "fall awake," that is, to bring attention to each part of your body, it is also okay to let your body do what it needs to do, and try again next time. If it happens regularly, perhaps it's important to look at whether you are getting enough sleep, and experiment with doing the body scan in a sitting position, or with eyes open."

Fred, a father of a boy with ADHD who struggled with attention difficulties him-self, described his impatience during the body scan: "The first leg was great, but by the second, I got bored, I had had enough!

T: What does being bored feel like in your body?
F: Gee, I never thought about it . . . I started daydreaming about more interesting things, thought about getting up to go to the bathroom, then I stretched my legs.
T: When we feel bored, and all of us have had that experience at one time or another, we can investigate what boredom feels like, in the moment, in our body. Then we can go back to whatever part of the body scan we were at, and try to bring the same curiosity to our body. How is the left leg different from the right one, or similar? Can I feel more than what I felt before? Can I feel different things?

By encouraging Fred to explore his reaction of "bored," we helped him to slow down his experience and really feel it in his body, instead of jumping first to action or fantasy. We also hinted at the boredom our children can experience and especially children with ADHD. By study-ing our own boredom, and our automatic patterns of reacting to it, we can understand the boredom of our children and their automatic reaction patterns better.

Felicia, mother of a 7-year-old, found the body scan very enjoyable. She liked being in contact with her body and all the different sensations, and felt it gave her energy.

Mary complained that she was not able to feel anything in her body during the body scan—she always had to think about each part in order to be aware of it. When the teacher asked her to clarify, she explained, "I could feel my foot, but when you asked me to feel my five toes, I had to think about it—I couldn't just feel it." The teacher asked Mary what happened next. "I thought—I can't do this." The teacher observed that she went from her body experience—feeling her foot, not feeling her toes clearly—to her thoughts—I can't do this. In fact, sometimes we feel nothing in some part of our body, and that's okay. We just notice that, and move on.

Carol's phone went off during the body scan and she felt embarrassed. She had real-ized during the body scan that she had forgotten to turn off her phone, and she was distracted by the worry that it would go off. The teacher noted that this kind of distraction is an excellent task for our practice. When we feel distracted by a pain, an itch, having to go to the toilet, or realizing we have not turned off our phone, we have a choice. We can either choose to simply be aware of the sensation and our impulse to do something about it, letting it be and noticing the effect. Or, we can

*take an action (change position, scratch, go to the bathroom, or turn our phone off),
but do so with full awareness, and noticing the effect in our body. The teacher noted
that distractions and interruptions are a part of meditation, and also good practice
for the rest of the group to notice their reactions. For example, one participant felt
irritated by the interruption, whereas another felt sympathy for Carol. The practice
for everyone involves noticing the effect it has on us, and then gently, and with an
open and friendly attitude, bringing our attention back to our body.*

8. REVIEW OF HOME PRACTICE

We go over the home practice with the group (see Handout 5.1).
We find it helpful to review the home practices one by one, clarifying any
questions. The home practice is divided in four categories: (1) reading of
handouts, which we advise to do mindfully, (2) mindful parenting practice, (3) formal practice (the daily standard meditations, which take time),
and (4) informal practice (the adaptation of mindfulness in daily life,
which generally does not take time, but attention—you have to think
about doing it; otherwise you forget). For the coming week, we ask parents to do the "child as raisin" exercise: observing their child once with
full attention, as if seeing the child for the first time. This is an important
exercise as "beginner's mind" is the theme of Session 2. Also, we ask
them to do the body scan once a day (six times a week), and we talk about
how to plan this in their busy lives, when and where to do it, and how to
make sure that they are not disturbed while doing the body scan. The
informal practices are an extension of the raisin meditation they did:
first, paying attention once a day to the first bite of one meal (some parents do this with the whole family together) and, second, choosing one
short daily routine activity to do with full awareness the coming week. It
is helpful to go around and let each person decide what routine activity
he or she is going to do mindfully this week and share it with the group.
Third, trying a nurturing informal meditation. This practice helps to
give parents an idea of how mindfulness can help them in taking care of
themselves.

9. CLOSING MEDITATION

We end with a brief meditation on the breath to close the session
and to make the transition to going back to the outside world of work,
family, and relationships. We like Sylvia Boornstein's "May I meet this
moment fully. . . . May I meet it with kindness" as it adds the element of
kindness which we so sorely need to bring to ourselves, as parents and as

human beings. This is a lovely phrase which reminds parents to bring an attitude of friendliness and kindness to themselves as they go back into their busy lives, reconnecting with their children or partners or arriving at work.

We invite participants to anchor themselves by noticing their body sensations, for example, noticing the feeling of contact with the cushion or chair and checking in with themselves ("What am I experiencing at this moment?"). We prepare to reopen to the world, seeing whether we can bring some of this present moment awareness to the next moments of our day.

May I meet this moment fully. May I meet it with kindness.

HANDOUT 5.1 Practice for the Week After Session 1

Reading

Read the handouts with full attention. Taking notes or underlining what is important for you may be helpful.

Mindful Parenting

"Child as Raisin": Observe your child with full attention, as if you are seeing him or her for the first time, or as if you have come down from Mars and have never seen such a creature before, as we did in the raisin exercise. Choose a moment when your child is not aware that you are watching him or her. Record your experience on the Practice Record Form, so that we can discuss it the next session.

Formal Practice

Do the body scan six times before we meet again (use the audio-recording and see Handout 5.4). See if you can remain open to whatever experience you have, noticing and letting go of judgments or expectations when they arise.

Informal Practice

Pay attention to the first bite of one meal per day, just as we did in the raisin exercise. What do you see, smell, feel in your mouth, and taste? What are the sensations of chewing and swallowing?

Choose one routine activity in your daily life, and make a deliberate effort to bring your full sensory awareness to that activity as you do it. Some possibilities include waking up in the morning, brushing your teeth, showering, drying your body, getting dressed, eating, driving, taking out the trash, shopping or other activities.

Try a nurturing informal meditation, such as drinking your first cup of coffee or tea in the morning with full attention. The ritual can begin with mindfully preparing your morning coffee or tea, sitting down on your favorite spot, feeling the warmth, the shape of the cup, the smell, the steam, and then the taste. Notice this doesn't take any extra time at all.

HANDOUT 5.2 Mindful Parenting

Raising children is one of the most intensive and challenging responsibilities in our lives. At times, it can be difficult and exhausting and at other times, richly rewarding and fulfilling. Sometimes we may become so busy in our lives that the richness of raising children becomes reduced to managing children and the family, instead of simply being with our children and family. When this happens, parenting can become just one of many tasks on our endless "to-do" list, and we lose touch with our experience of being in the moment with our children and families. We parent on automatic pilot.

One of the biggest challenges in modern family life is dealing with stress. Stress has a negative effect on our parenting. When we are tense or stressed, we may be less attentive to our children and to how we relate to our children. When we feel stressed, we may react more impulsively to our children, for example, becoming more easily angry and short tempered with them or worrying about them instead of having faith in their potential for growth.

Unfortunately, when we feel stressed, we react with our automatic survival patterns, which are evolutionary hardwired, automatic, and fast and which occur out of our awareness. This fast response is a *short route* in the brain, located in the brainstem. The brainstem helps regulate aspects of alertness and the bodily functions such as breathing and heart rate. The brainstem is also responsible for our fight–flight–freeze response, combined with the limbic area. This short route in the brain does not involve the prefrontal cortex, which is important for paying attention. A survival response such as fighting is functional in situation of real danger, as it is fast (e.g., grabbing your child's arm forcefully when he dashes out into traffic) but is ineffectual and potentially destructive for the parent–child relationship in cases where there is no real or immediate danger.

Stress can also have a very negative effect on our relationship with our partner. When stressed, couples may have the tendency to work against each other instead of supporting each other and may forget to make time for each other, to give each other attention, or to simply be with each other. And of course, problems in the couple relationship have a direct negative effect on parenting. When partners don't feel supported by each other, they may react by becoming more irritable towards their children or may withdraw from the children. Alternatively they may become too close to their children, so that children don't have the emotional space they need to grow.

Negative experiences from our own childhood can also have a negative effect on our parenting style. Without realizing it, we may react to our own children in the way that our parents reacted to us as children.

HANDOUT 5.2 Mindful Parenting (continued)

We may find ourselves going down the same negative path with our own children, despite our good intentions, because it's the most worn-out path in our brains, and we repeat it automatically, when under stress.

In Mindful Parenting, we learn to focus our attention to be more in the "here and now" and to shift to the "being mode" instead of the "doing mode" while parenting. Learning to focus our attention in this way can help us to deal better with stress in ourselves, in raising our children, in our relationship with our partner, and in our family. This can have many positive effects on parenting and on our contact with our children. We can be more present for the joys of parenting, as well as the difficulties. We can become more empathic towards ourselves and our children. When we parent with fuller awareness, we also slow down our automatic reactions. This gives us a chance to use the "longer route in the brain"—that is, to activate our frontal cortex which helps us to pay attention, organize, plan, and see things from multiple perspectives, instead of our automatic fast route via the limbic system. Training our awareness can also help us become more aware of our own negative automatic reactions stemming from difficult experiences in our youth, so that we are less likely to react in these automatic ways towards our children, partner, or family. When we become aware of these automatic reactions, we can choose to respond differently, in more effective ways. Finally, Mindful Parenting can help transform the quality of our relationship with our child.

We invite you to commit to this process by coming on time every week to the training sessions and to commit about 1 hour a day for the exercises, 6 days per week. We have found that participants who are able to commit to this schedule experience the most positive effects and are most satisfied with the training. You don't have to feel a particular way while doing the exercises or reach a particular goal; what's important is simply doing the exercises.

HANDOUT 5.3 A Definition of Mindful Parenting*

Mindful parenting is an ongoing creative process, not an end point. It involves intentionally bringing nonjudgmental awareness, as best we can, to each moment. This includes being aware of the inner landscape of our own thoughts, emotions, and body sensations, and the outer landscape of our children, our family, our home, and the broader culture we inhabit. It is an on-going practice that can grow to include

(1) *greater awareness of a child's unique nature, feelings, and needs;*
(2) *a greater ability to be present and listen with full attention;*
(3) *recognizing and accepting things as they are in each moment, whether pleasant or unpleasant;*
(4) *recognizing one's own reactive impulses and learning to respond more appropriately and imaginatively, with greater clarity and kindness.*

---

* Myla and Jon Kabat-Zinn, personal communication, Sept. 2012.

HANDOUT 5.4 Body Scan Meditation*

1. Make yourself comfortable lying down on your back, in a place where you will feel warm and undisturbed. You can lie on a mat or rug on the floor or on your bed. Allow your eyes to close gently.

2. Take a few moments to get in touch with the movement of your breath and the sensations in your body. When you are ready, bring your awareness to the physical sensations in your body, especially to the sensations of touch or pressure where your body makes contact with the floor or bed. On each out-breath, allow yourself to sink a little deeper into the mat or bed.

3. To set the appropriate intention, remind yourself that this will be a time for "falling awake" rather than falling asleep. Remind yourself as well that the idea here is to be aware of your experience as it is unfolding, however it is. It is not to change the way you are feeling or to become more relaxed or calmer. The intention of this practice is to bring awareness to any and all sensations you are able to be aware of (or lack of sensation) as you focus your attention systematically on each part of the body in turn.

4. Now bring your awareness to the sensations in the belly, becoming aware of the changing patterns of sensations in the abdominal wall as the breath moves into the body and as it moves out of the body. Take a few minutes to feel the sensations as you breathe in and as you breathe out, as the belly rises on the in-breath and falls on the out-breath.

5. Having connected with the sensations in the belly, now bring the focus or spotlight of your attention down the left leg, into the left foot, and all the way to the toes. Focus on each of the toes in turn, bringing a gentle, interested, affectionate attention to be with and investigate the quality of the sensations you find, perhaps noticing the sense of contact between the toes, a sense of tingling, warmth, perhaps numbness, whatever is here, perhaps even no sensations at all if that is the case. It is all okay. In fact, whatever you are experiencing is okay; it is what is here right now.

6. When you are ready, on an in-breath, feel or imagine the breath entering the lungs and then passing all the way down the body, through the left leg, to the toes of the left foot. On the out-breath, feel or imagine the breath coming all the way back up from the toes and the foot, right up through the leg and torso and out through the nose. As best you can, continue breathing in this way for a few breaths, breathing down into the toes on each in-breath and back out from the toes on each out-breath. It may be difficult to get the hang of this—just practice this "breathing into" as best you can, approaching it playfully.

*From *The Mindful Way through Depression* by Williams, Teasdale, Segal, and Kabat-Zinn (2007), pp. 104–106. Copied with permission of Guilford Press.

HANDOUT 5.4 Body Scan Meditation (continued)

7. Now, when you are ready, on an out-breath, let go of the toes and bring your awareness to the sensations in the bottom of your left foot—bringing a gentle, investigative awareness to the sole of the foot, the instep, the heel (noticing, for example, the sensations where the heel makes contact with the mat or bed). Experiment with "breathing with" any and all sensations—being aware of the breath in the background, as, in the foreground, you explore the sensations in the bottom of the foot.

8. Now allow the awareness to expand into the rest of the foot—to the ankle, the top of the foot, right into the bones and joints. Then take a deeper and more intentional breath in, directing it down into the whole of the left foot, and, as the breath lets go on the out-breath, let go of the left foot completely, allowing the focus of awareness to move into the lower left leg—the calf, shin, knee, and so forth, in turn.

9. Continue to scan the body, lingering for a time with each part of the body in turn: the left shin, the left knee, the left thigh; the right toes and then foot and ankle, the right lower leg, the right knee, the right thigh; the pelvic area—groin, genitals, buttocks, and hips; the lower back and the abdomen, the upper back and the chest and shoulders. Then we move to hands, usually doing both at the same time. We rest first with the sensations in the fingers and thumbs, the palms and the backs of both hands, the wrists, the lower arms and elbows, the upper arms; the shoulders again and the armpits; the neck; the face (jaw, mouth, lips, nose, cheeks, ears, eyes, forehead); and then the entirety of the head.

10. When you become aware of tension or of other intense sensations in a particular part of the body, you can "breathe in" to those sensations in the same way as you can to any others—using the in-breath to gently bring awareness right into the sensations, and, as best you can, have a sense of what happens in that region, if anything, as each breath lets go and releases on the out-breath.

11. The mind will inevitably wander away from the breath and the body from time to time. That is entirely normal. It is what minds do. When you notice it, gently acknowledge it, noticing where the mind has gone off to, and then gently return your attention to the part of the body you intended to focus on.

12. After you have scanned the whole body in this way, spend a few minutes being aware of a sense of the body as a whole and of the breath flowing freely in and out of the body.

13. It is also very important to remind yourself that if you, like most modern people, suffer from low-grade chronic sleep deprivation, since the body scan is done lying down, it is very easy to fall asleep. If you find yourself falling asleep, you might find it helpful to prop your head up with a pillow, open your eyes, or do the practice sitting up rather than lying down.

HANDOUT 5.5 Practice Record Form Week 1

Fill in the record form after you practice each time (mindful parenting, formal or informal meditation). Write down what comes up for you during the practice, so that we can discuss it in the next session.

Day/date	Practice (Yes/No)	Comments

HANDOUT 5.6 Notes Informal Practice
and Mindful Parenting Practice Week 1

You may want to use this sheet to make notes about your experiences during the informal meditation practice and the mindful parenting practice. Or to make notes during or about the group session.

CHAPTER 6

SESSION 2: BEGINNER'S MIND PARENTING

Could there be any better way to get my nose rubbed in the truth of imper-
manence than to love a child in a jagged, careless world? Napping with Skye
in my king-sized bed—his head on my breast, my nose pressed against the
dark silk of his hair—I watch the heartbeat fluttering in the soft spot on
his skull. . . . And even if everything goes absolutely perfectly, I know that
this particular Skye—the one who warbles and passionately sucks on the bill
of his rubber duck as he splashes with me in the tub—it is going to dissolve
like bubble bath. Yesterday he was a kicking bulge in my belly as I swam laps
in the July sun; tomorrow he'll be a middle-aged man, weeping and scatter-
ing my ashes in a mountain lake.

Anne Cushman (2001)

Amanda had come to the group wanting to learn how to be calmer in parenting her
9-year-old daughter who was recently diagnosed with ADHD. In the second session,
she described her experience looking at her daughter with beginner's mind: "It was
a revelation to me. Normally I see her as my challenge. But while she was talking,
I noticed how sensitive and kind she is. She really is her own little person, separate
from me."

Frederica described taking a moment to observe her 4-year-old son, who was being
assessed for autism, curled up in her lap, as they both watched her daughter playing
on a swing. She described vividly the physical sensation of holding her son, feeling
his heart beating against her, smelling his hair, feeling a sense of how beautiful he
was, and a feeling of love.

Amanda and Frederica had become very focused on the difficulties
their children were having. When they let go of that for a moment, and

simply looked at the child before them, they saw and felt things which they had been overlooking, including qualities which had not been so obvious to them.

When we diagnose a child with a disorder, our attention is drawn to the ways in which he is struggling and the qualities which may make life difficult for him. This can be useful for a therapist to plan treatment or for parents to help children develop better skills. But if we become too focused on the problems, or if we lose sight of how these very same qualities can actually be strengths in other contexts, we don't see the whole child before us. We narrow our view, seeing only what is a problem and what needs to be fixed.

But what happens when we let go of having to change something, let go of our judgments about good or bad qualities? We can simply be with our child and take in the full experience. When Frederica felt the physical sensations of holding her son in her lap, she could savor the experience of being with him in that moment, and this brought her in touch with feelings of love and connection to him. In that moment, she didn't need to worry about his strengths and weaknesses. She didn't have to change anything at all. What a respite from all her worrying and trying so hard to help her son, to discover that she could rest in this moment of doing nothing with him and simply being with him!

BIASES AND PARENTING

Lets talk a minute about what happens to parents when we in the mental health profession give a child a diagnosis. As child psychologists, both of us have worn the hat of the diagnosing clinician, and as parents, both of us have experienced what happens when an expert labels your child with a symptom or diagnosis. Sometimes it can feel like that label becomes branded in your consciousness, in huge neon letters! For example, for years I would hear at parent-teacher meetings that my daughter was insecure. I came to dread these meetings. It didn't matter that her grades were great, that she got along well with others, had friends, and cooperated well. I came away with "My daughter is insecure. What have I done wrong?" I myself was shy and insecure as a child, so the last thing I wanted was for my daughter to have to go through this. But the point is that when my attention became too focused on this one comment, which was simply an observation by the teacher, I lost sight of the bigger picture. Our own emotional issues can lead us to focus too narrowly on certain issues of our child's. For a mother who had not struggled with feeling insecure herself, that label might not have stuck. But for me, it hit a sensitive spot, and I blew it out of proportion. This illustrates something we see in our groups, and something that the research literature confirms: when we struggle with our own emotional issues, we may become overly sensitive or biased to negative aspects of our child (Najman et al., 2001).

Furthermore, when our child struggles with difficulties, we may tend to overemphasize his weaknesses and overlook his strengths. Ironically, those of us who work in mental health settings may unwittingly foster this kind of biased perception when we focus too much on diagnosing a child's problems and not enough on his strengths. For example, as a child psychologist assessing children, my job was to look for problems and to see if they fit into a diagnosis. If a child had symptoms of ADHD, I would interview the parents about each of the symptoms. In this way, I trained parents to look for the symptoms, and often this led to parents noticing more and more of these qualities and labeling them as symptoms. In my desire to help, I was actually increasing parents' negative bias for these problems and increasing their worry about their child. I still remember one mother's comment after I had completed an extensive psychological assessment of her teenage daughter. I asked her if she recognized her daughter in my description. She said, "Well, sort of—I recognize my daughter, but only the negative side of her." Only later in my training, when I became a family therapist, did I learn to put the same effort into diagnosing strengths of the child and the family. Similarly, a friend of mine described what happened after her 3-year-old was diagnosed with autistic spectrum disorder. Before hearing the diagnosis, she had noticed how her daughter would line up all her stuffed animals in the hall way, and she found it adorable. But after she was told this was a symptom of autistic spectrum disorder, she felt anxiety when her daughter did this, which would trigger a cascade of worried thoughts: "She should stop this! There is something very wrong with her. What will happen to her?"

I had a similar experience with my son. My son has always had a remarkable eye for the tiniest details, zooming in and noticing with wonder a small insect on a leaf as we walk, an airplane in the sky, a piece of debris on the sidewalk which to him is a treasure. My husband and I have always taken pleasure in his natural beginner's mind, fantasizing about the artist or architect he will become. But when we consulted a psychologist, she was struck by how distractible he was and how easily his attention was drawn to all sorts of small details in her room. At once, something which I had observed with pleasure and pride was transformed into a problem. Being mindful does not mean valuing one view over the other but simply taking a broader view which encompasses both aspects. In the classroom, it may cause problems when my son eagerly attends to many things other than the teacher's lesson, whereas on a walk, such attention can bring richness to the moment.

So our view of our child and ourselves as parents can become quite narrowed and biased, either due to our own emotional issues or due to our child's emotional or behavioral difficulties. When we practice beginner's mind, we counteract this tunnel vision and open ourselves up to the whole universe of experience with our child.

Even if our child has not been diagnosed with a disorder, we may sometimes find ourselves labeling him or her. Think about it for a minute. If you are a parent of two children, have you ever noticed a tendency to think of one as "the easy one," one as the "difficult one"? Or the smart one and the athletic one? It's natural to compare our children, but sometimes we can get stuck in believing our own labels too literally, not giving each child the room to be however he or she is. And once we've decided our child is, for example, "not the scholastic type," how easy is it to notice the things that fit that description and overlook the things that contradict it? Since our child is literally growing before our eyes, these labels are not very reliable. We just don't know how he or she will develop. When we look at our child with beginner's mind, we also create room for our child to experience himself in a more expanded way, so that we don't limit his or her possibilities for growth. Part of how our children learn about themselves is through how they see themselves reflected in our eyes, so when we see them fully and openly with beginner's mind, they can also see themselves more fully.

This is especially important to keep in mind when children have been diagnosed with a particular disorder. Sometimes a child can become identified with her disorder and begin to view herself as a kid with problems, a loser, no good. We have all seen kids who have learned to act up because it brings them attention and because it fits their view of themselves as a "problem" child. Seeing our child with beginner's mind can help prevent our child from identifying with her problems and narrowing her view of herself to include only the negative.

HOW DOES MINDFULNESS PRACTICE HELP WITH OUR TENDENCY TO LABEL OUR CHILD?

We start by becoming aware that our "perceptions" of experiences and our child are not pure or even necessarily completely accurate. In Session 1, we used the morning stress exercise to illustrate how our per-

ception of an experience often includes thoughts, feelings, body sensations, and action tendencies which are merged together. When we begin
to separate these components of experiences, we can become aware of
how much of our perception of things is biased by our expectations or
interpretation of the situation. And we may become aware of things in
our perceptual experience which we have discounted or even failed to
register simply because they do not fit with our expectations or interpretation. Think, for example, of the video in which viewers see a brief film
of a basketball game, in which, in the middle, a person in a gorilla suit
saunters through. Although the video is shown in real time, the majority
of people completely miss the gorilla the first time they view the film,
because it is too anomalous. Our brains are simply not able to incorporate
this anomalous piece of information into our concept of a basketball
game, so, although we have "seen" it in the sense that the image was sent
to our eyes, we failed to process it. That is, until we view it a second
time, this time with the prior knowledge to expect a gorilla, we are
amazed at how we could have missed something so obvious! We use this
video to demonstrate to parents just how profoundly our expectations
shape what we perceive or more importantly, don't perceive.

Secondly, we use the practice of beginner's mind to intentionally
short-circuit our tendency to see only what we expect to see or make too
automatic interpretations of things. Beginner's mind helps us to expand
our experience of our child to include the totality of that child, in that
moment. In other words, we encourage parents to look for "gorillas" they
have missed—the anomalous features which don't fit into their view of
their child, but which are there for the noticing, when they open to them.
Beginner's mind is the practice of trying to see each new experience as
exactly that – a *new* experience, completely and utterly different from any
other, in the same way that this next breath coming in is completely and
utterly different from the breath before.

One reason why we fall so easily into the trap of seeing our children
in a stereo-typed or narrow way is that family life consists of so many
repetitive interactions and events, which occur hundreds if not thousands
of times. Think, for example, of waking your child up, helping him get
dressed, eating breakfast, brushing teeth, getting him to school, and so
forth. We like to turn these interactions into routines, predictable interactions which will go in a predictable fashion each day, to help our children know what to expect and to maximize our own efficiency. This
helps us to function and to get to school and work on time. However, the
downside of this predictability and sameness is that we lose our ability for
beginner's mind, to really see our experience unfold in *this* moment, on
this day, with *this* child, however he is *in this moment*, different than how

he was one moment ago, or the night before, when we put him to bed. As absurd as it may seem to view our child as being different in every single moment, therein lies the seed of change. From one moment to the next is the space in which each of us has the capacity to be different, to choose a different way of behaving. Mindfulness shows us that, if we take beginner's mind seriously, every moment literally contains the seed of change, in our child and in ourselves.

Of course, we should not beat up on ourselves for having brains that like to interpret reality for us. This tendency evolved because it helped our ancestors process complex information in their environment quickly, which helped them survive. We have evolved to have brains which don't need full perceptual information in order to interpret the world. As soon as our brain thinks, it knows what is happening, it doesn't waste any more time processing the raw perceptual data, and it makes meaning out of the situation (Blackmore, 2009). This bias is necessary, but we pay a price for it: sometimes we don't perceive what is before us, if our brain doesn't think it fits. We are all hardwired to have a bias for confirming our expectations and interpretations.

We're also not saying that identifying problems or making diagnoses is bad or unhelpful. On the contrary, it can be very useful for helping us to know how to help our child. For example, one mother found that when her child was diagnosed with autistic spectrum disorder, and the symptoms were explained to him, he felt relieved. He had always felt different, and now he understood why. It also helped his sister to understand his actions better and to be more patient with him. Still, we can be aware of some of the unintended effects of narrowing our focus and work to counteract this.

SPACIOUSNESS AND BEGINNER'S MIND PARENTING

It seems that often when problems arise, our outlook becomes narrow. All of our attention may be focused on worrying about the problem, and we may have a sense that we're the only one that is going through such difficulties. This can lead to a kind of self-absorption that can make the problem seem very intense. When this happens, I think that seeing things from a wider perspective can definitely help—realizing for instance that there are many people who have gone through similar experiences, and even worse experiences. The Dalai Lama (1998)

When we see our child with beginner's mind, we expand our view of the child, and we allow our attention to rest gently on all of our experience, not being pulled one way or another. This creates more space in our experience of our child.

But what exactly do we mean by spaciousness? Christina Feldman's use of the metaphor of a bowl of water with salt in it perhaps can convey the meaning best (C. Feldman, p.c., April 7–11, 2010). We changed it slightly by using the metaphor of a drop of red paint in a bowl of water. A drop of red paint in a small bowl of water turns it quickly red. However, the same drop of red paint in the ocean, once dissolved, is barely perceptible. As humans, we seem to have evolved to attend to negative features of our experience, the "red stains" of our experience, more so than neutral or positive experiences. This has a clear evolutionary advantage for avoiding danger or confronting difficulties but has the disadvantage that we are wired to give too much attention to negative features of our environment, including negative feelings, sensations, or thoughts. Spaciousness is the ability to broaden our perspective to include all aspects of our experience, negative, positive, and neutral, and to hold them lightly and equally, not giving any one aspect more or less attention. When we are focusing on a negative feeling, for example, our perception narrows, and our body muscles contract, so that our focus becomes more and more fixed on the negative feeling, as if we were looking into a microscope and enlarging the image until it fills our whole perceptual field. When we bring a more spacious view to bear on the experience, it's as if we bring the microscope focus back, broadening our view, so that we take in other aspects of our experience, and so that the negative feeling becomes smaller relative to the other things in our perceptual field. The negative feeling is still there, but now, it's smaller and surrounded by other aspects of the experience which may be negative, positive, or neutral.

Likewise, when we focus on a behavior of our child that we don't like, our attention narrows, and that problem behavior may fill the entire field of our perceptual and emotional awareness. We may forget about the other qualities our child has or we may not even notice them. When we expand our view, we may notice other things, just as Amanda noticed what a kind and sensitive daughter she had. When we view our child more spaciously, we become more accurate in our view of them, and we can become kinder and softer towards them and towards ourselves.

HOW DOES MINDFULNESS HELP US BECOME MORE SPACIOUS IN OUR EXPERIENCE?

How do the formal meditation practices help us become more spacious in our experience, especially our experience of our child? We begin with the practice of focusing the attention very closely on one thing, for example, the breath or body or sounds, in what is known as single-point concentration. In this practice, we focus on different aspects of our experience separate from the others, which strengthens our ability to concentrate on each one. With practice, we can focus our attention longer; we become more aware when our attention shifts and more able to go back to the focus of our attention. And, we become more flexible in directing our attention. In addition to this single-point attention, we cultivate the ability to have a wide, open attention which falls evenly across all experience. With this kind of attention, we are open to all aspects of experience simultaneously, without having a strong pull towards one or another aspect of experience. This is a form of spaciousness: that open, wide attention which can hold all of our experience, with kindness (Kabat-Zinn, 1990).

In Mindful Parenting, we use the formal practices to cultivate this ability, and we use the informal practices of observing our child with beginner's mind, savoring moments, experiencing gratitude, and bringing awareness to everyday moments, to begin to bring more spaciousness into our experience of our children and ourselves as parents. But we also accept that spaciousness fluctuates moment to moment. We all come equipped with a fabulous zoom lens that allows us to zoom in close to problems and to zoom out to get a broader perspective from a distance. What may seem like a disaster at one moment (e.g., my child being suspended from school) may at another moment be viewed in the fuller context of life's ups and downs and the gift of learning from experience.

GUIDELINES FOR SESSION 2

The main themes of Session 2 are beginner's mind parenting and bringing an attitude of kindness to ourselves. We explore beginner's mind parenting by asking parents to share their experiences of observing their child with beginner's mind, with an exercise in mindful seeing, and with a playful exercise which illustrates our tendency to miss seeing things which are right in front of our noses when we don't expect them (the gorilla video). A second theme is the attitude of kindness which we invite parents to embody in their experience as parents and in learning mindfulness. We first address this when we explore parents' attitudes towards themselves as they do the various practices and as they confront any obstacles to doing the home practice. We do an experiential exercise about parenting stress in a friend, in order to highlight our tendency to be kinder towards a friend than to ourselves, and we invite parents to bring this same kindness to themselves when they feel stressed. Finally, we do a brief practice in gratitude, in order to correct our bias for the negative in ourselves and our children.

We continue to build up the mindfulness practice by repeating the body scan and by adding a new practice, sitting meditation on the breath.

The home practice elaborates these themes. We ask parents to savor a pleasant moment, by noticing it, bringing attention to it, and fully experiencing the moment. This practice is a way of bringing beginner's mind to small moments throughout the day and of being kind to ourselves. We also invite parents to choose an activity to do mindfully with their child every day, to experience *being* with their child instead of doing, and to create space for more beginner's mind experiences with their child. Finally, we invite them to do the body scan each day and meditation on the breath as their formal meditation.

Box 6.1. Agenda Session 2

1. Body scan + inquiry, including discussing how the body scan went at home and informal meditation home practice—first bite, routine activity (50 min)
2. Observation of your child—discuss first in pairs, then in the group (20 min)
3. Morning exercise from the perspective of a friend (10 min)
4. Break (15 min)
5. Mindful seeing (10 min)
6. Gorilla video (15 min)
7. Gratitude practice (10 min)
8. Sitting with the breath + brief inquiry (20 min)
9. Discuss practice for the following week (10 min)
10. Closing meditation (5 min)

---

1. BODY SCAN + INQUIRY

We begin Session 2 with a body scan of about a half hour, led by the teacher (see Handout 5.4). We ask parents to share their experience of this body scan and ask how participants experienced the home practice of the body scan during the past week. Some themes which may arise are the difficulty making time for the home practice, not wanting to do the practice, or feeling bored, frustrated, or impatient during the practice, which we discuss below as obstacles to practice. Other parents may describe feeling relaxed during the body scan or surprised that something so simple can help them feel more calm. As teachers, we can embody beginner's mind by remaining open and curious about whatever arises in the group. We may simply note with curiosity the wide range of reactions possible: "Isn't it incredible—we all had the same assignment, yet look how differently we all experienced it?"

OBSTACLES TO PRACTICE

A common theme in Session 2 is dealing with resistance and obstacles to practice. During the week between Sessions 1 and 2, parents will have had their first experience with daily meditation practice. Many parents may express the concern that their lives are so busy and hectic that planning 45 min of practice per day is simply not possible, despite the fact they made a commitment prior to starting the training. We invite parents to explore all aspects of the practice, especially the difficulties they encounter, with an attitude of openness, curiosity, and kindness. Many parents describe a feeling of pressure ("I have to practice"), a "must" or a "should" ("I should be able to do this"), self-critical or judgmental thoughts towards themselves ("I'm constantly distracted"), as well as defensive or angry reactions against this ("I fell asleep every time I did the body scan," "You just don't understand how busy I am").

BRINGING KINDNESS TO OURSELVES

At this point, parents are beginning to see how we can be judgmental, critical, and harsh with ourselves when we don't live up to our own expectations. We introduce the idea of bringing a sense of kindness or self-compassion to ourselves. In the Buddhist tradition, open-hearted friendliness and kindness is the basic stance towards others and towards oneself. It has been compared to the stance of a mother towards her baby: warm, unconditional love. This stance of kindness and self-compassion is inherent to secular mindfulness practice as well. We invite everyone to notice our attitude towards ourselves when we do the practice, especially when we have difficulty or are unable to do the practice. We might ask, "When you were unable to do your home practice, what was your attitude towards yourself?" "Could you be kind to yourself, or were you critical and judgmental?" Participants are often so used to their critical, striving stance towards themselves that they are quite surprised to discover that they can choose to take a different, more kind, and supportive attitude towards themselves.

We like the simplicity of "kindness" as a basic attitude towards one-self and others. Kindness is a word deeply linked to childhood experience. As children we learn early to be kind to others. As parents, we try to be kind and loving to our children. This is such a pure, basic attitude, and we want to help parents make the emotional connection between kindness for others and kindness to themselves.

We often teach participants the seven attitudinal foundations of mindfulness which Kabat-Zinn (1990) describes: (1) nonjudging, (2) patience, (3) beginner's mind, (4) trust, (5) non-striving, (6) acceptance, and (7) letting go. We illustrate bringing these seven attitudes to difficult interactions with your child, by working them out using parents' examples. For example, I used them when my 8-year-old daughter would come out of bed for the umpteenth time. I would quietly recite to myself "Non-judging—okay, I'm not going to judge my daughter or myself. Patience—let me have the patience to deal with this situation. Beginner's mind—let me look at my child as if she was coming out of bed for the first time. Trust—She will eventually sleep. Non-striving—I cannot make her sleep, neither can she. Acceptance—I have to accept that she is a difficult sleeper right now, and so was I at her age. Letting go—She will deal with it, not much I can do." Parents often recognize how much they were living their lives with the complete opposite of the seven attitudes. One parent quipped, "Yup, I guess I do all of them—but the opposite! I judge myself and my kids, I lose patience, I feel like it's the same old story, I don't trust myself, I'm striving to be better, I can't accept myself and my kid . . . ." Many parents have felt judged by their child's school, their psychologist or psychiatrist, and even by well-meaning friends. The attitudinal foundation of acceptance, nonjudging, allowing things to be as they are, gentleness, and kindness is a helpful antidote which helps parents begin to let go of their judgmental attitude towards themselves and their children.

Sometimes we find ourselves forgetting one or more of the seven factors when trying to teach them in the group. This invariably leads to much laughter and is a chance to model being imperfect and being non-judgmental when we make a mistake. But parents have limited time and attention, and one father complained that it was simply too much to remember all these factors. He asked, "Couldn't you just boil it down to one?" We asked "What would it be?" After thinking a moment, he replied "Kindness." If we try to remember the seven factors, we may go into our heads, but when we think of "kind," we are instantly transported back to our childhood hearts. Of course, however you decide to convey this stance, the most important way is by embodying yourself the basic attitude of kindness, openness, curiosity, and compassion towards yourself, towards the group members, and towards the unfolding process in the group.

WHAT IS THE TEACHER'S ATTITUDE TOWARDS PARENTS' DIFFICULTIES WITH PRACTICE?

The challenge for the teacher is to balance the tension between two dialectical poles. On the one hand, we ask for a strong commitment to practice, based on our experience that regular, daily practice helps parents develop the skills of mindfulness which they will ultimately use in their daily lives and in interaction with children and partners. On the other hand, we want to model for parents a mindful stance towards whatever their experience is, a stance which is kind and not judgmental, and at the same time, curious, and open. Parents may judge themselves harshly if they are not able to practice as much as the planned. The teacher embodies taking a nonjudging, accepting stance while at the same time being curious and investigating what made it so difficult to do the practice. Sometimes, despite our best intentions, parents may experience us as being judging or non-accepting. It helps when we are aware of our own reactions, for example, noticing if there are judgmental thoughts which have automatically crept up. For example, we have sometimes found ourselves feeling rather irritated when it becomes clear that parents have not practiced and have noticed thoughts such as "We told them in the intake they would need to practice one hour a day!" Or, "They could make the time for some practice, if they really set their minds to it." Being aware of our own tendency to judge can help us, paradoxically, respond in a nonjudgmental way to parents. When we let go of our judgment, we can better help parents to observe and be aware of what happens during the practice; what their experience is, whether negative or positive; and what difficulties arise. It is helpful to invite parents to become aware of their internal attitude towards themselves when they are not able to practice. For example, "When you were unable to practice the body scan this week, how did you react? Were you kind towards yourself, were you curious about it, or were you harsh, critical, or judgmental?"

It's also good to keep in mind that there is nothing sacred about sitting on a cushion. We all have the ability to be mindful, and being mindful as we give our child a bath, sit in a traffic jam, or wait in the grocery store is every bit as mindful as sitting on a cushion watching our breath

(M. Batchelor, p.c., March 2009). In fact, ultimately, it is these moments of awareness throughout our day that we wish to encourage and to expand. We should be cautious not to discourage parents who have trouble finding the time to do the formal practice but who nonetheless experience a moment of awareness while sitting in the garden with their child, noticing a blue jay in a tree. In this way, they can acquire a taste for mindfulness, which can help motivate them to cultivate their practice. This is also a way of meeting people wherever they are in their mindful practice. Parents have told us that being aware of these small moments throughout the day is one of the most helpful aspects of the course and that it helps them to parent with more awareness.

We also explore the paradox of doing mindful practice without a goal of achieving something as compared to doing mindfulness to relax or reduce stress. Of course, it's important to acknowledge that we would all love to feel less stressed and more relaxed, and we would all love to be free of our (often self-inflicted) suffering. The point is that the more we strive for relaxation as a goal, the more it may elude us. We return to the idea of accepting things the way they are, instead of trying to make them different than they are: Can I just rest in this moment now, with things being exactly as they are, not trying to make anything different? When we can embody this space of not trying to change, we often do experience a moment of peace or restfulness.

VOICES OF THE PARENTS: THE HOME PRACTICE

Amanda approached the first week's practice in the spirit of meditation as boot camp. Both she and her husband awoke one hour earlier every morning, so that they could both do the practice together before their two young children awoke. She talked about how difficult it was for her, and how exhausted she felt after a week of this, and she wondered how she could possibly keep this regiment up. Although Amanda had completed the practice "perfectly," she had done so in her usual driven, perfectionist and self-demanding manner, which led her to feel exhausted and stressed, and doubtful if she could go further after a week. While it was important for the teachers to acknowledge her "success" in pursuing her intention, it was particularly important to be curious about her manner of approaching this situation, as if she were running a marathon, and to explore what effect this approach had on her body, her thoughts and her feelings.

Simone reported that while she was able to do the formal meditation every day, she struggled to do the mindful activity. She had chosen to brush her teeth mindfully, but then immediately felt it was a mistake: she didn't want to brush her teeth mind-

fully, it was much too boring! She noticed that she felt angry and resentful, and observed that she was brushing her teeth very hard. She reported this as if she had failed the assignment, and she indeed felt self-critical. But we found it an excellent illustration of just how mindful she had been—she was aware of her feelings, her thoughts, and her physical sensations in her mouth. We helped her become more aware of her attitude towards herself: critical and judging.

Christine described how she intended to take a mindful bite, but in the time between lifting her fork and putting it in her mouth, she forgot!

Adrienne commented in frustration that she didn't have time to take a first mindful bite in the morning because it was too rushed.

Teacher: How much time do you think you need to be aware of a first bite?
Adrienne: Maybe three minutes.
Teacher: Do you think you could get up three minutes earlier to make time for this?
Adrienne: That won't work. My son comes into bed with us in the morning, and he gets up when I get up. Listen, I don't think you understand what it's like. While I'm eating, I'm also putting on my son's shoes and feeding him at the same time. I really don't have the time!

The group laughed as we recognized the feeling of not being able to spare even 3 minutes in the morning rush and also recognizing the absurd juggling act involved in getting our children out of the house in the morning. The shared humor of these kinds of moments is very helpful in setting a light, accepting, and warm atmosphere in the group.

At the same time, the teacher used this as an opportunity to illustrate how meal-times with children can so often be rushed, and we may go into automatic pilot, losing contact with ourselves and our children. These are exactly the moments when we need to slow down and become mindful of our actual experience. In fact, being mindful of anything— the first bite—doesn't actually take any additional time, just the intention and remembering the intention in the moment.

Yet, on a process level, something different was going on. Adrienne was in essence saying, "You don't understand, I literally do not have the time, I am juggling three things at once." The teacher was questioning her in order to open up the possibility of bringing awareness to this hectic moment, but Adrienne experienced it as if the teacher were asking the impossible of her, and she felt angry and misunderstood. This theme, that there isn't enough time to be mindful, comes up throughout the group, and here it is important to closely watch the process between teacher and parent. What is intended as open, curious investigation by the teacher can be experienced by the parent as trying to convince or judge them. As teachers, we may notice that we are talking too much, problem-solving, or feeling irritated by the participant, and we may notice judging thoughts. When we notice our own judging thoughts or expectations, we can more easily let go of them. This frees us to be able to help the participant explore with curiosity her own reaction. When participants feel that we are genuinely trying to help them investigate their experience (rather than trying to make them practice more), they can take ownership of their experience. They can wonder why they react in a particular way, and they can ask themselves—What do I want to do with this practice? How do I want to incorporate this into my life?

BEING WITH STRONG EMOTIONS

Joy had chosen to do mindful cycling as her routine activity. She was feeling very sad one day, and thought that mindful cycling would help her feel less sad. At the same time, she didn't really feel like biking mindfully. She decided not to, but then ended up feeling even sadder.

On one level, this illustrates a common experience we all have—we forget to be mindful, or we actively resist it, exactly at those moments when we need it the most. But on another level, Joy was still trying to solve her problem using the doing mode: "If I cycle mindfully, I can get rid of these sad feelings." The teachers asked what it would be like to simply let the sad feelings be there and pay attention to what she was feeling in her body and mind. This was new for Joy. Later, Joy's soft "Let me feel it" became a sort of mantra for the whole group to remind us that it's okay to just feel emotions as they are, instead of trying to make them go away.

When painful or distressing body sensations, feelings, or thoughts come up during the practice, as they did for Joy, they can become obstacles to practice. Most of us try to avoid distressing feelings, by distracting ourselves, pushing them away, or denying them. For some of us, sad and vulnerable feelings may be more difficult to experience than angry feelings; others of us may tend to avoid anger. If we have suffered from depression or anxiety, we may avoid or actively fight against negative emotions. Psychologist Campbell-Sills and colleagues did an experiment to investigate this. They asked participants to watch a film that provoked strong emotions. While all participants responded with the same degree of negative emotions, anxious and depressed participants judged the negative emotions as less acceptable, and they suppressed them more than the others (Campbell-Sills, Barlow, Brown, & Hofmann, 2006).

Similarly, if we have struggled with physical difficulties such as chronic pain or physical injury, we may feel afraid when we experience uncomfortable bodily sensations, and we may try to suppress or avoid these sensations. Unfortunately, this can cause us to tense up in our body, leading to more pain or risk of injury.

Fears of strong emotions or physical pain may be intensified when we become parents. We may feel surprised at the intensity of our emotions, and it may be difficult to admit when we feel negative emotions such as anger, disappointment, or sadness with our children. Many of us feel self-critical or ashamed of the anger we sometimes feel towards our children, and we may have difficulty even recognizing these feelings. If we feel depressed, we may worry about the effect of our sadness on our children, and we may try to hide it from them. Some of us may fear "losing control" by experiencing strong negative feelings and body sensations, especially if we equate being competent as a parent with being in control of our household, our children, and our emotions. We are confronted with idealized images of parenthood in our society, especially of mothers. When our actual experience as mothers and fathers is discrepant from this idealized image, it may be hard to admit this to ourselves. The irony is that right at the moment that we are dealing with the increased demands and stress that parenthood brings, we are faced with images which reflect only part of our experience. This can make it hard for us to acknowledge the other parts.

I remember that when my daughter was an infant, I was surprised at how frustrated and angry I could feel when she wouldn't take her nap. I was so desperate to have this 2-hour break from being "on" as a parent that I would feel panicked when she would cheerfully pop up in her crib after 5 minutes, ready to go. The intensity of my feelings surprised me. I wondered if it meant I was not a good mother or that I didn't love my baby enough. Everyone had told me how much I would love my baby, and I did indeed love her to bits, but no one had ever prepared me for the anger I would sometimes feel.

We work with intense emotions or sensations by simply listening for the range of reactions parents may have to sitting with their emotions and bodily sensations and encouraging parents to explore not only these reactions but also the stance they take towards them, perhaps by asking, "What was your attitude towards the sadness (or fear, anger, pain, discomfort)? Could you let it be there? Did you notice yourself judging yourself or trying to move away from it in some way? What was that like?" It may help to acknowledge that we are inviting them to have a different stance towards their experience than usual. We are inviting them be open to their sensations and emotions, as well as to notice their habitual way of reacting to them.

In exploring the first attempts at mindful practice, we come back again and again to the attitude we bring to the practice: Whether we are in doing mode or being mode, whether we are judging ourselves, whether we are kind to ourselves or critical, whether we can accept our experience, or whether we are striving for things to be different than they are. No matter how much or little someone has practiced, we can explore mindfully their experience of trying to do the practice.

2. OBSERVATION OF YOUR CHILD: CHILD AS RAISIN EXERCISE

We began informally calling this exercise "child as raisin" because it often elicits the same kind of wonder and appreciation for the fullness of experiencing for our child as the raisin exercise does for a raisin. We ask the participants to pair up in twos to describe their experience observing their child as if for the first time. We then invite parents to describe their experiences in the full group. We often find this to be a very moving moment in the session, as parents reconnect emotionally with their feelings of amazement, love, and joy for their child. At the same time, this exercise can be very difficult, and parents can become aware of just how hard it is to see our child with beginner's mind. As teachers, we make the intention to be open and curious as we listen to the experiences.

VOICES OF THE PARENTS

Lizzy was struggling with her 15-year-old daughter, diagnosed with the oppositional-defiant disorder, whom she experienced as "closed." She described what happened when she went to observe her daughter with beginner's mind, without talking, simply being attentive from moment to moment. To her surprise, she noticed that something different happened. Her daughter, who usually would not say very much, started to share a lot of experiences, and Lizzy simply kept listening in astonishment. Lizzy realized that she herself was "closed," and that being attentive opened herself, and her daughter. She even observed that her own being "closed" caused her daughter to close up.

When Joy observed her two boys, her heart was filled with such love for them. Then she noticed the feeling went away, and she tried to get it back, but it was gone.

As precious as these beginner's mind moments are, they will inevitably be replaced by other moments. If we try to hang on to them, they slip through our hands, and we can fall into the trap of being disappointed with what there is. Our experience is ever changing, ever unfolding, and everything eventually changes, so moments of feeling love will be replaced by other moments. This can be hard to accept, because we want to prolong the good feelings and stave off the bad feeling. But allowing them to come and go naturally means less resistance to the reality of our experience and also less stress. The goal of this exercise is not to see our children as little angels but rather to expand and open our view of them to include more of what is there.

It's helpful to ask who had difficulty with this assignment or who had different experiences. For example, sometimes parents become aware of just how difficult it is to see their children with beginner's mind.

Pamela discovered her high expectations for herself and her child when she tried to do the exercise: "I kept trying to do the observation of my child the whole week, but it never seemed to work. I would start observing her, then think no, this isn't a good moment. I guess I had expectations about what I would see—I was hoping I would discover again the innocent and pure love I felt for her when she was a baby. But instead I couldn't keep out the criticisms I have of her, and the worries I have about her."

Irene reported "I couldn't do it—I kept thinking about how her hair was a mess, how this wasn't right, how that wasn't right."

John tried to observe his adolescent daughter while she was supposed to be studying for an exam but was instead hanging out in front of the TV. He was so full of judgments and irritation about her behavior that he could not observe her with beginner's mind.

Many of us can relate to these experiences. It's not easy to open to our child with beginner's mind. What's important is the intention of seeing our child anew, our awareness of what we are experiencing when we do that, and a healthy dose of self-kindness when we realize just how hard it is. Fortunately, every day we have the chance to look at our child with beginner's mind. We encourage parents to repeat this exercise often, if only for a brief moment. It's also a great one to do with our partners, and they will be grateful for it as well!

3. MORNING STRESS FROM THE PERSPECTIVE OF A FRIEND

The goal of this exercise is to introduce kindness and compassion as qualities that we all possess and that we can bring to ourselves in moments of parenting stress.

"Sit comfortably and close your eyes. Imagine the following scene as if it is happening to you, paying attention to your body sensations, feelings, thoughts, and any action tendencies which arise"

You've just dropped off your child at school, when you see a friend running frantically onto the schoolyard, dragging her child by the hand. When the friend returns, she says, "You wouldn't believe what a morning I had. First my daughter refused to get dressed because her favorite shirt wasn't clean, then she threw a temper tantrum right before we left because her hair was not just right, screaming she would not go to school anymore. Then I just completely lost it: I started screaming that if she didn't get up off the floor right now I was going to school without her, and finally I just dragged her out of the house, while my other two children were watching the scene from the car. It was horrible. It's a miracle we got here in one piece."

INQUIRY

We ask, "What do you notice in your body? What feelings do you notice? What thoughts are there? What do you want to say or do?"

On a whiteboard, we write the following:

What do you notice in your body? Some responses we have heard:

Goose bumps
Fast breathing
Tension
Calm

What do you feel? For example:

Sympathy.
Pity.
Warmth.
Worry.
Compassion.
I feel bad for my friend.

I see the humor of the situation.
I feel as if it's happening to me.

Thoughts? For example:

Poor parent.
Poor kid.
I know what she's going through.
How can I help?
Glad it wasn't me!
I'm not the only parent who can't get my kid to school on time!
She should get up earlier.

What do you want to say or do to your friend? (Action Tendencies) For example:

Hey, I've been there too.
How I can help?
Give her a hug.
Put my arms around her.
Take her out for coffee.

We ask the group: What's going on here? What do most of these responses have in common? We write down the various responses: *compassion, understanding, embracing, empathy, kindness, friendship*, or other words that come up in the group.

We then ask parents to compare these responses to the responses they gave last week when they imagined a similar parenting stress had happened to them. How did they feel towards themselves in the last exercise? Parents immediately see how easy it is for them to be kind and compassionate towards a friend, and how much they judge themselves. We invite them to embody a different attitude by asking, "Can you become as good a friend to yourself as you are to your friend? That's what self-compassion is about. During stressful and difficult moments with our child or others, we can tell ourselves: 'We're only human, we can give ourselves a hug, get ourselves that coffee, etc.'"

It's important to note that although the most common reactions we get are ones of empathy for the "friend" under stress, some parents may offer a judgmental or critical response. For example, one parent said, "She should be more organized in the morning!" and another felt critical towards the mother because of what she was doing to her child. We acknowledge all the reactions which come up with a spirit of openness and curiosity.

4. BREAK

Break for tea or coffee and cookies, with full awareness for the first sip or bite.

5. MINDFUL SEEING

In mindful seeing, we try to see without using our usual knowledge or concepts to shape our perception or interpretation. We invite the group to find a place to stand in front of one of the windows in the room, in order to do a seeing meditation. We ring the bell. We ask participants to look the way a painter would look at the scene or the way a filmmaker would look at a scene. We ask them to sense shape, color, shadow, and movement, without interpreting, with evenly distributed attention, noting whether any judgments, interpretations, and prior knowledge affect what we see (see Box 6.2).

It becomes immediately clear that we cannot "see" purely, without our brain organizing our perceptions or without our prior knowledge influencing what we see. For example, if we look at a tree, we may immediately think "a tree" (concept) and then notice a judgment ("beautiful, I like it"). Through awareness of perception, concepts, and interpretation, we can sometimes have glimpses of the basic elements—color, form, shape, contrast—that we actually see, before our concepts and judgments come in.

The point of this exercise is to help participants become aware of these automatic processes at work and to help them realize that when we look at our child, we also "see" many things based on our prior knowledge, concepts, or interpretations. Seeing our child with beginner's mind, over and over again, means consciously letting go of our ideas about her and seeing what is actually there in this moment.

VOICES OF THE PARENTS

Ken reported that he was looking at an electrical outlet on the wall, and noticed the difference between the white and the shadow, which gave it a perception of depth. He commented that this is already a perception, since according to Zen teachings, all we can see is light and dark, and all else is interpretation.

Box 6.2. Seeing with Fresh Eyes
(Adapted from Segal, Williams, & Teasdale, 2002)

We stand comfortably, bringing our attention to our posture, noticing any tension in the body and deliberately softening, allowing our arms to hang loosely along our body, and feeling the contact between our feet and the ground, aware of the movement of our breath in this position.

Then, bringing your attention to seeing with a beginners mind. Imagine you're from Mars and have never seen this scene before . . . shapes, lines, colors, light/dark, shades, far or close, movements . . . as if you are a painter, or a filmmaker. Or you may imagine you are a cat looking outside, what do you see? Try as best as you can to look at everything, without judging, labeling, or categorizing. So instead of noticing: car, tree, cloud, or man, look deeply at the object, noticing shape, light and dark, color, movement, form. What is your eye drawn to and what you tend to ignore? With the eyes of a beginner, observe in this new way.

This is an interesting moment of choice for the teacher. On the one hand, Ken is describing his experiencing of seeing white and shadow of the outlet, and at the same time, he is observing his brain's need to perceive this as depth. On the other hand, he quickly moved into a long, rather intellectual discourse about Zen philosophy, which took him away from his here and now experience. One could feel the other parents in the group becoming restless while listening to this. How does the teacher remain open to Ken's experience, while intervening to help Ken elucidate his here and now experience rather than give a discourse on Zen philosophy? There are many options, and as teachers, we each develop our own style of responding. One option is to comment and simply ask for more details about the moment to moment experience: "Interesting, you were aware of your experience seeing the outlet, and at the same time, you were aware of your mind's automatically interpreting that as depth. Tell us more about your experience." In this way, the teacher acknowledges Ken's attention to both the seeing and the process of seeing, while also redirecting back to his experience of seeing and away from a conceptual discussion of Zen practice.

Annette described how she felt drawn to looking out of the window, and how she noticed also the window frame, as if it was the frame of a painting which made her think of modern paintings which depict the frame in the painting. She noticed a slight shadow on the window sill. She looked at the scene as if she were going to paint it, really looking at what form and color were there. Despite this, she found herself labeling what she saw—"a tree, a cloud"—and she found herself judging ("how beautiful, this is nice to look at, this is not"). She thought of her cat looking out of the window, how he is endlessly fascinated without having words or concepts, and tried to look with his eyes. She then deliberately choose to focus on a point inside, instead of looking outside the window which was more pleasurable. Looking up at the ceiling, she noticed for the first time that is was quite high, and rounded, actually rather grand. She also noticed the fluorescent lights which she had not noticed before.

Annette's experience highlights several themes that often arise in this exercise. One theme is simply how difficult it is for us to separate our concepts from our direct sensory experience. Like Ken, Annette was able to experience more of the sensory aspect of seeing: she saw the frame of the window as well as the view outside, noticing the shadow on the window. By imagining she was going to paint or that she was seeing like a cat, she was able to focus on shapes, colors, light, and darkness. Nonetheless, she noticed conceptual labels popping up in her mind— "tree, cloud" and judgments about what she liked and did not like. She also noticed her mind being drawn to look out the window, which she found pleasurable, and had to consciously choose to look inside the room, which she found less interesting, here again catching her mind judging "pleasurable" and "unpleasurable." Finally, she had a beginner's mind experience when she focused on looking inside the room, in that she noticed things which had been there all along—the high rounded ceilings and fluorescent lights—but which she had not noticed before, perhaps because it was not interesting to her.

Perhaps what this exercise demonstrates most clearly is how difficult it is for our minds *not* to interpret or judge. Our brain wants to interpret and does so automatically. In fact, we are constantly interpreting our experience in line with our prior experiences, expectations, and biases. Mindful seeing helps us to notice these biases, allowing us to see things in a new way.

6. GORILLA IN THE MIDST

We introduce this video by saying that we will show a short film clip of a basketball game and that we would like them to count how many times the team in black catches the ball (see www.youtube.com/watch

?v=vJG698U2Mvo). Afterwards, we ask whether they noticed anything unusual. Then we tell them that a man in a gorilla suit walked through the game. We show the video again, and parents are usually shocked at having missed the gorilla. This is a great demonstration of how we sometimes do not see literally what is in front of us, if it doesn't fit our expectations. The obvious lesson is what do we miss seeing in our children (or our partners, or ourselves) because it doesn't fit into our view of them? What do we miss when we focus on . . . ? For example, we can talk about how when we look for problems, we certainly find them, but we may overlook other important things. Using our beginner's mind is a way to become more spacious and see more of our child.

7. GRATITUDE PRACTICE

We do a brief practice to remind ourselves of what we feel grateful for in our child (or children) and ourselves as parents. We borrowed this exercise from Chris Germer because we find it a lovely antidote to our biased attention to our child's problems and to our own flaws as parents. As the Dalai Lama points out, when we struggle with problems, it is all too easy to let the problems fill up our entire experience and for us to forget, or take for granted, how much our children enrich our lives.

For example, if our child had a rough day and felt bad about a friend slighting him, we may focus on that, forgetting about the strengths and resources he has to deal with these inevitable ups and downs. If we were impatient with our child and snapped, we may remember that more than the hundred other caring things we did for our child. When we deliberately open our attention to things that we feel grateful for, in ourselves or our child, we can view the difficulties we face as parents and the difficulties our children face in a more spacious and forgiving light.

A colleague once told me a story that brought this home poignantly. She had seen a family with three young children with serious behavior problems. The parents were at their wits' ends and felt desperate for help. My colleague felt at a loss herself to know how to guide the family as the children seemed so out of control. Several weeks later, the family returned. In the meantime, there had been a fire in the home, and one of the children had died. All of a sudden, the "crisis" of the previous weeks was inconsequential compared to the devastating loss. It brought home for my colleague how easy it is to let our focus on our problems overshadow what we have and cherish.

Box 6.3. Gratitude Practice

(Adapted from C. Germer, p.c., November 12–13, 2011)

Sit comfortably, close your eyes, and bring your awareness to your body posture . . . sensations . . . and now to your breathing. (*Wait a few moments until everyone is settled.*) Let an image of your child come up, Asking ourselves, What do I feel grateful for in my child? Opening our minds and hearts to three things we feel grateful for, however small, without thinking too much. (*Allow a few minutes*). And now, bringing our attention to ourselves, imagining ourselves in our role as parent. And asking, What do I feel grateful for in myself as a parent? Three things, however small, about myself as parent? Allowing the answer to bubble up spontaneously without too much thinking. And now, when you're ready, opening your eyes.

Parents can write down the three things they are grateful of in their child and in themselves as parents in their workbook, if they like. Then they can share one thing they are grateful for in their child and in themselves as parent with the person sitting next to them, in a small group of three persons, or, if there is time, with the group as a whole. As with all practices, but especially with practices in which we intentionally acknowledge the positive, we remain open and curious to whatever experiences arise in the group, including parents who can find nothing to feel grateful for in themselves or their child at that moment. The teacher can be curious about how that feels and acknowledge that we all struggle to feel grateful at times. We might talk about how when we feel depressed, or hopeless, or critical, or alone, it may be hard to get in touch with feeling grateful. If no one spontaneously mentions having difficulty feeling grateful, we may ask "Was there anybody who had difficulty with this or who had other feelings come up?" It's so much in our human nature to focus on negative events or feelings that it's important to remind ourselves that it's okay if we don't always feel grateful. In fact, this is why we do this practice, because it *doesn't* come naturally to us.

One mother shared the following experience:

It was easy to think about three things in my child that I'm grateful for: initiating, social, kind. Thinking about three things I am grateful for in myself, nothing came, not a single thought. And from nothing it came up and I could not suppress it; tears, sadness, a tight throat. Well, that was clear. I found nothing to be grateful for in myself. Yes if I thought longer, but that came from far. Sadness from a far past, I knew that, but that it would be brought up like this I had not expected.

8. SITTING MEDITATION: THE BREATH

The teacher guides the group in a sitting meditation on the breath, for about 10 min (see Handout 6.4). For this first sitting meditation, it's helpful to devote some time to helping people find a comfortable position on the cushion, bench, or chair. The teacher can go around and help adjust people, for example, by adding more cushions for support if needed.

INQUIRY

In the inquiry following the first formal sitting meditation, parents often mention difficulties they encounter such as painful sensations, thoughts, difficulty going back to the breath, feeling bored or tired, and feeling distracted by thoughts, feelings, noises, itches, or other body sensations. Some parents feel they are not doing it right. The most important thing we want to communicate as teacher is that whatever we experience is okay—there is no right or wrong when it comes to meditation. In fact, all of the difficulties or obstacles to practice are simply experiences to become aware of. The moment we are aware that we have been distracted, our awareness is back. It is also helpful to acknowledge that it is difficult and that it is completely normal for our minds to wander and become distracted: "That's what minds do, they wander." Another nice metaphor is "monkey mind"—the tendency of our minds to jump from one branch of thought to the next. What we are doing is creating spaciousness with compassion. We normalize the experience as simply part of being human, and this creates a feeling of acceptance and compassion. When participants can bring that acceptance and compassion to their own experience, they open to it more and can watch their experience unfold with less self-judgment. And they will begin to notice their self-judgments as well and begin to bring acceptance to that experience.

In the inquiry, we try to model bringing open, nonjudgmental curiosity to all of our experiences. We might ask: What did you notice in your body? How did you recognize that you were distracted? Was it possible to return to the breath? Did anyone notice any judgments? We can also ask questions to help participants explore their *reactions* to their experience. For example, when you noticed you were very distracted, what happened next? Did you notice any thoughts or feelings coming up? Or, when you felt sleepy, or tired, how did you react? Here we are listening for the attitude towards their experience—whether they respond with self-judgments or with self-compassion. We also listen for reactions to emotional or physical pain—what did you do when you became aware of the painful sensations? Here we listen for the whole range of reactions—from immediately shifting position to sitting like a martyr with extreme discomfort. It's also interesting to explore what we do with emotional pain—do we avoid it by quickly changing the subject or do we stay with it? What happens when we stay with it? Do we notice a kind of contagion to other thoughts and feelings? We also can ask, where did you feel it in your body? This is helpful for anchoring experience in the here and now. We can also reflect for the whole group some key points in practice, such as "That's what the meditation is about, again and again noticing that we're distracted and bringing our attention back to the breath, the body . . . . Pain, boredom, falling asleep, hunger, and thoughts (or anything else mentioned) are all examples of experiences we may notice while meditating. All we have to do is simply be with our experiences, investigating them rather than wanting them to go away or judging ourselves harshly when we notice them." It is also helpful to add that when we notice we are wanting some experiences to go away, or that we are judging ourselves harshly, that is also okay.

9. REVIEW OF HOME PRACTICE FOR NEXT SESSION

We review the home practice and answer any questions about it (see Handout 6.1). We ask parents to choose now a short routine activity with their child to do with full attention this week. If time allows, it is helpful to take a moment to let each person decide what routine activity with the child he or she is going to do mindfully this week and share it with the group. We also ask them to practice again the body scan once a day and, at another time once a day, the mindfulness of breathing sitting meditation. Finally, we ask them to record savoring moments that are related and unrelated to parenting.

10. CLOSING MEDITATION

We do a brief meditation, for example, Sylvia Boorstein's "May I meet this moment fully. . . . May I meet it with kindness," or just a few minutes of sitting in silence, or any other brief meditation of your choosing.

HANDOUT 6.1 Practice for the Week After Session 2

Reading

Read the handouts mindfully

Mindful Parenting

Choose a new routine activity to practice with full awareness but now a routine activity with your child. Make a deliberate effort to bring moment to moment awareness to that activity each time it happens. Some examples are dressing your child, combing your child's hair, reading a story to your child, asking your child how his or her day was, waking your child up, putting him or her to bed or another activity that you prefer.

Formal Practice

Practice the body scan every day, six times a week. Practice also at least once without audio recording. Record your experiences on the Practice Record Form.

At other times, practice 10–15 min mindfulness of breathing for 6 days. Being with your breath in this way each day provides an opportunity to become aware of what it feels like to be connected and present in the moment without having to do anything. Use the audio recording or just set a timer, but in that case, first read Handout 6.4.

Informal Practice

Complete the Savoring Pleasant Moments Calendar (one entry per day). Savoring moments can be really small things, such as really savoring the first sip of coffee, enjoying when someone smiles at you, and listening when your child is singing. You can savor experiences which are related and unrelated to parenting or your child. Use recording those events as an opportunity to become really aware of the thoughts, feelings, and body sensations around one savoring event each day. Notice and record each event as soon as you can, in detail (e.g., record the actual words or images, body sensations, feelings).

HANDOUT 6.2 Beginner's Mind Parenting

When we look at our child with the eyes of a beginner, we may be surprised at what we see. When we open ourselves to experience our child more fully, we expand our view of him. If our child has had difficulties, or been diagnosed with a psychological disorder, this new perspective can be truly revelatory.

Our image of our child has been shaped through the history of our interactions with him going a long way back. For example, if our child was a colicky or born premature, years later we may still remember the anxious start we had with this child, and this memory may influence the way we interact now with our child. If our child has been diagnosed with a mental disorder such as ADHD or autism, this may influence how we look at him, what we expect, and how we interact with him. We may view our eldest child as the "mature one" and the youngest child may be our "baby" who we love to cuddle and joke with. These labels can limit both of them from fully developing if they are too rigid.

When we label our child, either with a diagnosis or a label of our own making, we pay more attention to behaviors which fit that label, and we may overlook behaviors which do not fit the label. When this happens automatically, we lose our beginner's mind and can become stuck in rigid or negative ways of seeing our child. When rigid labels narrow our attention, we may miss subtle changes in our child's behavior and miss opportunities to respond in new or creative ways. Our interactions can become automatic and repetitive, with less room for growth and change.

We may also have trouble seeing ourselves with beginner's mind, instead judging ourselves based on our entire parenting history or our partner's or child's view of us. Or we may view our partner in a rigid way, not seeing him or her fully.

Seeing our child, ourselves, and our partner with the mind of a beginner opens the door a crack for the possibility of change, in every moment. When we see something new in our child, something unexpected, out of character, or fresh, we offer him the gift of experiencing him more fully and giving him the space he needs to grow and change.

HANDOUT 6.3 The Attitudinal Foundation*
of Mindfulness Practice

1. Non-judging
2. Patience
3. Beginner's mind
4. Trust
5. Non-striving
6. Acceptance
7. Letting go

*Adapted from *Full Catastrophe Living* by Kabat-Zinn (1990).

HANDOUT 6.4 Mindfulness of Breathing—Sitting*

Settling

1. Settle in a comfortable sitting position, either on a straight-backed chair on a soft surface on the floor with your bottom supported by cushions or on a low stool or mediation bench. If you use a chair, sit away from the back of the chair so that your spine is self-supporting. If you sit on the floor, it is helpful if your knees can actually touch the floor, although that may not happen at the beginning; experiment with the height of the cushions or stool until you feel comfortably and firmly supported.
2. Allow the back to adopt an erect, dignified, and comfortable posture. If sitting on a chair, have the feet flat on the floor with legs uncrossed. Gently close your eyes if that feels comfortable. If not, let your gaze fall unfocused on the floor four or five feet in front of you.

Bringing awareness to the body

3. Bring your awareness to the level of physical sensations by focusing your attention on the sensations of touch, contact, and pressure in your body where it makes contact with the floor and with whatever you are sitting on. Spend a minute or two exploring these sensations.
4. Now bring your awareness to the changing patterns of physical sensations in the belly as the breath moves in and out of the body, just as you did lying down.
5. Focus your awareness on the wild sensations of stretching as the abdominal wall gently expands with each in-breath and on the sensations of gentle release as the abdominal wall deflates with each out-breath. As best you can, stay in touch with the changing physical sensations in your abdomen for the full duration of the in-breath and the full duration of the out-breath, perhaps noticing the slight pauses between an in-breath and the following out-breath and between an out-breath and the following in-breath. As an alternative, if you prefer, focus on a place in the body where you find the sensations of breath the most vivid and distinct (such as the nostrils).
6. There is no need to try to control your breathing in any way—simply let your body breathe by itself. As best you can, also bring this attitude of *allowing* to the rest of your experience—there is nothing that needs to be fixed, and no particular state to be achieved. As best you can, simply surrender to your experience as it is without requiring that it be any different.

*From *The Mindful Way through Depression* by Williams, Teasdale, Segal, and Kabat-Zinn (2007), pp. 78–79. Copied with permission of Guilford Press.

HANDOUT 6.4 Mindfulness of Breathing—Sitting (continued)

Working with the mind when it wanders

7. Sooner or later (usually sooner), the mind will wander away from the focus on the breath sensation in the belly, getting caught up in thoughts, planning, or daydreams, or just aimlessly drifting about. Whatever comes up, whatever the mind is pulled to or absorbed in things is simply what minds do; it is not a mistake or a failure. When you notice that your awareness is no longer focused on the breath, you might want to actually congratulate yourself because you've already come back enough to know it. You are, once more, aware of your experience. You might like to briefly acknowledge where the mind has been (noticing what is on your mind and perhaps making a light mental note: "thinking, thinking" or "planning, planning" or "worrying, worrying"). Then, gently escorting your attention back to the breath sensations in the belly, as you bring awareness to the feeling of *this* out-breath, whichever is here as you return.

8. However often you notice that the mind has wandered (and this will quite likely happen over and over again), each time take note of where the mind has been, then gently escort your attention back to the breath and simply resume attending to the changing pattern of physical sensations that come with each in-breath and with each out-breath.

9. As best you can, bring a quality of kindness to your awareness, perhaps seeing the repeated wanderings of the mind as opportunities to cultivate greater patience and acceptance within yourself and some compassion toward your experience.

10. Continue with the practice for 10 min, or longer if you wish, perhaps reminding yourself from time to time that the intention is simply to be aware of your experience moment to moment, as best you can, using the breath as an anchor to gently reconnect with the here and now each time that you notice that the mind has wandered off and is no longer in touch with the abdomen, in touch with this very breath in this very moment.

HANDOUT 6.5 Savoring Pleasant Moments Calendar

Be aware once a day of a pleasant moment *at the time it is happening.* See if you can savor these moments by deliberately bringing awareness to the pleasant sensations. Notice moments related and unrelated to parenting. Use the following questions to focus your awareness on the details of the experience as it is happening. Write it down later.

What was the experience?	Were you aware of the pleasant feeling *while* it was happening?	What happened in your body, in detail, during this experience?	What moods, feelings, and thoughts accompanied this experience?
Example: *My daughter crawling into bed with me in the morning*	*Yes*	*Warm, relaxed, stretching out, smiling; enjoying the contact with my daughter, enjoying the feel and smell of her body*	*Joy, pleasure, love. "She is so loving and sweet." "I'm glad she still lets me cuddle her"*

HANDOUT 6.6　Home Practice Record Form Week 2

Fill in the form each time you do the formal practice. Note whatever comes up for you during the formal practice, so that we can talk about it next session.

Day/time	Practice (Yes/No)	Comments

HANDOUT 6.7 Notes Informal Practice and Mindful Parenting Practice Week 2

You may want to use this sheet to make notes about your experiences during the informal meditation practice and the mindful parenting practice. Or to make notes during or about the group session.

CHAPTER 7

SESSION 3: RECONNECTING
WITH OUR BODY AS A PARENT

Don't go outside your house to see the flowers.
My friend, don't bother with that excursion.
Inside your body there are flowers.
One flower has a thousand petals.
That will do for a place to sit.
Sitting there you will have a glimpse of beauty
inside the body and out of it,
before gardens and after gardens.

Kabir (1971)

How OFTEN do we really inhabit our own bodies? Think about it. How often do you actually feel what is going on in your body, while it is happening? Our bodies are our homes, we live in them and through them, yet more often than not, we treat them dismissively, only reluctantly heeding their signals that we are tired, in pain, or reaching our limit. Instead, we live in our heads, dwelling in the cockpit of our being, directing our experience with our rationale thoughts, goals, and plans, only occasionally dropping down to the lower floors to check out what's going on below.

We live in this disembodied way, until something forces us to pay attention to our bodies. More often than not, we only truly listen to our body when it screams out in pain, or grinds to a screeching halt, saying in effect: "I'm not going any further." This may be a point of crisis: a point when we realize we are driving ourselves too hard, losing the forest for the trees. Our body may shut down in physical or emotional pain, or less dramatically, we may become aware of physical discomforts such as back or neck pain, stomach upset, heartburn or digestive track problems, headaches or migraines, and fatigue. Or we may suffer a near-fatal incident, such as a heart attack or stroke.

Why is it so important for us to reconnect with our bodies, especially when we become parents? Our body provides a very simple way to return our attention to the immediate experience of the present moment. Functioning as a parent requires a tremendous amount of doing mode. Adrienne's description of feeding her son while simultaneously tying his shoes and eating her own breakfast is a recognizable example of how we can automatically go into doing mode, losing touch with ourselves and our bodies. It is not uncommon for parents to say that they are so busy taking care of their young children that they forget to eat, or forget to go to the bathroom, as if they are in a trance of doing mode. It's as though we put our bodies off to the side to be attended to later when our children's needs have been met.

Bringing our attention back to our body, either to the breath or other sensations in our body, breaks through that trance and connects one immediately to the present moment as it is felt in the body. When we step back into our body, we might notice that our shoulders are tensed up to our ears, our stomach is in knots, or that our chest is tight. Often in that first moment of reconnection with the body, we experience a release of tension, a slowing down of breathing, and a slowing down of our reactions. It seems to help initiate the movement from doing mode to being mode. We may then spontaneously notice thoughts and feelings arising as well, which further helps us connect with our immediate experience with ourselves and our child.

For example, when Joy took a moment to "check in" with her body while she was rushing to get her child ready for school, she noticed how her head, neck, and shoulder muscles were tensed, and she became aware of feelings of irritation at her daughter, as well as worries that she would be late for an important meeting at work. Her body sensations were like a barometer helping her to feel what was going on with her in that moment of stress. Recognizing the tension in her body, she spontaneously thought to herself "let go" and felt some of the tension leaving her body and an ebb in her irritation. Becoming aware gave her a moment to think about how she wanted to handle this moment, and she decided to let go of the pressure she was feeling to get her child to school on time. With her relaxing, she could focus more on attending to her daughter in that moment and was able to ask herself, "What does my daughter need in this moment?" As she slowed down and stopped rushing her daughter, her daughter was able to dress herself and became more cooperative.

When we step back into our bodies and fully experience their sensations, we tune into ourselves, which is the first step to tuning into our children (Siegel & Hartzell, 2003). After all, if we are completely out of touch with ourselves, how can we possibly tune in to our children? As Joy noticed, tuning into her own needs and taking the pressure off herself helped her to tune into what her daughter was needing in that moment.

By the time they come to the training, many parents have already had years of ignoring their bodies' signals and ignoring their own physical and personal boundaries and limits. This is often encouraged in the achievement-oriented culture we live in. At work, we are expected to work as long and as hard as possible to achieve our goals, without regard to the psychological or physical toll it may take on ourselves or our families. At the gym, we may try to push our bodies to their limit and beyond, trying to become fitter, thinner, more muscular, and more limber, rather than accepting our bodies for how they are and tuning in to the wisdom of our bodies.

Unfortunately, ignoring our body can have serious consequences for our physical and emotional health such as chronic pain, injury, medical illness, or depression. By the time we experience pain, we have already gone past our own bodily limits. If we can get to know these limits, we can use the wisdom of our body to take better care of ourselves. When we learn to tune in and listen to our bodies, we can learn a lot about what we are experiencing in the here and now.

When we practice yoga mindfully, we become more familiar with our body: what it feels like when we make certain movements, what it feels like when we approach a limit, and what it feels like when we go over a limit. Practicing yoga mindfully is also an antidote to striving. It's not about doing the movement perfectly or increasing flexibility or strength. It's simply about experiencing the physical sensations arising from our body; appreciating what our bodies actually can do, whatever our physical condition; and learning to listen to and respect our bodies' limits. When we can pay attention to our bodily limits, we become better able to pay attention to our emotional or psychological limits as well, which is important for taking care of ourselves and for setting limits on children.

When we respect our bodies' limits, we are accepting them as they are and letting go of wanting them to be different. This can be a physical metaphor for accepting ourselves and our experiences. Our body is as it is, and it's okay. We don't actually have to change it at all. All we have to do is listen more closely to what it has to tell us. Our physical limitations also offer us a concrete confrontation with reality in the here and now.

This is what there is, right now. We can try to deny or ignore it, but that eventually leads to stress, injury, or suffering. Since so much of our suffering comes from wanting things to be different from how they are, accepting our body's limitations can help us let go of wanting things to be different in other respects.

Something else happens when we tune into our bodies—we can also experience the small pleasures of life. I like to shower mindfully, and I really enjoy the sensations of the warm water rushing over my body. But often I will feel pulled to start planning my day, which takes me out of my body and into potentially stressful territory. My day has barely started, and I'm already mentally stressing out! So when I notice this happening, I remind myself to just enjoy my shower and leave the planning for later. There are probably hundreds of such small moments throughout the course of one day which if we tune into our bodies, we can actually enjoy: the first sip of steaming hot coffee, feeling a cool autumn breeze, relaxing the tension in your shoulders when you notice it, and feeling the breath come into your body. Life is full of these small moments of pleasure—why would we want to deprive ourselves of enjoying them fully?

Returning to our body during stressful interactions with our child or our partner can also help us deal with stress better and short-circuit our automatic parental reactivity. When we feel stressed and we deliberately pay attention to our body sensations, we become grounded in the present moment. Whatever is happening, we are now at least experiencing it fully. Ironically, when we ignore our body sensations, we are more likely to go into a stress reaction without realizing it. When we pay attention to what's happening in our body, we can feel the physical sensations as our stress reaction begins. Just paying attention may slow down this reaction, or we may need to ride it out with awareness. Most importantly, when we become aware that we're having a stress reaction, we can pause before reacting, which is crucial for de-escalating stressful interactions with our child or partner.

In Session 3, we invite parents to re-inhabit their bodies, especially when parenting or with their children, during pleasant moments, moments of physical challenge, and during parenting stress. We invite them to befriend their bodies, to go back to them as if to an old dear friend whom we have neglected but who is still there for us, waiting patiently. We do this by introducing yoga practice and sitting meditation on the breath and body sensations. We invite parents to begin to pay attention to bodily sensations while they are happening. For example, paying attention to what is happening in the body when experiencing something pleasurable and savoring the experience. We also invite parents to give the same attention to their bodies when they are under stress. Often when we feel stressed, we seek refuge in our heads—we try to work things out rationally or make a plan. But instead of a refuge, we create a hell for ourselves and actually increase our stress. So we invite parents to experiment with dropping back into their bodies when they noticed they are beginning to feel stressed.

EMBODIED EMOTIONS

Our emotions begin in our body. So another reason it's important to get in touch with our bodies is to get in touch with our emotional states, which often originate as rumblings in our abdomen, or the appropriately named "gut feelings" that fuels our intuition. When we are emotionally upset, we can also go back to our body. What does this sadness actually feel like, in my body? Where do I feel it? What can I notice about it? Does it change or shift? Get more intense? The body can be a safe haven for experiencing emotions, much safer than our thoughts, which can whisk us back to past sadness or future worries. When we experience strong emotions like sadness or anger, and we feel them in our bodies, we are allowing ourselves to be with the emotions, with nothing else extra on top. Using the breath to guide us through the body sensations, we may find we can stay with painful emotions longer, with more gentleness and curiosity towards ourselves, than when we stay in our heads. Staying present with the feelings offers us a chance to explore them, not with words, but with sensations, to give them more space and perhaps to view them from an expanded, larger perspective.

Try this experiment: the next time you feel sad or another strong emotion, try paying attention to where you feel it in your body. You may find that you feel it more intensely, maybe tears will start rolling down your cheeks. But it's just as important what you're not doing—you're not trying to solve the sadness, push it away, or deny it—all of which take energy and are more likely to make you get stuck in feeling sad or even depressed. So learning to be in our bodies and really paying attention to all of our body signals is also helping us to develop the ability to be with our emotions, which we will talk more about in Session 5.

BODIES AND CONNECTING WITH OUR CHILD

Our bodies also connect us with our child in so many ways. For mothers, our child starts out as part of us. But also for fathers and adop-

tive parents, holding our child up close to our body is such a basic experience—when we feed, comfort, or just hold our child. For young children,
our bodies are a playground. Think of the sheer delight children experience climbing up on our body, being held aloft in our arms, resting on
our belly, pushing or pulling us, and testing their strength against ours.
When we connect with our own bodies, we can connect with our children. And when we are able to be more in touch with our bodies and our
emotions, we are more able to be emotionally in touch with our children.
Simply put, we cannot tune into another person's emotional state unless
we are in tune with our own, which starts when we connect with our
bodies (Siegel & Hartzell, 2003).

SELF-COMPASSION

Another them of Session 3 is self-compassion. In the first two sessions, parents explored their responses to imaginary parenting stress
situations. We noted in Session 1 how we tend to react with strong body
sensations, emotions, and self-critical thoughts when under routine parenting stress. In Session 2, we saw how we react with more kindness and
compassion towards a friend under stress. In this session, parents call to
mind a stressful parenting situation of their own and become aware of
their bodily sensations, thoughts, feelings, and action tendencies. Then,
we invite them to apply the same compassion that they felt towards their
friend to themselves, and we use this as a springboard for teaching the
skill of self-compassion.

Self-compassion is a simple but powerful antidote to our tendency
to strive for perfection as parents. Self-compassion does not depend on us
achieving particular goals, living up to a particular standard or a particular view of ourselves. On the contrary, self-compassion is what we give
ourselves at our most difficult times—when we feel we have failed, when
we feel ashamed, disappointed, or upset with ourselves. Self-compassion
involves being fully aware of our present moment experience, rather than
fleeing from it by defending a particular view of ourselves.

Often when we struggle, we judge ourselves harshly and feel so
alone. Self-compassion practice reminds us that all human beings suffer
at times and, in this way, brings us closer to others at times of suffering,
rather than isolating us. When we come face to face with our shortcomings, as parent, as spouse, as friend, as worker, we can remind ourselves
that "To err is human" and that being imperfect just means we're human
and brings us into the fold of all humanity. Kristin Neff, a developmental psychologist and lifelong meditator who studies the effects of self-

compassion, teaches self-compassion by first asking us to think about how we respond naturally when we notice a friend is in distress. Our natural compassionate response to a friend is exactly what we need to do for ourselves during stressful times. When we contrast our tendency to judge ourselves harshly and our desire to be compassionate towards a friend, parents immediately get the contradiction, and they open to the possibility that they can be kinder towards themselves (Germer, 2009; Gilbert, 2009; Neff, 2011).

GUIDELINES FOR SESSION 3

Box 7.1. Agenda Session 3

1. Sitting meditation: breath and body sensations (20 min) + inquiry (20 min)
2. Discuss home practice (first in pairs, then in whole group): savoring *events calendar* (20 min)
3. 3-min breathing space + inquiry (10 min)
4. Discuss other home practice (in pairs or in group): body scan, sitting meditation, and routine activity with child (10 min)
5. Break (15 min)
6. Yoga (lying down) (25 min) + inquiry (15 min)
7. Discussion: watching the body during parenting (stress) (10 min)
8. Parenting stress: bringing kindness to ourselves (20 min)
9. Review of home practice (10 min)
10. 3-min breathing space (5 min)

1. SITTING MEDITATION: BREATH AND PHYSICAL SENSATIONS

In Session 3, the sitting meditation is expanded to include the body sensations (see Handout 7.4). We invite parents to expand their attention from their breath to their whole body breathing. It can be hard to experience your whole body, sitting and breathing. Some participants notice themselves switching back and forth between awareness of breath and awareness of bodily sensations. Other people have an easy time experiencing whole body awareness. Just listen for the various different reactions. In fact, we can notice how many different ways we can experience our bodily sensations: we can be aware of a focused area of our body, for example, if we feel pain or an itching sensation or if we focus on muscle groups which work together such as face muscles, back muscles, shoulder muscles, or stomach muscles. Many people can easily sense their legs and feet as they are sitting, feeling the pressure of their buttocks and legs against the cushion, or sensations of pressure in their feet. All of this can be experienced as body sensations. We can also notice to what places our attention is pulled—do we find a particular pain drawing our attention? It often takes more deliberate effort to experience the entire body as a whole, but with practice, this can become easier.

I often struggle to experience my body as a whole—I find my attention is often drawn to specific parts of my body, especially my poor feet, which have a bad habit of falling asleep during sitting meditation. I console myself with the fact that we have probably evolved to be more quickly aware of sensations, especially pain, in specific areas of our body, which direct us to parts of our body needing attention. But I've come to think of whole body awareness as a kind of spaciousness within our bodies. Just as we may focus on negative experiences, narrowing our focus of attention, and losing the broader more spacious perspective, when we focus on painful sensations in our bodies, we may lose the big picture of our body as a whole, which includes many areas which do not have pain or discomfort. When we learn to move back and forth between the uncomfortable sensations that pull at our attention, and the sensation of the whole body, we can "hold" the more difficult physical sensations. Christina Feldman describes that when she works with people experiencing a lot of physical pain, she asks them to find a part of their body that doesn't hurt at the moment—maybe their left earlobe, the tip of their nose (C. Feldman, p.c., April 7–11, 2010). Even when we are in pain, there are still parts of our body that are free from pain, and we can intentionally move our attention to these parts as well.

In addition to attending to the bodily sensations during the sitting meditation, we can also notice our mind's reaction to the difficult sensations, such as resistance, frustration, anger, or wanting the discomfort to go away. As Kabat-Zinn (1990) noted in his groundbreaking work with patients with chronic sickness, injuries, or pain, it is often not the pain itself that causes people so much suffering, but the reaction to the pain—fear, avoidance, worries that the pain will never go away, anger, frustration. By not accepting the painful sensations, we make our suffering worse. Accepting uncomfortable sensations or even pain is therefore the first step in healing our own suffering, because it eliminates the unnecessary suffering caused by our fighting against what there is. For many people, it comes as a revelation that they are in fact increasing their own suffering through their reaction to painful sensations.

When we sit with difficult body sensations, notice our own reactions of resistance to them, and gradually let go and simply experience the discomfort as it is, we may discover some surprising things: the pain may not be as intense as we feared or it may wax and wane. Or it may be intense, but still bearable, in contrast to our fear that we won't be able to bear it. We learn to ride the wave of the painful sensations and experience that they can change, diminish, and eventually go away in some cases. In this way, we free ourselves from the grip that pain has on us; it becomes more manageable, less frightening, and less powerful. Once we have had this experience of sitting with painful sensations, the next time they arise, we may be able to react more openly to them, accepting them instead of tensing our bodies against them.

Accepting painful or distressing sensations does not mean we have to like them or that we don't want to feel better. It is only natural that we seek to avoid pain, and certainly we have an "evolutionary right" to our habits of pain avoidance. It simply means accepting the reality that in this moment, here and now, there is pain. By acknowledging what there is now, and accepting it rather than fighting it, we can begin to see possibilities of change.

Being able to be with physical pain is a power metaphor for the many types of emotional pain we experience in our lives or our children's lives. Again, it is only natural to want to avoid emotional pain, but when we get in the habit of avoiding painful feelings or fighting against them, it only adds to our suffering. In addition to the suffering from the pain, we then experience the suffering from fighting against the pain, which in itself can be more debilitating than the original pain.

So sitting with difficult body sensations is a good practice for learning to sit with difficult emotions. We can also notice our reactions to emotional states and to bring a softer and more accepting stance of allowing them simply to be as they are, instead of fighting, denying, or avoiding them. In later sessions, we will apply this same skill to sitting with difficult emotions. When we are able to sit with difficult emotions, we may feel less frightened of them.

VOICES OF THE PARENTS

During the sitting meditation, Sue described having an itch, and feeling an intense urge to scratch it. When she scratched it, however, it seemed to just move to another part of her body, which she then needed to scratch. So as she scratched, she watched the itch move around her body.

Rachel described having pain in her bladder and uterus, an area where she had had surgery. Normally she would have immediately gotten up to go to the bathroom, but in this case she decided to experiment with seeing what would happen if she stayed meditating. To her surprise, the sensations did not increase, and in fact they eventually diminished, so that she felt she could finish the meditation. Having described this to the group after the sitting meditation, she stood up, saying "And now, I really do have to go to the bathroom," eliciting some laughter from the group.

Miriam described having intense pain in her lower back and legs during the sitting meditation. She decided to "stay with" the pain, despite the fact that it was becoming increasingly painful as the position exacerbated her sciatica. By the time the meditation was finished, it was as if she had endured torture.

The examples above illustrate the dialectical stance the teacher tries to embody with regard to reactions to bodily sensations. On the one hand, the teacher encourages participants to experiment with sitting with difficult emotions rather than reacting immediately to them.

On the other hand, Miriam's pain became almost excruciating, and forcing herself to stay in that position despite the pain had a quality of striving for some idea of perfection. The point is not to be a martyr or achieve some ideal but to sit with bodily reactions long enough to explore them and, if necessary, consider some action. For example, after becoming aware of the body sensations of pain, and any accompanying thoughts or feelings, Miriam could have chosen to do something to alleviate the pain, such as shifting to a more comfortable position. The crucial point here is allowing enough time to become fully aware of our experience, so that we make a deliberate, conscious response, instead of automatically reacting.

In our daily lives, we often react quickly and automatically to difficult or stressful situations, particularly with children or other intimates. When we react quickly, we lose the opportunity to explore the situation as it unfolds and to consider different ways we might respond. By first sitting with painful feelings, instead of immediately trying to get rid of them, we allow ourselves to experience the natural course of them: how they arise, build up, perhaps ultimately fade away, move to another part of the body, or become more or less intense. We can also observe how we react—whether we feel aversion, frustration, anger, and resistance or whether we can open to the sensations with curiosity, kindness, and acceptance. We can also observe our action tendencies—what we feel like doing or actually do.

Sitting with difficult body sensations can help us develop a more accepting stance towards ourselves and our children. Accepting difficult sensations can become a metaphor for accepting the difficult in our children—in ourselves—and in parenthood, accepting the messiness of parenthood and the emotions that it stirs up, and accepting our children's pain and not trying to make it go away. We all have the tendency at times to want things to be different than they are—wishing our child didn't have the particular difficulties she has, wishing we could be different as a parent, wishing our partner was more supportive, wishing parenthood was easier, and wishing we wouldn't feel such anger or frustration with our children. Sitting with difficult bodily sensations is a practice which can teach us tolerating what there is, seeing it for what it is, and instead of fighting, denying, or avoiding it, bringing a curious and open stance towards it.

2. HOME PRACTICE REVIEW: SAVORING PLEASANT MOMENTS

We review the home practice of savoring pleasant moments in pairs and then come together as a group to discuss. As Hanson (2009) notes, when we savor an experience, we help to sustain and intensify it, so that it can be registered deeply in our emotional memory. When we discuss this in the group, we ask about the bodily sensations parents experienced. The teacher draws a chart on the board, *Event/Aware at the moment?/Bodily sensations/Emotions, and thoughts*, and invites parents to share their savoring moments in the group. As parents describe a savoring moment, the teacher asks "What made it pleasant?" and "How did you know it was pleasant?" in order to focus awareness on the bodily sensations involved in pleasure, joy, and other positive experiences.

VOICES OF THE PARENTS

Amy recounted enjoying the smell of mowed grass, and noticed how her body relaxed and she felt happier.

Mia had had a difficult week, but remembered at some point to tune into pleasant experiences. When she did, she noticed the wind on her face, and found it very pleasant. The teacher asked her where she felt it in her body, and she recalled: "I felt the wind on my face, and felt the pleasure also in my upper body and my chest."

Joe described savoring making fresh orange juice: the physical sensations in the muscles of his hand, the smell, the anticipation of the taste, the feeling of happiness and contentment, the thought of the sun in the orange.

Karen felt touched when she saw her 8-year-old son spontaneously laughing while watching the Muppet show. Her son has been diagnosed with autistic spectrum disorder, and he usually laughs in a way that feels fake, imitating others. She felt tears in her eyes and goose bumps.

Rachel described having a pleasant experience, but complained that she felt "nothing," a complaint she often had.

*Rachel: "I bought a book for myself, and I was allowed to have it, without feeling
    guilty. But I didn't feel anything."*
T: Did you realize it while it was happening?
R: Yes, I did.
T: What moment was it?
R: When I was taking it off the shelf.
T: What did you experience?
R: I thought, "It's mine!"
T: Okay, you felt, aaah, it's mine, and then what?
R: That's it—I didn't feel anything else.
*T: Did you feel anything at all in your body—can you put yourself back in that
    moment?*
R: Yes, I can remember exactly.
T: What do you feel in your body?
R: I felt something here, by my chest (pointing to her chest), like a string pulling.
*T: Where your heart is—okay, our heart is where we feel what we want, what we
    desire, so there was something going from your heart to the book—"I want this
    book."*
R: Yes.

For Rachel, her initial idea that she felt "nothing" changed when she focused on the physical sensations in her body when she took the book off her shelf. The teacher could then "translate" the bodily sensation into a metaphor of her heart's desire. For people who have difficulty recognizing or experiencing emotions, awareness of body sensations offers a way into their emotional reactions.

For Allison, the savoring events calendar brought up feelings of dissatisfaction with her life, as she began thinking "I haven't done anything pleasurable this week!" This led to self-critical thoughts "Why haven't I done more enjoyable things?" "There is nothing enjoyable for me in my life." As she described these thoughts in the group, she realized that her expectations were so high that she was not paying attention to smaller, potentially pleasant events. She then remembered one moment. She had to serve as volunteer lifeguard at the pool. Initially her thought was "What a pain that I have to waste 2 hours with this." But while at the pool, she became aware of the physical sensations while walking around the pool: "The air felt pleasantly cool on my skin. The sun broke through the clouds now and then, warming my face. When I looked up, I saw the blue sky streaked with clouds, and the tops of the large trees swaying gently in the breeze. I breathed in and felt glad to be able to enjoy the nature in this park, instead of being stuck indoors somewhere. Actually, when I put aside my irritation or resentment of having to be there instead of having free time, I could experience it as quite pleasant." The teacher asked her where she felt it in her body, and she remembered, "On my skin and my face, and in the movement of my body."

This is a good example of how our thoughts can sometimes get in the way of our experiencing pleasant experiences, because we may have certain concepts which dictate how we think we should feel. For example, Allison thought she should feel irritated because she had to volunteer 2 hours of her precious time. Had she not, in the moment, been able to focus on her physical sensations of walking and enjoying the sun and breeze on her face, she may have completely missed this moment of pleasure!

3. 3-MIN BREATHING SPACE

The 3-min breathing space, developed by Segal, Teasdale, and Williams (2002) in their groundbreaking work applying mindfulness to depression, helps us to bring mindfulness into our everyday lives and to bridge the gap between our usual experience and being mindfully aware. The structure of the breathing space is like an hourglass: we start with our attention wide to all of our experience, then we gather and focus our attention to the breath, and then we expand our attention once again to the entire body.

In step 1 of the breathing space, we check in with what's going on in this moment: what thoughts, feelings, or sensations do I notice? It's like checking in on the weather, and our body is the barometer. In step 2, we bring our attention to our breath and the movement of our belly. This anchors us in the present moment and creates some space before we react. In step 3, we broaden our attention to take in the entire body and its sensations, opening us up to the world in a more spacious way.

The 3-min breathing space serves as a bridge to help parents go from doing mode to mindful awareness, by stopping a moment to go into their body sensations. This can bring a sense of spaciousness, an enlarging of possibilities, and a pause in which to reflect before responding. It allows all the feelings, thoughts, and action tendencies to be held in the body itself, which can have a calming and centering effect (see Handout 7.5).

4. OTHER HOME PRACTICE REVIEW

We discuss in pairs or in the whole group the other home practice: the body scan, sitting meditation, and doing a routine activity with the child mindfully (see Handout 6.1). Parents may be surprised with the experience of doing a routine activity with their child, such as dressing, doing the hair, and asking how the day was, with full, beginner's mind attention.

VOICES OF THE PARENTS

Trish describes how something as simple as giving her young son a few minutes of attention when waking him up turned out to make a world of difference for how smoothly the morning went. Gently saying "Good morning, wake up sleepy head," in his ears, and watching his face while he slowly woke up (she mimics the movements of his face as she whispered good morning to him) helped him to come down on his own, cleaned and dressed without Trish having to keep telling him to hurry up.

Jill had a similar experience with her adolescent daughter. She works at home, and normally when her daughter comes home from school she says hello from behind her computer. This time, she closed her computer and, looking at her daughter with her full attention, she asked her how her day was. This simple act took only five minutes, but made a difference for the whole afternoon: her daughter listened better, did her homework and Jill felt more connected with her.

Other parents may bring up less positive experiences:

Sue expected that by saying good morning attentively "This would be our special moment," but the opposite happened: her son pushed her away saying: "Go away!" and Sue felt rejected and disappointed.

Paul paid attention to his adolescent daughter when she came home from school, but she went upstairs to her room yelling, "Leave me alone!"

The challenge for Sue and Paul was to be aware of the painful feelings, to notice how it feels to be pushed away despite our good intentions, and to let go of high expectations. When parents share these kinds of disappointing or difficult experiences, it is very helpful for the group, because it reminds everyone that mindfulness is about being present with whatever is going on, including difficult or frustrating experiences. In fact, we make a point of routinely asking about difficult experiences, and volunteering our own examples, to give full expression to the range of experiences and to counteract the tendency of group members to talk more about positive experiences than negative.

5. BREAK

A short break takes place, for tee, coffee and a snack brought by one of the group members, and to chat.

6. YOGA (LYING AND SITTING)

The goal of mindful yoga is to experience the bodily sensations arising during the practice, rather than achieving a particular goal of increased flexibility or muscle strength (although these may be side benefits). Because of its active nature, and because it involves muscular contraction and stretching, yoga practice helps us experience our body sensations more vividly, which is especially helpful for people who have trouble feeling their body sensations. Yoga practice also helps us to become more aware of our physical limits. During the yoga, we pay attention to our body's limits which may be felt as stretching, discomfort, or pain. We tune in to even the most subtle sensations that suggest we are reaching our body's limit, noticing mild stretching sensations, tension, or slight discomfort. Our goal is not to push the limit or to expand our body's potential but just to recognize and accept the signals our body sends us telling us we are coming to a limit of what we can comfortably do. In a larger sense, we open ourselves to experiencing the wisdom of our body, learning to trust in our body's ability to tell us what's going on in this moment.

Yoga is more challenging physically than the body scan, and it can elicit difficult sensations such as restlessness, impatience, discomfort, frustration, or even pain. This mild physical challenge provides an opportunity for us to get to know our bodily sensations more intimately, to practice becoming aware of these sensations, and to practice a curious, open, accepting, nonjudgmental, and friendly stance towards whatever is happening in our body, while at the same time paying attention to our limits and not going over them.

Yoga practice also helps us get in touch with our body's ability to balance itself. When we practice yoga mindfully, we become aware of the fact that even in the simplest position, our body is constantly making small adjustments to balance itself. This happens on its own, without our having to consciously do something, until we reach a point where we are about to lose our balance. Then suddenly, our body will make more marked shifts to try to regain balance. This natural balancing act that our body performs is a nice metaphor for our work as parents. We are constantly balancing ourselves in relation to our children, our partners, and our work, whether we are aware of it or not. We are also constantly making slight adjustments to how we relate to our children, based on their changing developmental needs. When things are going smoothly, we're not aware of these constant adjustments. It's only when things get really out of balance—when there are problems with how we're balancing all the demands of family, partner, children, and work or when children are having difficulties—that we may notice feeling out of balance, and we may feel the need to make stronger, more conscious adjustments in our lives.

The teacher guides the group in simple lying yoga postures for about 25 min (see Handout 7.6 for general instructions and drawings of the practices). We invite participants to try to experience the body sensations fully and to pay attention to when they feel they are approaching their own physical limits. The emphasis is on doing the yoga in "being mode," that is, fully experiencing all the sensations in the body, rather than achieving anything. If a participant is physically unable to do a movement or posture, they are invited to do it in their imagination.

VOICES OF THE PARENTS

Mary's increased awareness of her physical limits and stress reaction helped her to set limits for herself during a busy week at work where she was asked to do too many tasks. In the past, she would have taken the work on, feeling she "had to" do it, but this time she used her awareness of her body's limits to help her communicate her needs to her boss.

Respecting one's own bodily limits can feel empowering to parents who have had difficulty asserting their own needs with others. Often people who have difficulty acknowledging their own limits or boundaries also have difficulty asserting themselves with colleagues, bosses, friends, partners, or with their children.

Helga had to meet an important work deadline and realized that she would not be able to pick up her children and make dinner. In the past, she would have tried to do both, but with more attention to her own limits, she asked her husband for help, and avoided going over her own limit.

Karen's reaction to the yoga practice was: "I didn't like it at all. It was painful and too difficult," adding "I guess I need to lose 10 pounds." She had pushed herself to do all the poses, even though some were too difficult for her. This led to negative thoughts that she was too fat and a failure. The teacher asked her "What would it feel like to just accept your body as it is right now, and not have to change anything about it?" With that, Karen began to cry, as she recognized her own striving for perfection and lack of acceptance of her body.

7. WATCHING THE BODY DURING PARENTING STRESS

In this exercise, we pay attention to what happens in our bodies, thoughts, and emotions when we feel stressed. We begin by asking participants, "How do you know when you are feeling stress? Where do you feel it in your body? What emotions do you notice? What thoughts?" We write a few examples on the board and invite participants to describe in as much detail as possible their experience.

Event	Body sensations	Emotions	Thoughts
Daughter lying to me I see it in her eyes	Tension in head, chest high fast breathing fast heartbeat	Anger, pity, fear, guilt feeling	I cannot deal with this any longer, I should believe her, I don't know what to believe anymore
Working all night to make a deadline	Intense headache cold, tense shoulders pain in right arm	Fear, lonely	I'm stupid that I'm doing this, I should organize my work better, I will be judged negatively if I don't make it

We might start the discussion by asking: "Why it is so difficult to watch the body while under parenting stress?" and "Why it is important to watch the body in such moments?" Parents are sometimes surprised at the intensity of their physical reactions during stressful situations. Many of us have particular areas of the body where we habitually experience stress, such as butterflies in the stomach, tightness in the chest, head and neck pain, flushed face, or racing heart. We can connect these physical reactions to the fight–flight–freeze stress reaction that we discussed in Session 1. Becoming aware of our parenting stress in our body is the first step to being able to be with it and accept it, rather than fighting it. Being aware of stress in the body can also feel less personal than all the stories we attach to our stress. When we go into our body, we notice, for example, "there is tension in my face," "my stomach is knotted up," and "my neck is sore." These bodily experiences are less personal than the thoughts we might have when we are stressed, so going to the body helps to neutralize that unnecessary negative chatter.

8. PARENTING STRESS: BRINGING KINDNESS TO OURSELVES

In this exercise, we ask parents to call to mind a recent stressful interaction with their child or partner and to notice their bodily sensations, feelings, and thoughts, similar to the exercise before. But now we go one step further—we ask them to notice what is your attitude towards yourself? For example, we may feel guilty, judge ourselves harshly, or criticize ourselves. When parents have had time to experience this, we then ask them to deliberately bring an attitude of kindness and compassion to this moment in the same way we did for our "friend" in the previous week and to notice how that feels. Some parents describe that when they deliberately adopt a self-compassionate attitude, they feel an immediate release of tension in their body, and their automatic reaction seems to dissolve. Many parents are surprised at the contrast between their habitual reaction of getting down on themselves and the empathic reaction which they would normally reserve for a friend or loved one. The idea that they can choose to respond kindly and compassionately to themselves feels liberating and surprisingly easy for some parents. Some parents have told us they find it helpful to do something physical to comfort themselves, like giving themselves a little hug or rubbing their neck and shoulders. This makes a lot of sense: research has shown that physically comforting ourselves releases oxytocin, just as being physically comforted by someone else does. So we really can comfort ourselves and experience the physiological benefits as well (Neff, 2011).

Sometimes parents feel that being compassionate to themselves is equivalent to making excuses for behavior that they find unacceptable. But being self-compassionate does not mean we are justifying or excusing something we've done which we feel is wrong or hurtful. In fact, it's when we've done something objectionable to ourselves when we most need self-compassion. When we've done something we regret or hurt someone, even unintentionally, we feel bad. This is normal and reflects our moral conscience. When we are compassionate with ourselves instead of judgmental, we are tending to the part of ourselves that is suffering, comforting ourselves in our moment of pain, in the same way we might be kind to a friend who has done something she regrets. In that sense, self-compassion lies closer to forgiveness; it is accepting that, being human, we cannot help but make mistakes or have difficulties in our interactions with loved ones.

Self-compassion is not self-justification or saying, "It's okay, it's not really so bad, you really didn't mean any harm." It's simply acknowledging the pain of your own suffering and being compassionate towards yourself in that moment of suffering, instead of heaping more criticism on yourself.

We use this exercise as a springboard for describing the three aspects of self-compassion which Kristin Neff has elaborated. According to Neff (2011), self-compassion involves:

1. Awareness (that this is a moment of suffering)
2. Self-kindness (responding with kindness to your own suffering)
3. Connecting with our common humanity (all parents have made mistakes)

As Neff points out, when we feel upset, we often do the opposite: we don't pay attention to our feelings, we judge ourselves harshly, and we tend to feel isolated and alone. Teaching parents to notice their moments of suffering, respond kindly as a good friend would, and remember that our imperfection just makes us human helps them to respond in a way that emphasizes our common humanity, helping us feel closer to others rather than isolated. She also points out that, contrary to popular belief, being compassionate with ourselves makes us more open to facing our own faults, rather than less open. In fact, the evidence suggests that people are more able to admit faults the more they are self-compassionate. This should come as no surprise. Imagine you have a kind and compassionate boss versus a harsh judgmental boss. To which boss would you be more willing to admit you had made a mistake?

Neff recommends that couples can take a self-compassion break in the middle of a fight when they see that things are getting out of hand or destructive. Each partner can go to their separate corners, taking some of the oxygen out of the fight and giving each a chance to lick their wounds and comfort themselves. This is important, because when in conflict with a partner, it may not be possible to get the normal support from them, so we need to be able to provide that for ourselves. For the same reason, we invite parents to take a self-compassion break when they are in a difficult interaction with their child. Even more so than with our partners, with our children, we need to be able to sustain our sense of emotional balance when upset; we cannot expect them to comfort us, especially in difficult interactions. At the same time, children can say and do things that evoke very strong emotions in us, including strong anger and feelings of vulnerability. It's important that we can take care of ourselves emotionally when we feel triggered by the things our children say and do, so that we don't react back in kind. With children, it's not even necessary to tell them you need a self-compassion break but simply telling them you need to take a little break from the conversation to cool down or collect yourself and that you will come back to them shortly. In addition to giving parents a chance to give themselves some self-compassion, this break also helps to interrupt the negative escalation that can often lead to the automatic, "low-road" emotional reactions that we have talked about.

Box 7.2. Parenting Stress Exercise: Bringing Kindness to Yourself
(Adapted from Neff, 2011 and C. Germer, p.c., November 12–13, 2012)

Sit comfortably, letting your eyes close. Imagine a difficult or stressful parenting interaction which you feel did not go well. Imagine the situation as vividly as possible, as if it is happening right now. Who is there, what are they saying or doing, and what are you saying or doing? [*The teacher asks whether those who don't have a situation yet raise their hands, and if so allows a few moments more*]. When you have a clear picture, bringing your attention to this moment, checking in: how are you right now, noticing whatever comes up. Are there bodily sensations, emotions, thoughts, tension? Saying to yourself: whatever it is I'm feeling, it is okay, let me feel it. Just noticing whatever comes up . . . are there critical or judgmental thoughts? Feelings of sadness, anger, guilt? Tension in the body? *(allowing a couple of minutes)*

And now, seeing if you can bring an attitude of kindness and compassion for yourself, the way you would toward a friend. Recognizing this is a moment of suffering for you. Comforting yourself, for example, by saying to yourself *"This is really hard"* or *"My dear [NAME], you try so hard to be a good parent, but sometime it's too hard."* If you like, experimenting with comforting yourself physically by placing both hands over your heart, feeling the warmth of your hands on your chest (allow a few moments). Or hug yourself by placing your arms around your shoulders (allow a few moments). Or try stroking yourself wherever if feels comfortable for you, arms, face . . .

And now, can you remind yourself that all parents struggle, make mistakes, or feel they failed their children at times? Perhaps remembering other parents who struggle or regret things they've done? Reminding yourself that making mistakes is part of being human, and connects us with all other parents who struggle to do their best and yet make mistakes along the way.

VOICES OF THE PARENTS

During the exercise, Joy felt self-critical towards herself when she remembered an interaction with her son where she lost her temper. When she deliberately shifted to giving herself compassion, she felt her body relaxing, and the judgmental thoughts fell away. She was amazed at how quickly she was able to let go of the judgmental thoughts, once she gave herself compassion.

Marie found herself massaging her neck and shoulders during the exercise, because that is where she feels tension and stress.

Rachel found that wrapping her arms around her shoulders in a kind of embrace felt very comforting to her. It reminded her of a recent fight with her husband, where she was very angry at him. He began stroking his own arm. At the time, she found it strange, but now she realized that he was probably trying to soothe himself.

Mary asked "What if I feel that what I did was wrong? I don't want to be compassionate to myself if I've done something with my child that I don't think is right—I don't accept what I did." The teacher asked, "If a friend of yours had done the same thing, and felt bad about it, what would you say or do?" Thinking for a moment, Mary said, "I guess I would comfort her, tell her everyone has their bad moments as a parent, that I know how that feels. And give her a hug." "Can you do that for yourself?" asked the teacher. Mary struggled, "Somehow it's harder to do that for myself. I get stuck on thinking how wrong I was. (she sighs) But yes, I see how I have a double standard—for my friends I am much kinder and understanding."

For Mary, the practice brought into relief her own high standards and judgment for herself, in contrast to her spontaneous impulse to hug her friend. It will take some deliberate practicing of self-compassion for Mary to be able to befriend herself in the way she does so naturally with a friend.

9. REVIEW OF HOME PRACTICE

We ask parents to one time this week do an activity with their child with full awareness, for about 10 min. We also ask them to watch their body this week in moments of parenting stress and fill in the Stressful Moments Calendar afterwards. We invite them to choose one difficult or stressful parenting moment to try a self-compassion break, as we have practiced in Session 3. The formal practice involves lying/sitting yoga and sitting meditation, including the breath and body. Finally, they do the 3-min breath space three times a day.

10. CLOSING MEDITATION

We do a 3-min breathing space.

HANDOUT 7.1 Practice for the Week After Session 3

Reading

Read the handouts with full awareness, letting the words drop into your body and mind.

Mindful Parenting

Do one mindful activity with your child, for about 10 min. It can be anything, such as playing football, imaginary play or storytelling, reading together, playing a computer game together, drawing, or anything else you or your child likes. Practice moment-to-moment awareness in the same way that we did with the raisin. Try being aware of your child, yourself, and the interaction between the two of you. Make notes in your diary afterwards about your experience.

Take a self-compassion break at least one time this week during a moment of parenting stress or suffering or during a difficult interaction with your child or partner (see Handout 7.3 for further instructions). Make notes in your diary.

Observe your body during moments of parenting stress. Notice whatever is happening in your body, without judging. Fill in the Stressful Moments Calendar once a day.

Formal Practice

Day 1, 3, and 5: Yoga exercises (lying) (three times a week), see Handouts 7.6 and 7.7.
Day 2, 4, and 6: Sitting meditation on the breath and bodily sensations (three times a week), see Handout 7.4.

Informal Practice

Do the 3-min breathing space, three times a day; see Handout 7.5. It helps to set times in advance, for example, by setting an alarm on your cell phone, or putting up post-it stickers to remind you, or choosing set times of the day. Record each one on the record form.

HANDOUT 7.2 Watching the Body During Parenting Stress

While practicing the sitting meditation or yoga, you may notice physical discomfort, pain, or tension in certain areas of your body. Or you may notice tiredness, sleepiness, hunger, an itch, or other physical sensations. See if you can be aware of whatever bodily sensations come up from moment to moment, without trying to change the way things are at that moment. Also notice your reaction to the feelings of discomfort—do you feel irritated by it, impatient, feel the urge to get up, wish the pain would go away? This is part of the practice too—noticing our mind's reaction to our body sensations.

Of course, if we pay attention, we can notice tiredness, pain, tension, stress, or discomfort in many moments of our busy lives. For example, while typing this at 11.45 at night on my laptop in my bed, I notice tension in my neck, in my legs, and around my eyes, and I notice that my face is warm and my hands are cold.

When we become aware of our bodily discomfort at a particular moment, we may have the urge to judge this or take action. For example, when I just noticed my physical discomfort while typing this text, I thought: "I should go to bed earlier. I should not be working in my bed. I should get reading glasses." Here the doing mind is coming in, planning to take action, to get rid of the discomfort.

When you notice your doing mind coming in this way, see if you can just observe it, instead of taking action. The mind is always busy making plans to take action. If we act impulsively, we may do something we regret. On the other hand, if we don't take action, we may feel guilty. So our practice is to take a third path: simply watch the body in these moments, and watch the activity of the mind. Sometimes, though, we might choose to take action. For example, let's say you are late for work, and you see the train about to pull out of the station. You decide to make a run for it. You can still notice what happens in your body when you speed up and what happens in your body after you catch the train (or miss the train).

When we are under parenting stress, watching the body and not taking action is particularly difficult. Notice what happens in your body and your breath when you race to school to pick up your children in time. Or how your body feels in the evening when you are trying to get your children to bed. Or in the morning when you are trying to get your children to school in time. Or when you are angry with your child or worried about her or feeling anxious or critical with yourself as parent. Or any time you notice the sensations in your body which tell you that you're feeling stressed.

HANDOUT 7.2 Watching the Body During Parenting Stress (continued)

We can also notice how our body feels during different parenting tasks. For example, what does my body feel like when I . . . bathe my baby? Help my son dress? Cook dinner for my family? Read to my daughter in her bed? Help my son with his homework? Put my daughter to bed? Lie in bed waiting for my teenager to come home late at night?

In fact, we can reconnect with our body sensations, and ourselves, *every* moment of the day.

HANDOUT 7.3 Compassion with Yourself as Parent*

Compassion is the desire to alleviate suffering. For most of us, feeling compassionate towards others comes naturally. When we notice that our child, a loved one, or a friend is in distress, we naturally feel sympathy and want to help alleviate their pain. Just as we console our child or a friend in distress, we can comfort, console, and soothe ourselves in difficult times and through difficult emotions.

Yet often we do not treat ourselves very compassionately when we are in distress. We may judge ourselves harshly when we feel we've made a mistake, or blame ourselves when something goes wrong in our lives. As parents, we may be self-critical when we find ourselves reacting impatiently to our children, or making the inevitable parenting mistakes. In contrast, if we were talking with a friend about the same situation, we would probably take a much more compassionate stance, even if we felt our friend had made a mistake.

In fact, it is exactly in these moments of suffering, when we've made a mistake, feel disappointed in ourselves, or when things have not gone as we hoped, that we are most in need of self-compassion. Many of us, however, have learned to be critical of ourselves in these moments. We may feel that a self-critical attitude is necessary to keeps us performing at a high level, or that we deserve criticism when we've made a mistake or failed in some way. Being kind and compassionate to ourselves may feel self-indulgent, or we may feel we don't deserve it.

Self-compassion practice means deliberately bringing kindness and compassion towards ourselves when we are suffering, especially when we feel we have made mistakes or done something wrong. To understand self-compassion, it helps to think of how we would comfort a loved one who is feeling distressed.

For example, imagine a friend is going through a divorce, and she comes to visit. What happens? First, you might notice that something is wrong—you see in her face that she is upset. Second, you would probably be kind and compassionate towards her, perhaps asking her what is wrong and offering support and encouragement. Finally, you might express empathy for her situation, sharing how you or others have been in a similar boat, and that she is not alone in her suffering. In this natural reaction, you will have experienced the three key ingredients to self-compassion:

1. **Mindfulness**—noticing your friend's suffering
2. **Kindness**—being kind to your friend
3. **Connection to common humanity**—pointing out you or others have experienced this, that she is not alone

*Adapted from *Self-Compassion* by Kristin Neff (2011).

HANDOUT 7.3 Compassion with Yourself as Parent (continued)

When we practice self-compassion, we can use these three steps to guide us. We first have to notice we are suffering or in distress, by being mindfully aware: "This is a moment of suffering." We notice body sensations and any reactions such as judging ourselves, feeling guilty, etc. The second step is to deliberately bring an attitude of kindness to ourselves, *because* we are suffering. We can say kind and comforting words, such as "This is really hard right now" or any other words. We can even comfort ourselves physically by putting our hands over our heart, giving ourselves a gentle hug around the shoulders, or massaging our neck. Research has shown that this kind of physical self-comfort releases oxytocin, the attachment and comfort hormone. Finally, we can remind ourselves that we are not alone in our suffering, that all parents struggle, and that it just means that we are human. To summarize, self-compassion involves three steps:

1. **Bringing mindful awareness to your suffering:** "This is moment of suffering." Notice any habitual reactions, especially self-judgment.
2. **Bringing kindness to yourself:** "This is really hard" or choose your own words, or try comforting yourself physically.
3. **Reminding yourself that this connects you to other parents:** "All parents struggle at times or make mistakes or have regrets. It's only human. All parents have suffered at some time."

HANDOUT 7.4 Sitting Mediation:
Mindfulness of the Breath and Body*

1. Practice mindfulness of the breath, as described earlier (Handout 6.4) for 10 min in an erect and dignified sitting posture, whether in a chair or on the floor.

2. When you feel you have settled to some degree into feeling the breath moving in and out of your body at the belly or at the nostrils, intentionally allow the field of awareness to expand around the breath to include as well a sense of the body as a whole sitting and breathing. You may even find you get a sense of the breath moving throughout the body.

3. If you choose, include together with this wider sense of the body as a whole, and of the breath moving in and out of the body, awareness of the more local, particular patterns of physical sensations that arise where the body makes contact with the floor, chair, cushion, or stool— the sensations of touch, pressure, or contact of the feet or knees with the floor, the buttocks with whatever is supporting them, the hands where they rest on the thighs or together in the lap. As best you can, hold all these sensations, together with the sense of the breath and of the body as a whole, in a wide and spacious awareness.

4. Of course, in all likelihood, you will find the mind wandering repeatedly away from the breath and body sensations. Keep in mind that this is a natural tendency of the mind and is in no way a mistake or a sign of failure or "not doing it right." As we have noted before, whenever you notice that your attention has drifted away from sensations in the body, you might want to let it register that to be aware of that fact means that you are already back and awake to what is going on in the mind. In that very moment, it can be useful to gently note what was on your mind ("thinking," "planning," "remembering") and then to reestablish your attention on the breath sensations and a sense of the body as a whole.

5. As best you can, resting in a gentle attending to the actuality of the field of sensations throughout the body from moment to moment, and being aware of any feelings of pleasantness, unpleasantness, or neutrality as they arise.

6. The longer the session continues, the more you may experience sensations arising that are particularly intense in one region of your body or another, perhaps in the back or in the knees or in the shoulders. With greater intensity of sensations, especially if they feel unpleasant and uncomfortable, you may find that your attention is repeatedly drawn to them and away from your intended focus on the breath or the body as

*From *The Mindful Way through Depression* by Williams, Teasdale, Segal, & Kabat-Zinn (2007). pp. 130–131. Copied with permission of Guilford Press.

HANDOUT 7.4 Sitting Mediation:
Mindfulness of the Breath and Body (continued)

a whole. In such moments, rather than shifting your posture (although you are always free to do that, of course), you might experiment even briefly with intentionally bringing the focus of attention right into the region of greatest intensity and, as best you can, exploring with gentle and wise attention the detailed pattern of sensations there—what, precisely, are the qualities of the sensations; where, exactly, are they located; do they vary over time or shift around in the body from one place to another? This exploration is undertaken in the realm of sensing and feeling, rather than through thinking. Again, as best you can, opening to feeling whatever is already here to be felt, allowing yourself to know what you are feeling via directly experiencing it. As in the body scan, you may play with using the breath as a vehicle to carry awareness into such regions of intensity, "breathing in" to them, and out from them.

Whenever you find yourself "carried away" by the intensity of physical sensations, or in any other way, as best you can reconnect with the here and now by refocusing attention on the movements of the breath or on a sense of the body as whole sitting in a balanced and dignified posture, even in the midst of the intensity of sensation, grounded in the present moment. Notice how much we create "pain" out of discomfort through the thoughts we have about it and especially our thoughts about how long it is.

HANDOUT 7.5 3-Min Breathing Space*

The breathing space provides a way to step out of automatic parenting and reconnect to awareness in the moment. We begin with our attention wide, then focus it in on our breathing, then expand it again at the end, like an hourglass.

1. Checking in

Bringing yourself in the present moment by deliberately adopting an erect and dignified position. If you like, closing your eyes. Asking yourself: What is my experience right now? What thoughts are going through my mind? What feelings are here? What body sensations do I notice? What action tendencies am I aware of?

2. Breathing

Then, gently turning your full attention towards your breathing. Following each breath all the way in . . . and all the way out . . . maybe also aware of the pause between the inbreath and the outbreath. Using the breath to anchor you into the present, and help you tune into a state of awareness and stillness.

3. Expanding

Now expand the field of awareness around your breathing, so that it includes a sense of the body as a whole, your posture, and facial expression. A sense of this breathing body, in this moment of time, in this space.

---

*Adapted from *The Mindful Way through Depression* by Williams, Teasdale, Segal and Kabat-Zinn (2007).

HANDOUT 7.6 Mindful Yoga Instructions

The goal of mindful yoga is to experience your body sensations as they arise during the different positions as fully as possible, rather than achieving a particular goal like becoming more flexible or stronger (although these may be side benefits). Yoga practice helps us experience our body sensations more vividly. It also helps us to become more aware of our physical limits. During the yoga, we pay attention to our body's limits which may be felt as stretching, discomfort, or pain. We tune in to even the most subtle sensations that suggest we are reaching our body's limit, noticing mild stretching sensations, tension, or slight discomfort. Our goal is not to push the limit or to expand our body's potential but just to recognize and accept the signals our body sends us telling us we are coming to a limit of what we can comfortably do. In a larger sense, we open ourselves to experiencing the wisdom of our body, learning to trust in our body's ability to tell us what's going on in this moment.

Yoga practice may sometimes elicit difficult sensations such as restlessness, impatience, discomfort, frustration, or even pain. This mild physical challenge provides an opportunity for us to get to know our bodily sensations more intimately, to practice becoming aware of these sensations, and to practice a curious, open, accepting, nonjudgmental, and friendly stance towards whatever is happening in our body, while at the same time paying attention to our limits and not going over them. If we feel pain, we have gone over our physical limit. With more practice, we can learn to recognize when we are approaching our body's limits so that we don't go over them.

Yoga practice also helps us get in touch with our body's ability to balance itself. When we practice yoga mindfully, we become aware of the fact that even in the simplest position, our body is constantly making small adjustments to balance itself. This happens on its own, without our having to consciously do something, until we reach a point where we are about to lose our balance. Then suddenly, our body will make more marked shifts to try to regain balance. This natural balancing act that our body performs is a nice metaphor for our work as parents. We are constantly balancing ourselves in relation to our children, our partners, and our work, whether we are aware of it or not. We are also constantly making slight adjustments to how we relate to our children, based on their changing developmental needs. When things are going smoothly, we're not aware of these constant adjustments. It's only when things get really out of balance—when there are problems with how we're balancing all the demands of family, partner, children, and work or when children are having difficulties—that we may notice feeling out of balance, and we may feel the need to make stronger, more conscious adjustments in our lives.

HANDOUT 7.6 Mindful Yoga Instructions (continued)

If you are having physical difficulties, contact your physician as to whether or not it's wise to do these practices and which adaptations may need to be made. Always listen to the wisdom of your body: only you can feel what a practice does or does not do for you. Be especially gently with your neck, for example, with neck rolls.

We advise to start practicing with the aid of an audio recording of the yoga practices, to also get a sense of the pace in which to practice. The yoga practices are described in the book *Full Catastrophe Living* (Kabat-Zinn, 1990) and for audio recordings see www.mindfulnessCDS .com.

1. It's helpful to wear loose-fitting clothes and to have a mat or carpet to lie on.
2. Lie down, and bring your attention first to the sensations of contact with the mat or floor. Bring your attention to your breath coming in and out of your body, at your chest or belly, and notice the rising and falling of your chest or belly. This will help to bring you into "being mode"—experiencing fully the physical sensations in the here and now. You might make the intention to bring an attitude of kindness and acceptance to this practice.
3. As you practice, notice when you have become distracted, and gently bring your attention time and time again back to the bodily sensations you are experiencing in the moment.
4. Notice any sense of striving or competing—a wish to do better, be stronger, or push yourself beyond your limits—and see if you can let go of this striving and return to the present moment experience in your body.
5. Notice what is happening to your breathing. For example, if you may notice that you are holding your breath during a difficult pose, gently remind yourself to keep breathing.
6. Pay attention to your own bodily limits. When you feel that you are approaching a limit (e.g., you notice a slight stretching feeling), investigate that limit with curiosity, but do not go over it. If you feel pain, or have difficulty breathing, you have gone over your limit. This is an important part of the practice. If we push ourselves over our own physical limit during the yoga, we may injure ourselves. Often we may push ourselves over our own limits in parenting or other situations and end up feeling stressed, exhausted, or even physically ill. So learning to stay within our limits is very important.
7. If you are physically unable to do a movement or posture, you can do it in your imagination.

HANDOUT 7.6 Mindful Yoga Instructions (continued)

8. After each posture, pause a moment to feel the effect on your body and on your breath.
9. Do the posture on both sides, even if only one side is shown in the picture.
10. See if you can bring an attitude of gentleness, kindness, and acceptance to your experience, whatever it is, and to your body and yourself. When you notice judgmental or self-critical thoughts, give them space to be there, but return back to your body, and see if you can bring this kinder and gentler attitude to your experience.
11. Savor any pleasant feelings! Although this is also not the goal, many people experience a sense of relaxation during or after the yoga practice. By tuning into you're here and now sensations, you can fully savor these pleasant moments.

HANDOUT 7.7 Lying Yoga Postures

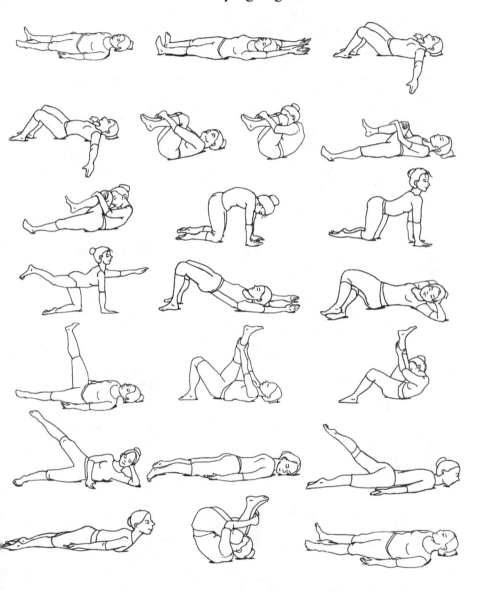

Sequence of postures adapted from *Full Catastrophe Living* by Jon Kabat-Zinn (pp. 106–109), copyright © 1990 by Jon Kabat-Zinn. Used by permission of Dell Publishing, an imprint of The Random House Publishing Group, a division of Random House LLC. All rights reserved.Redrawn by C. Bögels. In Bögels and Restifo (Springer, 2013)

HANDOUT 7.8 Stressful Moments Calendar

Be aware once a day of a stressful moment *at the time it is happening.*
See if you can be aware of these moments by deliberately paying attention to physical sensations. Write down stressful moments that are related and unrelated to parenting/your child. Use the following questions to focus your awareness on the details of the experience as it is happening. Write it down later.

What was the experience?	Were you aware of the stress *while* it was happening?	What happened in your body, in detail, during this experience?	What moods, feelings, thoughts, and action tendencies accompanied this experience?
Example: *My teenage son stayed out past his curfew*	*Yes*	*Tense, pain in neck/ shoulders, restless*	*Irritated, inpatient, worried "Why does it have to be so difficult?" "Doesn't he understand that I'm worried?" Tendency to call him and get angry*

HANDOUT 7.9 Home Practice Record Form Week 3

Fill in the record form each time after you practice (mindful parenting, formal or informal meditation). Write down what comes up for you during the practice, so that we can discuss it in the next session. Circle a 3 each time you have done a 3-min breathing space.

Day/time	Practice (Yes/No)	Comments
	3 3 3	
	3 3 3	
	3 3 3	
	3 3 3	
	3 3 3	
	3 3 3	
	3 3 3	
	3 3 3	

HANDOUT 7.10 Notes Informal Practice and
Mindful Parenting Practice Week 3

You may want to use this sheet to make notes about your experiences during the informal meditation practice and the mindful parenting practice. Or to make notes during or about the group session.

CHAPTER 8

SESSION 4: RESPONDING VERSUS REACTING TO PARENTING STRESS

She [Vanja, 4 years] is already practiced in the ways of the world and can be so cheeky that I completely lose my head and sometimes shout at her or shake her until she starts crying. But usually she just laughs. The last time it happened, the last time I was so furious I shook her and she just laughed, I had a sudden inspiration and placed my hand on her chest. Her heart was pounding. Oh, my, how it was pounding.

Knausgard (2012), pp. 30–31

PARENTING STRESS can bring out the worst in us. Those moments when we "lose it" with our children, and erupt in anger and frustration, are the moments we regret most as parents, as we know they leave traces, just like the traces we struggle with from our own youth, our interactions with our parents. In *My struggle*, Karl Ove Knausgard describes such moments of a father with his young daughters, wondering why it is that he gets so out of control.

Why do parent–child relationships seem so ripe for these moments when we "lose it," finding ourselves in a different mind state, angry, self-righteous, and no longer aware of our child? As discussed in Chapter 2, we have evolved to react first, think later in situations of perceived danger. LeDoux (1996) describes the fast, automatic reaction to perceived threat which is mediated by the limbic system and amygdala and bypasses higher cortical involvement. LeDoux gives the example of a person mistaking a stick on the road for a snake, and reacting with fear, stopping in his tracks. Moments later, his higher level thinking catches up, and he realizes it's only a stick, and there's no need to panic. From a survival point of view, it's much better that we err on the side of reacting as if we are in danger first ("the fast route") and then later cognitively evaluating the situation ("the slow route").

But when our "fast-route" or "low-road" reaction is triggered by a stressful interaction with our child, we can end up enraged and out of control with our child, (Siegel & Hartzell, 2003). Ironically, there appears to be something inherent to intimate relationships that primes us to be more easily emotionally triggered than in other situations, making the risk of "losing it" highest in exactly the context where they can do the most damage—our relationship with our children, who are vulnerable and dependent upon us. An evolutionary perspective can help make sense of this apparent paradox. Like all mammals, we have evolved to protect our offspring from threats. Reacting first and thinking later is thus an evolutionary strategy which made our forbearers more likely to survive but leaves us vulnerable to emotional overreactions when under stress. Furthermore, the emotional meaning we give these stressful parent–child interactions, based on our past experiences with our own parents, also contributes to our emotional overreactivity. (This will be addressed in Session 5 when we discuss parents' own early childhood schemas.)

The core theme of Session 4 is becoming aware of what happens to parenting when we are under emotional stress so that we can learn to respond more wisely. In Sessions 2 and 3, we focused on increasing our awareness of our bodies' reactions to stressful as well as pleasant events. Becoming aware of our body's reaction to stress is the first step in learning to respond differently. In Session 4, we examine our automatic behavioral reactions when under stress. These automatic reactions may stem from several sources, including (1) evolutionary survival mechanisms, (2) our tendency to grasp at what we like and reject what we dislike, (3) how we experienced our relationship with our own parents (which we will take up in Session 5), and (4) our lack of self compassion, as well as lack of felt partner support (which we will address in Session 7).

In Session 4, we help parents explore their habitual patterns of reacting to parenting stress in several ways. We do a sitting meditation focusing on sounds and thoughts. Our automatic responses to sounds (labeling, pushing away, startling) are a good example of automatic reactions. Our tendency to add thoughts to stress or discomfort ("I can't take this any longer"), and thereby multiplying our suffering, is another good example of habitual reactions to parenting stress. Parents discuss stressful parent–child reactions which they have observed in the past week and written down in the parental stress calendar, including their body sensations and action tendencies. We use a demonstration (the fight–flight–freeze/dance exercise) to illustrate in an action-oriented and humorous manner how we often react to stressful situations in ways which only compound our difficulty. In this nonverbal exercise (described below), parents can recognize immediately their own typical way of reacting to stress. In a second experiential exercise, we ask parents to call to mind a stressful parent–child interaction, become aware of their bodily sensations, and experiment with bringing an attitude of compassion and acceptance to their reactions. Thus, the first step is awareness and acceptance of parenting stress.

Having recognized our parenting stress, we turn to the question of how we find wiser, more skillful ways of dealing with our stress, instead of compounding our stress with our automatic reactions. In other words, how can we find a way to dance with our problems, instead of ending up in a futile struggle with them or avoiding them? Batchelor (2007) calls this "creative engagement"—using mindfulness to create the space we need to view our difficulties with fresh eyes and to be able to come up with solutions which we may have been unable to see before. We demonstrate this with the "dance," and we do the "doors" exercise, in which parents can experience creative solutions and new ways of responding coming up once we take a breathing space. We practice using the 3-min breathing space as a way to hit the "pause" button on our automatic reactions. Taking a mindful breath is always the first step to interrupting the automatic reactions to stress. When we become aware that we are feeling stressed, even *one* mindful breath can be enough to create this pause between stress and reactivity.

THOUGHTS

Adding thoughts to a stressful moment is one way in which we are reactive under stress. Robert Sapolsky (1994) points out in his book *Why zebras don't get ulcers* that although we share with animals our innate tendency to fight, flight, or freeze under stress, we do something that animals don't do and which may explain why they don't develop the same stress-related diseases as we do: we add thinking. We ruminate. Worry. Catastrophize. Make ourselves more miserable than we already are by adding thinking.

Let's look at the kind of thoughts that parents may have when something difficult or stressful happens with their child or in their relationship with their child.

I recently went with my daughter to the dentist, to have yet another cavity filled. The cavity turned out to be much deeper than expected, and she needed anesthesia, which she refused, as this was one of her fears. [She had suffered from dentist fears.] It took a lot of persuasion on the part of the dentist before my daughter accepted the anesthesia and having her cavity filled. Afterwards, the dentist found another cavity which would have to be filled, and she told my daughter that her teeth were full of plaque. The appointment ended with the dentist telling me that she would take care of teaching my daughter to brush better. On the way back home, I lost it. I felt my heart beating, my blood boiling; I biked faster than usually, unaware of my environment, with a narrow attention span. I expressed how angry I was that she does not remember to brush her teeth by herself. I said that if she continues like this, she would end up with artificial teeth at the age of 18. When I threatened that I would take away her allowance until she brushed her teeth at school, she told me to shut my mouth, put her fingers in her ears so as not to hear me and eventually jumped off the back of my bike, to go home on her own. On my own, I calmed down, following my breath, feeling my stress and the whole range of my emotions: fear, anger, despair, and loneliness. I also realized that part of my anger was towards other people than her, her father, her dentists, and myself. Back home, I apologized to her for my explosion and realized how dependent she still is on me and how brave she had been in overcoming her fear of anesthesia. The thoughts that had gone through my mind were "the damage is irreversible," "she will lose all her teeth," "she will never be able to take care of her own life," "I'm a bad mother because I did not manage to make her brush better," "my dentist will think badly of us," and "I have to do it all alone, nobody is helping me."

Stressful moments are universal; they happen to all parents, but our thoughts add to the stress. Our thoughts are an automatic response when under stress, just as our fight–flight–freeze response is. But thoughts have great power over us as we tend to take them as reality and do not treat them as simple automatic responses when under stress. I cannot predict the future of my daughter, including her teeth; I don't know what our dentist was thinking; I did my very best the last years to make her brush better and more often; and I'm not alone, as at least the dentist was offering help, and there are more children in the world suffering from cavities and parents trying to fight it with them, and she is trying to do better. I was right in thinking that the damage done to her teeth was irreversible but so is the damage of my losing it. Being able to watch thoughts as thoughts, images as images, and not getting taken away by them as if they were reality, is what we practice over and over again during meditations.

PAUSING

The pause between experiencing bodily sensations of stress and reacting is a crucial skill that mindfulness training helps develop. From a neuropsychological point of view, we are developing our brain's ability to inhibit impulsive responding, to observe and judge the situation, and to plan a response. These are all aspects of executive functioning which are critical to how we react in situations "off of the cushion," that is, in our day-to-day lives. In particular, they are critical for developing the core skills required for *nonreactive* parenting. When we sit with stress or pain instead of reacting immediately to it, we are practicing *being* with the situation instead of *reacting* to the situation. Being with the situation as it is allows us to explore it, and to consider what kind of response, if any, is needed from us at this moment. The pause, however brief, also allows us to engage our executive functioning system, to allow the processes of observation, judging and planning to be engaged. Quite simply, this pause can be the difference between reacting impulsively in a way that we may later regret and responding wisely. After impulsively reacting, we may realize that we've made a mistake and regret it, but by then, the consequences of our action may already be set in motion. For example, a conflict which was beginning may have escalated, instead of moving towards resolution.

Nowhere is this more obvious than in intimate relationships, particularly parent–child relationships, where automatic or impulsive responding sometimes seems to rule the day. While as parents we seek to teach our children to inhibit reacting, delay gratification, and think before acting, we may often find ourselves reacting impulsively and even explosively to our children, especially in "hot" moments—moments of high emotional arousal or conflict which can trigger older emotional reactions. We know we're losing it when we find ourselves reacting, usually loudly and explosively, without pausing to reflect on what we are doing or the potential effects, as if there is a temporary power outage in our frontal lobe. In fact, we may find ourselves defiantly thinking or even shouting something like "I don't care if I am out of control. . . . I'm so fed up with you!" Ironically, we may often model exactly the kind of behavior we wish to discourage, and yet somehow, we expect a child to be able to "do as we say, not as we do" even if we have not mastered this skill as adults.

The following description from Karl Ove Knausgard's novel *Father* nicely illustrates such moments of reactive parenting in a father with three young children, as well as the need to create distance:

> *As I write, I am filled with tenderness for her [Heidi, 2 years]. But this is on paper. In reality, when it really counts, and she is standing there in front of me, so early in the morning that the streets outside are still and not a sound can be heard in the house, she, raring to start a new day, I, summoning the will to get to my feet, putting on yesterday's clothes and following her into the kitchen, where the promised blueberry-flavored milk and the sugar-free cereal await her, it is not tenderness I feel, and if she goes beyond my limits, such as when she pesters and pesters me for a film, or tries to get into the room where John [the baby] is sleeping, in short, every time she refuses to take no for an answer but drags things out ad infinitum, it is not uncommon for my irritation to mutate into anger, and when I then speak harshly to her, and her tears flow, and she bows her head and slinks off with slumped shoulders, I feel it serves her right. Not until the evening when they are asleep and I am sitting wondering what I am really doing is there any room for the insight that she is only two years old. But by then I am on the outside looking in. Inside, I don't have a chance.*
>
> *My Struggle, Book One.* Karl Ove Knausgard, p. 34

Notwithstanding situations where immediate action is required, such as when a child is in actual danger, most situations parents are confronted with are not life or death situations. The reactive parenting which may be the vestige of our ancestors (see Chapter 2) is more often a hindrance rather than a help and more often can lead to parent–child interactions that parents later regret, such as the ones described above, and even to potentially damaging parent–child interactions such as emotional or physical abuse. Hence, the need to help parents develop the ability to insert a pause between feelings and action. Tolerating what there is, in the moment, in the body, and developing a nonreactive stance to whatever is there, is the most important step in this process. The 3-min breathing space can help us with this.

GUIDELINES FOR SESSION 4

Box 8.1. Agenda Session 4

1. Sitting meditation including sounds and thoughts (20 min) + inquiry (15 min)
2. Read Koan (5 min)
3. Discussion stressful moments calendar in pairs (10 min)
4. Grasping and pushing away (10 min)
5. Fight, flight, freeze, and dance (10 min)
6. Group discussion of further home practice (15 min)
7. 3-min breathing space under stress (5 min)
8. Break (15 min)
9. Imagination: awareness and acceptance of parental stress + doors (15 min) + inquiry (15 min)
10. Standing yoga (15 min)
11. Halfway evaluation (20 min)
12. Review home practice (10 min)

---

1. SITTING MEDITATION, ADDING MEDITATION TO SOUNDS AND THOUGHTS

We sit for a meditation of about 20 min focusing first on breath, then the body, and we introduce the new element sounds and thoughts (see Handout 8.5 for a summary of the hearing and thinking meditation).

The inquiry starts as always with a general invitation to share experiences of this sitting practice, but the teacher makes sure that there is a discussion about our tendency to label sounds (= to judge) and what happens when we try not to label them. Generally, the experience is that when not labeling sounds, the sounds become richer and the attention for it longer and more intense. The teacher may talk about the evolutionary function of labeling sounds very fast (Snake in the grass! Jump!) and the function of our capacity to select which sounds are relevant and should be in the foreground, and which sounds are irrelevant and can be ignored. The labeling of sounds, thus, has important functions for survival and for shutting our attention system down for irrelevant sounds, so that we can sleep, focus, listen, or rest. In contrast, opening our awareness to *any* sound during meditation helps us to be in the present moment and experience it fully.

Participants may also share feelings of discomfort during this longer sitting, such as pain, tension, boredom, frustration, tiredness, and a tendency to push such feelings away and grasp at pleasant feelings (see Handout 8.2). When we have these uncomfortable experiences, we may tend to think: "How long will this last," "This is not working for me," "I'm wasting my time," "Let's shorten the exercise," "Let's stop this course." We add to our stress and suffering by adding thoughts. An important theme for the inquiry concerns how we relate to thoughts. Thoughts have enormous power in taking our attention away from the here and now of the present moment to the content of our thinking. We explore where the thoughts take us to and what wakes us up and brings us back. Recognizing the types of thoughts and giving them labels is helpful: for example, planning thoughts ("about shopping and cleaning," "picking up children," "getting to work in time," etc.), catastrophizing thoughts ("I'll never learn to mediate," "My child will never make friends"), self-depreciating thoughts ("I'm a bad mother," "I cannot cope with my workload"), judgmental thoughts ("This is boring," "My child is lazy"), decision-making thoughts ("Should I work less?" "Should I fire my au pair?"), and paranoid thoughts ("My child does not want to live with me," "My partner is using me"). Thoughts have the power to intensify our emotions, to increase our stress, and to affect our actions, including our parenting. Being able to recognize thoughts as thoughts, being able to observe the effects that certain (negative) thoughts can have on us, and being able to distance ourselves from our thoughts are therefore critical skills to lessen the grip that thoughts have on our parenting.

One typical experience that parents often report is while thoughts come up constantly during the sitting meditation, once the practice focuses on observing thoughts, no thoughts may come up, aside from thinking about the fact that no thoughts come up, which is a thought. This demonstrates how automatic our thinking is, and that once we pay deliberate attention to our thinking, it immediately changes.

The inquiry may end with an invitation to discuss how the sitting meditation at home went in the past week.

2. READ KOAN

Koan illustrates the "train of thoughts" parents can get caught up in (see Handout 8.4).

3. DISCUSSION OF STRESSFUL PARENTING EVENT IN DYADS

We break up in dyads and invite participants to discuss the stressful event calendar, with a focus on *what* makes the event stressful and on bodily signals of stress. The teacher explains that he or she will ring the bell when the roles of speaker and listener are to be reversed, after 5 min.

4. GRASPING AND PUSHING AWAY

We discuss the stressful parenting events further in the entire group, with a focus on how our tendency to push away what is unpleasant, and to grasp at what is pleasant, enhances the stress. We invite parents to specifically look in their stressful event calendar for tendencies to push away what is unpleasant, and we write some examples on the flip chart.

VOICES OF THE PARENTS

Jill described how her 6-year-old daughter starts yelling when she starts to comb her hair in the morning. She immediately becomes tense, short of breath, thinking "Why is she so over-sensitive?" "Why can we never have a normal morning?," "Why doesn't she cooperate like the other children?" and feels angry and sad. This is a wonderful example of how the yelling is pushed away. Jill goes on to describe how having become aware of her stress helped her afterwards to take a moment of self-compassion, holding herself. Frank adds other morning stress examples: one child complaining about what is on his sandwich, another refusing to wear the clothes his wife selected for her. Sylvia found herself so angry and frustrated with her adult son lying on the couch the whole day, smoking pot, that she literally had turned all the pictures of the son that were in the house, backwards, pushing his image away.

The common experience here is that the defiant, willful, complaining, or difficult behavior of the children is not allowed or welcomed, and pushing what is unpleasant away adds stress to family life!

Thus, instead of (on the flip chart):

Unpleasant event + aversion/pushing away → stress → reactive parenting (fight–flight–freeze)

This:

Unpleasant event → staying present in the body → creating space → choosing to respond from a more spacious place

The same principle is true for pleasant things. Holding on to things that are pleasant, grasping, can lead to stress and suffering as well (see Handout 8.2).

5. DEMONSTRATION FIGHT, FLIGHT, FREEZE, AND DANCE

This exercise is meant to demonstrate in a lively and physical way our different reaction patterns when under stress (see Box 8.2).

Box 8.2. Dance

The teacher stands in the middle of the group circle and asks who wants to volunteer to be the teacher's problem. The teacher asks the group member to approach him or her physically pretending to be his or her problem. The teacher announces to the group that he or she will demonstrate four different ways of responding to the problem.

The group member approaches the teacher and the teacher first demonstrate a fight response, pushing back with both hands against the hands of the group member, both members of the dyad pushing towards each other with great force until a stalemate is reached. The teacher ends the first round, telling the group that this was the first way of reacting, and then invites the problem to approach again. Now the teacher demonstrates a flight response, running away from the group member who in turn will spontaneously pursue the teacher. The teacher runs out of the room, with the group member still following. The teacher then returns, notes that this was the second reaction, and invites his/her problem to approach again. Now the teacher demonstrates a freeze or submission reaction, curling up into a ball on the floor and covering the face with the hands, while the problem keeps hammering on the teacher. This is the third reaction. (The teacher can demonstrate the three reactions in whatever order he/she prefers, as long as all three reactions are demonstrated). Then, the teacher invites his or her problem to approach a fourth time. This time the teacher tries to dance with the problem, by finding a tango-like position together, for example, taking the right hand of the problem with his/her right hand and putting his/her arm around the waist of the group member and starting to dance. The teacher may start to softly sing along.

Usually, after some struggling in which the teacher uses the force of the problem by going with it instead of resisting it, and then takes over, the dance really takes place!

The teacher thanks the group member and both resume their places in the group. We begin the inquiry by first asking the group member about his/her experiences: What was it like for you as my problem? Often the "problem's" experience of the interaction is quite illuminating. Then, we invite the group members to identify the four ways of reacting and to talk about the effects. Fighting did not solve the problem and took a lot of energy from both parties. Avoiding did not solve anything either, the problem kept coming. Here I generally give the example of the tax form that I avoid filling in, but when you don't fill it in, it keeps coming back to you! Same with unpaid bills, they keep coming! Freezing: the problem keeps hammering! And dance: a creative use of energy, trying to create something new, something better, by engaging fully and directly with the problem. This is a physical metaphor for "creative engagement."

Parents almost always recognize their own habitual reaction patterns in this demonstration, but because of the very humorous manner of demonstrating them, it becomes easier for parents to be more accepting of their reaction patterns and to laugh about the futility of them. For example, Katy, a divorced mother who had been exposed to marital violence, and to violence by her father when she was a child, recognized her struggle with her adolescent son whose behavior she experienced as aggressive, and that she tended to respond in submissive ways.

After this discussion, the teacher goes back to the rationale of the first session (turning back the flip chart) connecting the three reactions, fight, flight, and freeze, to the short route in the brain while under stress. Dancing can be seen as the conscious response, taking the longer route in the brain. In order to engage this conscious response and to make space for a creative solution, we need to first use the breathing space to create a pause and to be able to stand back and observe our reactions to the problem.

6. GROUP DISCUSSION OF FURTHER HOME PRACTICE

Why is it that often participants find it more difficult to make space for the 3-min breathing space a day than for a 45-min body scan, sitting meditation, or lying yoga? When we raise this question in the group, parents talk about their busy schedules, that they feel there is literally no time. We encourage them to try the breathing space in the most rushed periods, for example, around breakfast in the morning, in the middle of a busy working day, before or during cooking in the evening, or while bringing the children to bed. The experience of a breathing space when the potatoes are cooking (they take 20 min at least), the children are tired from school or daycare, and the parent is exhausted from work, can be insightful. Another reason why it may be more difficult to do the breathing space than a longer meditation is that it is not part of daily routine and hard to remember. That's why we ask group members to exchange cell phone numbers in pairs, and to text each other once a day at a random time during the coming week, with the text ".b," which stands for "stop and breathe." This idea was developed by Burnett (2009) for his mindfulness in high schools project, but we have found it works with adults just as well as with adolescents (see Box 8.4).

The experiences with the lying yoga can be very variable; some participants completely enjoying it, saying this is really something for them, and much better than the body scan or sitting meditation; other participants may have more negative experiences. The inquiry should first focus on deepening the experiences, positive or negative. We ask questions about what they enjoyed, how that felt, what bodily experience, what effect the liking had on them, and what they concluded ("I should do this more often," "I should take a yoga course"). We ask similar questions about what others disliked, how that felt, what bodily experiences occurred, and what the result was of the disliking, what conclusion was drawn ("Yoga is really not for me"). Some of the themes that may come up in the inquiry are the comparing mind, comparing experiences to each other and judging (better, worse), rather than approaching each experience with a beginners' mind, and our tendency to grasp at what we like and reject what we don't like. The invitation is to try the yoga (now standing yoga) again next week and as best as we can, experience it all while noticing our tendency to compare and judge.

We also share experiences about the mindful activity with the child.

Lucy planned to bake cookies with her daughter mindfully. She was aware of her tendency to control the process so that it would succeed and not get messy, and letting go of that, she became aware of the knowledge and skills that her daughter already had about making cookies, and she noticed how her daughter enjoyed practicing her knowledge and skills.

Jill said that she was waiting every day for the right moment to initiate a mindful activity with her son, until her son came to her and said: Mom do you want to play tennis with me? She was watching him playing tennis for the first time, using his own rules, she observed his joy in his body and face, she was aware of her tendency to correct him but decided not to.

7. 3-MIN BREATHING SPACE UNDER STRESS

We sit for a breathing space with extended instructions, as it can be used when under stress or when there are intense emotions.

Box 8.3. 3-Min Breathing Space Under Stress
(Adapted from Williams, Segal, Teasdale, & Kabat-Zinn, 2007)

Bringing yourself in the present moment by deliberately adopting an erect and dignified position. If possible, close your eyes. Turning your attention inward. Asking yourself: How am I doing? What is my experience right now . . .

What thoughts are going through my mind? As best as you can, acknowledge thoughts as mental events, perhaps putting them into words, giving them labels: "self-critical thoughts are here," "ruminate thoughts," and catastrophizing thoughts."

What feelings are here? Turning towards any sense of emotional discomfort or unpleasant feelings, maybe putting them into words: "there is fear," "shame," "anger," or "sadness." What body sensations am I aware? Turning towards any physical discomfort, sensation of tightness, bracing, and pressure in the body.

What action tendencies do I notice? Becoming aware of a tendency to get up and move, getting angry, avoiding, and hiding.

You have connected to how you are right now; this is the first step.

Then, gently turning your full attention towards your breathing. Following each breath all the way is . . . and all the way out . . . maybe also aware of the pauses between the inbreath and the outbreath. Aware of the breath breathing itself. Using the breath to anchor you in the present and help you tune into a state of awareness amidst of the stress or intensity. Perhaps a sense of watching the turmoil from a place of stillness. This is the second step.

Now expanding your attention to the whole body, so that it includes a sense of the body as a whole, your posture, and facial expression. You may get a sense of the movement of the breath throughout the body, as if the whole body is breathing. This breathing body, in this moment of time, in this space. Embracing any sense of discomfort or tension in the body. Saying to yourself: "It's okay. Whatever it is what I'm feeling, it's okay. Let me feel it. It is already there." Staying a moment in this more spacious awareness.

8. BREAK

A short break takes place.

9. IMAGINATION: AWARENESS AND ACCEPTANCE OF STRESS USING THE BREATHING SPACE AND DOORS

Box 8.4. Awareness and Acceptance of Parenting Stress + Doors
The group takes its sitting position, and the teacher announces that we are going to do a short imagination practice. Group members are invited to sit comfortably in an upright position, shoulders relaxed, chest open. After participates have taken a moment to anchor themselves in this sitting position, they are invited to let a stressful event between them and their child come to the surface. It does not need to be very difficult situation, just a moment of stress. It can be an event from last week, perhaps described in the parental stress calendar, but it does not need to be. If another situation comes up, a less recent one, or situation with someone else than the child, such as partners, boss, or friend, that is okay too. Let the stressful even unfold, and imagine it as vividly as possible, as if it is happening right now.

Where are you? Who is present? What is happening? What are you doing, saying? What are you feeling and thinking at that moment? What is the other person (child, partner, etc.) doing, saying? What are they feeling? What is happening between you? The teacher asks group members to raise their hand if they have not found a situation yet and pauses a moment, in order to allow everyone to find a situation.

When you have a clear picture of the stressful situation, turn your attention to this moment, checking in, how are you right now, noticing whatever comes up . . . are there any bodily sensations you are aware of right now? Are there any thoughts you notice? What is it you are feeling right now. . . . What emotions are coming up . . . sadness, anger, fear. . .? Do you notice any action tendencies? Describe your experiences in words, labeling them, for example, saying in yourself: "A feeling of anger is arising," "Hopelessness thoughts are here," "Sensations of nervousness are in the stomach," "A tendency to step up and walk away." This is the first step. Becoming aware of what is going on in your body and mind right now.

Now, gently redirecting your full attention to the movement of the breath in your body. Following every breath the whole way in and the whole way out . . . maybe also noticing the pauses between each inbreath and each outbreath. Following the movement as if you're on a swing, riding the waves of your breath. That is the second step.

The third step, allowing your attention to expand to your body as a whole—especially to any sense of discomfort, tension, or resistance. Aware of whatever you experience in the body. If uncomfortable sensations are there, then bring your awareness to it by "breathing into them" on the inbreath. Then, breathe out from those sensations, softening and opening with the outbreath. Saying to yourself on the outbreath: it is okay. Whatever it is that I'm feeling, it is okay. It is already there. Let me feel it.

Now imagine you enter a large mansion, you open the door and enter into a wide corridor with many doors. . . . Imagine that, on the left side, behind every door, you find ways of taking care of yourself. Choose which way you go, open one door, look at what possibility is offered, and try it out. . . . Try not to judge the possibility but see how it feels for yourself. . . . Then, move to other doors, at your own pace, trying out other possibilities, even if they appear crazy or wrong.

If the image of the doors does not work for you, you can simply see whatever possibilities come to mind and try them out . . .

We are coming to the end of this exercise. . . . When you hear the bell, take a moment to stretch your body or do whatever feels good for your body.

INQUIRY

Participants may experience strong emotions during this practice, and it is important to share this with group members or hear about similar experiences of others. The teacher may want to clarify that there is no need to share the details of the situation imagined with the group but rather the experience of what it was like to imagine the stressful situation, doing the breathing space and trying out different responses to the situation.

One parent put it like this after having done the exercise: "I noticed I was able to embrace the stress."

VOICES OF THE PARENTS

Lynn described a stressful situation with her partner and the children of her partner, who have been both diagnosed with ADHD. The four of them are playing a game, but the children are moving a lot, throwing the chips in the air, unable to wait for their turn, and not paying attention to the game when it is not their turn. She noticed how restless she felt as a result of watching their restlessness, and how she felt irritated with her partner for not correcting them, stressed because she constantly felt an urge to correct them, and sad because of the lack of connectedness she felt. Paying attention to the children she realized how they liked doing what they were doing, and that for them it was a moment of connectedness. She went to the doors on the left, and tried asking her partner to correct them, tried reprimanding them herself, tried getting out of the situation by reading in a corner while they continued the game, and tried behaving as wild as they did. While trying out these different possibilities, she realized that she wanted to feel connected to these children that are so different from her, and that trying to control them made her feel disconnected to them.

Mary imagined a situation with her autistic son, who has difficulty with change: the continuous battle in the weekends of him refusing to go out. She first tried a door on the right side, she felt like crying and being held by her partner. Then, she went to the left side, and was surprised to find several new possibilities to work with this issue behind the doors: setting a specific time every weekend with him where he has to go out, or agreeing how long he can play inside, and then going out.

Mark tried several doors on the right side. Behind one door, there was a swimming pool and he went for a swim. The other door offered a cold beer. The third door opened to a wide forest and he took a walk. He felt replenished and calm.

When parents explore the possible scenarios coming up behind the doors, sometimes extremely rejecting or aggressive scenarios come to their mind's eye. For example, one parent mentioned putting an advertisement in the newspaper to give the child away for adoption. Trying out such a scenario, next to all others, felt good for that parent. The key point of this exercise is that when we are able to hold our emotions and stress, moving into it rather than away from it, and not trying to change the situation, we also open up to the emotions of others, make space for them, and feel that we are connected.

10. HALFWAY EVALUATION

We have found it helpful to evaluate halfway through the course how everyone is doing, and where each participant is in the process of following this course. The teacher invites group members to share with the group where they are in the process and how things are going. Participants are free to choose if and when they want to speak. We tend to not look at group members in particular, and generally do not ask further questions, but thank each person when they are finished. There may be silent moments during this evaluation, and it is okay if group members do not want to speak.

VOICES OF THE PARENTS

Jill, who had gone through postnatal depression after the birth of her daughter (and has been diagnosed and treated for bipolar disorder), describes how she enjoys being with her daughter since she is in the group, whereas before she experienced it more as something she had to do. Group members notice how she smiles more.

Arthur, diagnosed with Autistic Spectrum Disorder, notices that he feels more, physically and emotionally, whereas he used to be much more cognitive.

Martha tells that she is so much more aware of daily stress, and as a result experiences that she can deal better with the stress of raising an autistic child.

Group members may also describe that things are pretty difficult; that they have become more sensitive; that they have become more aware of intense emotions, such as sadness, anger, and stress; that they have more nightmares; etc. It can be helpful to describe the four stages of learning: (1) unconscious not capable, (2) conscious not capable, (3) conscious capable, and (4) unconscious capable. Becoming aware of suffering is phase 2 in the learning process.

11. STANDING YOGA

Going through the 8 weeks, we want meditation to become more and more part of daily life. Standing yoga, and in the next session, walking meditation, helps make the transition from being aware of our body while lying and sitting to standing and walking, to bringing awareness to when we are upright, often in our doing mode.

The group stands in a circle, or facing the teacher, with enough space between each member so that each person can stretch their arms without touching their neighbor. For the drawings of the standing yoga practices, see Handout 8.5.

In the inquiry, the teacher may focus on how we relate to our limits and of our tendency to compete. That is, what happens when you are confronted with pain, stiffness, or balance problems? What do you feel in the body, what thoughts come up ("I cannot do this," "I should be able to do this as others are doing it too," "I used to be able to bend much further," "I should be going to gym classes," "I am awful at this"), what action tendencies (going further than what is wise for the body right now, focusing on others rather than on own body, or challenging limits too little).

12. REVIEW OF HOME PRACTICE

This week's home practice (Handout 8.1) consists of practicing the 3-min breathing space in two ways: when under (parenting) stress and three times a day at random moments, including the help of a group member; see Box 8.5 for instructions for .b. The formal practice includes sitting meditation including sounds and thoughts, and lying yoga, on alternative days.

Box 8.5. .b

We ask group members to exchange cell phone numbers in pairs (people who prefer not to be with a particular person can choose another person) for the following practice. In the coming week, send each other a text message once a day at a random time with the text: .b, meaning stop and breath (obviously not in the middle of the night). The receiver of the text message has to do the breathing space at the moment he or she sees the text message (if the phone is off as soon as the phone is on) and the sender after sending the .b. Participants may share fun moments the week thereafter about when they received the .b and what effect the breathing space had.

HANDOUT 8.1 Practice for the Week After Session 4

Reading

Read the handouts mindfully.

Mindful Parenting

Practice the 3-min breathing space under stress, or follow three breaths mindfully, whenever you notice unpleasant feelings and particularly when you notice parental stress. Don't expect any result, such as your stress to diminish; the goal of the 3-min breathing space under stress is to slow down your automatic reaction (to push away what is unpleasant and the fight–flight–freeze reaction) and instead be aware of, be with, move towards the stress, and connect to the body.
Fill in the parental stress calendar: breathing space.
Write a brief autobiographical description of your relationship with your parents when you were a child and the relationship between you and your child now. Afterwards, do a 3-min breathing space.

Formal Practice

Do the sitting meditation including breathing, body sensations, the body as a whole, and sounds and thoughts every other day (so three times this week).
Try this simple experiment when you are meditating and notice an itch. Experiment with doing nothing at all. What happens to the itch? Notice the intensity, also the location, and notice your action tendencies—what you want to do (but try to delay reacting!). See what happens, and write it in your journal.
On alternate days, do the standing yoga practice (so three times this week).

Informal Practice

Practice the 3-min breathing space, one time a day on a standard, pre-scheduled moment, namely, _____ and once a day when the random .b text message comes in and when you send a .b once a day (so three times a day)

HANDOUT 8.2 Grasping

I hold something dear, a small Korean golden bowl, for example. Because it is mine and because it is precious. I grasp at it. So physically I hold it in the palm of my hand and tighten my fist around it. If I do this for some time, I will get a cramp in the arms. But also I will not be able to use my hand for anything else, which means that I am stuck to what I am grasping at. The solution to the grasping pattern upon contact is not, of course, to get rid of the hand that grasps or to get rid of the object being grasped at. That is too drastic. The object has not asked to be grasped at, even if advertising and packaging made it incredibly alluring. Meditation can help me open my hand gently and have the object rest lightly upon my palm; in this way there is the possibility of movement and freedom.

From: Martine Batchelor, Let Go: *A Buddhist Guide to Breaking Free of Habits,* 2007

All of us have the tendency to want to hang on to pleasant experiences and to avoid unpleasant experiences. We "grasp" at pleasant experiences, emotions, fantasies, and bodily sensations and try to hold on to them. Grasping is one of the first actions a baby can perform and has a clear survival value.

But what happens when we rely too much on grasping? Although of course we all like pleasant experiences, they cannot last forever, and by grasping at pleasant experiences, we open up the divide between what we are experiencing, here and now, and the pleasant state we are longing for. This discrepancy usually makes us feel distressed or uncomfortable, and we lose touch with what we actually are experiencing. We become less free, open, and creative, and we lose spaciousness. Note the difference between grasping and savoring positive events. Savoring the good things of life, for example, looking over the pictures of our past holidays, our developing children, revisiting beautiful memories, and feeling grateful, helps us enjoy our life.

Grasping can also be seen in our tendency to reject or avoid unpleasant experiences or feel aversion. It may seem second nature to us that we would try to avoid unpleasant experiences, but this is a kind of negative grasping. Aversion is another form of wanting things to be different, of not wanting things to be the way they are. For example, I have this stress—I don't want to feel it! So I avoid the stress, deny the stress, push the stress away, distract myself from the stress. This can work for minutes, hours, and even days, but eventually, the more we try to push the stress away, the more it returns. One of the parents in a Mindful Parenting group found himself so frustrated with his adult son

HANDOUT 8.2 Grasping (continued)

lying on the couch the whole day, smoking pot, that he literally had turned backwards all the pictures of his son that were in the house, pushing his image away.

Mindfulness offers a third way—instead of grasping and aversion, can we hold the experience lightly, gently, with openness, curiosity, and compassion. Paradoxically, this light holding and allowing it to be can often change our experience of the suffering. We all experience feelings of stress, sadness, or anger which we try to push away or avoid, perhaps by telling ourselves it's silly to feel that way or that we don't have time to feel these things, or we shouldn't feel them, or by distracting ourselves, or by going into our thought—stream. We may experience momentary relief but at a high price—cutting ourselves off from our feelings and our very selves and leaving us exhausted from the effort to hold back the tide of emotions. When we allow feelings of stress, sadness, or anger to be there, staying present with them, we no longer have the tension between how things are and how we wish things were. When we open to these feelings, we can create space for them to be, which in itself can be transformative. The feelings don't necessarily go away, but our ability to tolerate and be with them changes. We have a chance then to look at them with curiosity instead of fear and eventually to choose a new way to respond to them, instead of reacting automatically.

HANDOUT 8.3 Staying Present with Parental Stress

When we try to push away our pain, we add stress to our experience. Instead of just experiencing pure pain, we now experience pain + stress, which multiplies our pain.

For example, one day recently, my children had the day off from school, and I had planned to do something special with them—go to a museum, a park, etc. But I woke up with a headache, and what I really felt like doing was resting in bed. Somehow I kept grasping at my image of myself as a wonderful mindful mother, spending special time with my children at a special place. The more I grasped, the worse I felt, since the morning was slipping away, and so far, no wonderful plans had materialized. I found myself feeling very irritated and unhappy, and when I felt this, I immediately tried to push it away—this did not fit my picture of the happy mother spending quality time with her delightful children. Meanwhile, my children were becoming less and less delightful as the day wore on. They were bored, hungry, and tired, wanting me to play with them, not wanting to go outside, etc. My irritation increased, as did my self-criticism (what a terrible mother! I'm useless!). Meanwhile, my intention to stay present with myself and my children had gone completely out the window. Finally, I found myself snapping at them over something small, making me (and them) feel even worse.

What went wrong here? What would have happened if I had been able to acknowledge and stay present with my bodily sensations of fatigue and headache, and my feeling of irritation, instead of trying to avoid it, deny it, judge myself harshly for it, or make it go away. What would have happened if I had been able to let go of the fantasy of the perfect outing with my children and instead had tuned into what was actually going on with myself and my children, and what we each were needing in this moment. Perhaps if I had made space for these feelings, I would have been able to respond with more kindness and acceptance to my own feelings, and I might not have felt so stressed by the situation. I might not have lost my temper and yelled at my children. Instead, I might have made a deliberate decision to make a different plan, given how I was feeling. Maybe I would have suggested that we all stay home in our pajamas and eat pancakes, which would have suited all of our needs much better!

Paying attention to our body can help us to stay present with difficult emotions instead of pushing them away. All emotions resonate somewhere in the body, although we are often not in touch with these bodily sensations. When we experience strong negative emotions, we can gently turn our focus inward to the body, asking ourselves, "Where do I feel this sadness? What exactly does it feel like?" Instead of going into an automatic pattern of negative thoughts ("Why do I feel this way?

HANDOUT 8.3 Staying Present with Parental Stress
(continued)

What's wrong with me? I always feel this way. Things will never be different.") which only increase our distress, we ask, "What am I feeling in my body? Where do I feel it? How do the sensations change?" This puts us in touch directly with our feelings on a bodily level; furthermore, it helps us avoid the trap of going into ruminative or problem-solving mind. Using the breath to guide us through the body sensations, we may find we can stay with painful emotions longer, with more gentleness and kindness and curiosity towards ourselves, than when we stay in our heads. Staying present with the feelings offers us a chance to explore them, to give them more space, and perhaps to view them from an expanded, larger perspective. From this perspective, we can eventually decide how to respond, rather than reacting automatically.

HANDOUT 8.4 A Zen Koan for Parents*

Question 1:
What is the sound of one hand clapping?
Answer:
The sound of one hand clapping is the sound of one hand clapping.

Question 2:
What is the sound of a child misbehaving?
Answer:
The sound of a child misbehaving is the sound of a child misbehaving.

Question 3:
What is the sound of *my* child misbehaving?
Answer:
The sound of "I cannot control my child," the sound of "I should be able to," the sound of "I am a bad parent," the sound of "I don't know what to do," the sound of "I hate this child," the sound of "I should not feel this way," and the sound of my failure

*Coyne and Wilson, 2004

HANDOUT 8.5 Mindfulness of Hearing and Thinking*

1. Practice mindfulness of breath and body as described in Handout 7.5 until you feel reasonably settled.
2. Allow the focus of your awareness to shift from sensations in the body to hearing—bring your attention to the ears and then allow the awareness to open and expand so that there is a receptiveness to sounds as they arise, wherever they arise.
3. There is no need to go searching for sounds or listening for particular sounds. Instead, as best you can, simply open your mind so that it is receptive to awareness of sounds from all directions as they arise—sounds that are close, sounds that are far, and sounds that are in front, behind, to the side, above, or below—opening to the whole space of sound around you. Allow awareness to include obvious sounds and more subtle sounds. Allow it to include the space between sounds and silence itself.
4. As best you can, be aware of sounds simply as sounds, as bare auditory sensations. When you find that you are thinking *about* the sounds, reconnect, as best you can, with direct awareness of their sensory qualities (patterns of pitch, timbre, loudness, and duration), rather than their meanings or implications.
5. Whenever you notice that your awareness is no longer featuring sounds in the present moment, gently acknowledge where your mind has drifted off to and then return your attention back to hearing sounds as they arise and pass away moment by moment.
6. When you are ready, let go of featuring sounds and instead feature thoughts center stage in your awareness. Just as you were aware of whatever sounds arose—noticing their arising, lingering, and passing away—so now, as best you can, allowing your awareness to discern any and all thoughts that may arise in the mind in just the same way, noticing thoughts arise, as they linger in the space of the mind and as they eventually dissolve and disappear. There is no need to try to make thoughts come or go—just let them come and go on their own, in the same way that you related to the arising and passing away of sounds.
7. You might find it helpful to bring awareness to thoughts in the mind in the same way that you would if the thoughts were projected on the screen at the movies—you sit, watching the screen, waiting for a thought or image to arise. When it does, you attend to it so long as it is there "on the screen," and then you let it go as it passes away. Alternatively, you might find it helpful to see thoughts as clouds moving across a vast spacious sky. Sometimes they are dark and stormy;

*From *The Mindful Way through Depression* by Williams, Teasdale, Segal, and Kabat-Zinn (2007), pp. 166–168. Copied with permission of Guilford Press.

HANDOUT 8.5 Mindfulness of Hearing and Thinking (continued)

sometimes they are light and fluffy. Sometimes they fill the entire sky. Sometimes they clear out completely, leaving the sky cloudless.

8. If any thoughts bring with them intense feelings or emotions, pleasant or unpleasant, as best you can, note their "emotional charge" and intensity and let them be as they already are.

9. If at any time you feel that your mind has become unfocused and scattered, or it keeps getting repeatedly drawn into the drama of your thinking and imaginings, see if it is possible to come back to the breath and a sense of the body as a whole sitting and breathing and use this focus to anchor and stabilize your awareness.

HANDOUT 8.6 Standing Yoga Postures*

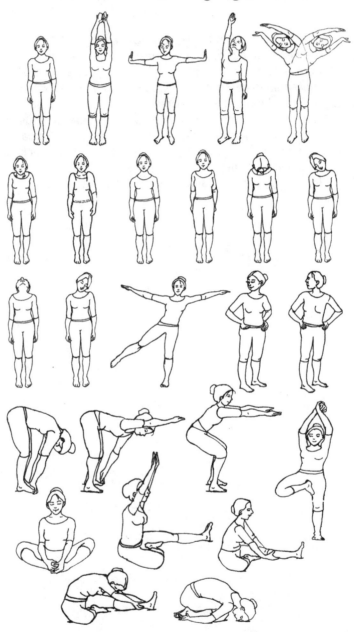

*Sequence of postures adapted from *Full Catastrophe Living* by Jon Kabat-Zinn (pp. 110–113). copyright © 1990 by Jon Kabat-Zinn. Used by permission of Dell Publishing, an imprint of The Random House Publishing Group, a division of Random House LLC. All rights reserved. Redrawn by C. Bögels.

HANDOUT 8.7 Parental Stress Calendar: Breathing Space

Be aware once a day of a stressful event between you and your child, or you and your (ex)partner about your child, *when it occurs*. If possible, take a 3-min breathing space at some point during the stressful event, or afterwards, or in anticipation. Write down your experiences at a later moment using the chart below.

Describe the stressful parenting situation	What made you notice the stress (body signals, thoughts, emotions, action tendencies?)	Did you react out of habit? If yes, describe your (automatic) reaction	Or did you take a breathing space? (How) did that change the chain of reactions?

HANDOUT 8.8 Home Practice Record from Week 4

Fill in the record from each time after you practice (mindful parenting, formal or informal meditation). Write down what comes up for you during the practice, so that we can discuss it in the next session. Circle a 3 each time you have done a 3-min breathing space.

Day/time	Practice (Yes/No)	Comments
	3 3 3	
	3 3 3	
	3 3 3	
	3 3 3	
	3 3 3	
	3 3 3	
	3 3 3	
	3 3 3	

HANDOUT 8.9 Notes Informal Practice and Mindful Parenting Practice Week 4

You may want to use this sheet to make notes about your experiences during the informal meditation practice and the mindful parenting practice or to make notes during or about the group session.

CHAPTER 9

SESSION 5: PARENTING PATTERNS AND SCHEMAS

At the moment of giving birth to a child, is the mother separate from the child? You should study not only that you become a mother when your child is born, but also that you become a child.

Dogen Zenji (edited by Tanahashi, 1985)

PARENTING CAN be one of the most emotionally rich and satisfying experiences in our lives. As parents, we are privileged to revisit ourselves as children, as we are present for our own child's unfolding experience. The joy and wonder that our child experiences as he or she discovers a ladybug nestling on a new green leaf in the springtime becomes our joy and wonder as well. When our child eagerly anticipates the coming of the tooth fairy, we too feel the excitement and joy of her imminent arrival, temporarily suspending our disbelief. These experiences touch us at such a deep level, which gives raising our child an intense emotional richness.

In addition to *re-experiencing* our own childhood through our children, parenting gives us the chance to experience some things for the first time. A father of a girl who grew up without a sister gets to experience firsthand the world of girlhood and of braiding long hair, girlish fantasy, and soaring emotions. The mother of a boy gets to experience firsthand the world of "boyness" vicariously through her son: the world of boy friendships, of rough and tumble play, and of boy sweetness, hidden behind the veneer of boy toughness.

We also get a chance to do things differently than our parents, correct some of the perceived mistakes, or give our children experiences we never had. A mother raised in an emotionally cold family tries to create a warm and loving home. A father raised by an abusive father tries to be calm and patient with his own children. This is perhaps the most transcendent aspect of parenthood: the possibility that we can give our children something we didn't experience ourselves, something better, and in so doing, experience a kind of healing for our own childhood experience. This can occur on a concrete level—for example, a father who grew up poor taking pleasure in being able to provide materially for his children due to his financial success—or on an emotional level, as the previous examples illustrate. It is this double experience—experiencing our child and reconnecting with our own experience as a child—which gives parenting the unique emotional pull that it has.

This emotional pull which brings such intense joy can also be our downfall. The emotional intensity of our relationship with our child can make all our emotions stronger, not only joy and happiness, but also anger, sadness, fear, and disgust. Our ability to share in our child's experience and to empathize with him and understand his world also has a darker side—we can at times become lost in our identification with our child. When that happens, we can find ourselves acting in ways we never thought possible. How many times have we found ourselves saying or doing something to our child which we swore we would never do, or literally heard our mother or father's voice coming out of our mouths, as if an alien had temporarily taken over our body? This is so commonplace that we don't give it much thought. But this phenomenon is central to our experience of being a parent and may in fact be more important than all of our conscious beliefs and attitudes about parenting. It is especially important for us to become aware of these automatic patterns, because often they run *counter* to what we may believe we are doing or the values we hold. Our belief about the kind of parents we are may sometimes get in the way of seeing how we actually interact with our child; mindfulness helps us to see the reality more clearly.

The core theme of Session 5 is to recognize when we are emotionally triggered during interactions with our child or when under stress, and to recognize when we shift into more childlike states or schema modes. Parents learn to use mindfulness to become aware of and investigate different patterns in their relationship with their child and to see whether they are similar to patterns from their own childhood experience. We use the concept of schema modes to help parents recognize when a current interaction with their child is triggering an old emotional reaction from their past. When parents can recognize that they are being emotionally triggered, they can often disengage from emotional overreactions to their children.

The second theme of this session is to practice holding our reactions to stressful parent–child interactions in an open and accepting way. Being able to hold the strong emotions, thoughts, body sensations, and action tendencies which are evoked in stressful interactions with our children is key to our being able to recognize them and ultimately change them. After all, if we cannot admit when we become locked in dysfunctional ways of reacting because we are too judgmental of ourselves, we are likely to remain in denial about the interaction. We practice holding your emotions like a baby in Session 5. The 3-min breathing space when your child behaves in the worst possible way, plus adding self-compassion if needed, is a home practice that supports parents in holding strong reactions and emotions.

EFFECTS OF OUR OWN CHILDHOOD EXPERIENCE ON PARENTING

How do our childhood experiences affect how we parent our own children? On an intuitive level, we may recognize the myriad ways our own experiences growing up have affected our parenting style and our relationship with our child. Sometimes we may embrace this heritage, as when we choose to raise our children in the same religious or cultural background as we were raised. Other times we may consciously reject this background, for example, by choosing to be less strict or more involved than our parents.

But sometimes when things between us and our children heat up emotionally, we may feel the influence of our own childhood experience when we least expect it or intend it. In these moments, we may not be aware of that influence. Marinus Van IJzendoorn, a psychologist who studies attachment between parents and children, has examined this phenomenon for many years. In a meta-analysis of many studies, he found that how mothers thought about their close attachment relationships was the best predictor of the kind of attachment their own children had with them. In fact, mothers' "attachment representations"—how they experienced themselves in close relationships—was better at predicting their children's attachment to them than how they actually parented their children. Van IJzendoorn calls this the "transmission gap" in our knowledge of how parents' attachment patterns are translated to their children. As parents, we seem to transmit something very important to our children which cannot necessarily be measured or even observed in our interaction with our child (van IJzendoorn, 1995). How can we understand this, and, more importantly, what can we do about it?

SCHEMAS

One way that we may "transmit" our own attachment or relation-ship patterns from our youth to our own children is through how we mentally represent those relationships or our "schemas." Jeffrey Young (1994) describes how schemas are formed in early childhood through a child's internal representations of his relationship with his parents. This representation includes cognitive, emotional, and bodily representations and is often experienced automatically and out of conscious awareness. We tend to experience schemas as a totality: we simultaneously experi-ence thoughts, feelings, and body sensations which together make up the schema. Schemas organize the way in which we experience and interpret the world, and they organize how we tend to respond. According to schema theory, schemas can be adaptive or maladaptive. Young described the maladaptive schemas of people with personality disorders. For exam-ple, a person with the abandonment schema, when triggered by real or imagined abandonment, may feel scared and vulnerable, have thoughts that he will be alone forever; feel painful bodily sensations in his gut; and act by trying to prevent the abandonment from occurring. Maladaptive schemas are transient: they are triggered by particular interpersonal events, or by feelings, thoughts, or body sensations. They don't last for-ever, but when a schema is triggered, a person's entire mode of thinking, feeling, and acting is transformed, so that he is in a different mode of processing his experience.

SCHEMA MODES

When an early schema of ours is triggered, we may shift into this different mode of experience, which reflects more childlike ways of being. Young calls these *schema modes*. When we are in a schema mode, we may experience ourselves as being in a child role or a parent role. The child modes as described by Young include "angry child" and "vulnerable child," and the parent modes include "punitive parent" and "demanding parent." The hallmark of being in a schema mode is the intensity of emo-tion, as well as the accompanying thoughts, body sensations, and actions.

To illustrate, let's return to the example of my "losing it" after the dentist visit. I was aware of my mounting anger towards my child, and although I did not realize it at that moment, my angry child mode was triggered and I had an "adult temper tantrum." What is important here is the *mode* of processing and responding, not the particular content that triggered the mode: the emotions, thinking, and body sensations are strong and not modulated by the healthy part of ourselves that understands our child's perspective or recognizes that we are overreacting. Our ability to take perspective is limited, so our actions are not checked: we hurl full force into the action dictated by our angry feelings and thoughts. Another feature of schema modes is that they can shift rapidly. Angry child mode is often preceded by vulnerable child mode, but we may first become aware of the angry child mode. Furthermore, child modes can often elicit parent modes: since schemas are internalized representations of the parent–child relationship, every child schema mode includes a parental mode as well. Going back to the example with my daughter, after "losing it" with her (angry child mode) I shifted into punitive parent mode: I yelled at her, threatened to punish her, and threatened that her teeth would all fall out! When my daughter jumps off the bike and allows us to have time separate from each other, I follow my breath and start to calm down. I think about my child's suffering (nobody likes going to the dentist, particularly not when it ends with the parent having an outburst), her brave behavior, her willingness to do better, and our ruptured connection. I also feel compassion for myself, for having tried so hard to take care of things and having failed in some ways. I have shifted from the angry child and punitive parent mode to the healthy adult mode. When I calm down and soften, this leads immediately to my being able, for the first time in this interaction, to take perspective on the whole situation, see things from my daughter's perspective, remember my daughter's emotions, empathize with those emotions, and think about the experience from my daughter's point of view and from the point of view of our relationship together. When I arrive home, and see my daughter again, I am in healthy adult mode: looking at the situation from multiple perspectives, taking into account my own emotions and thoughts as well as my daughter's, and understanding the interaction in terms of our relationship history, our dentist history, as well as the wider context of our relationships with others.

HOW DOES MINDFULNESS HELP WITH SCHEMA MODES?

In Session 5, we use mindful awareness to become aware of the child and parent modes, labeling the modes, to create distance. We bring an attitude of acceptance to the child modes: it's okay for them to be there. We recognize the parent modes that may get activated under stress, which we have internalized from our own relationship with our parents. We relate to the child modes with kindness and compassion, allowing the child emotions to be there, comforting the child part, and reassuring the child part that the healthy adult part can care for the child. In essence, we are taking a self-compassion break, but we are directing our self-compassion at our most vulnerable, childlike part.

When parents are able to recognize their own schema modes, as well as what types of situations tend to trigger them, they can use this awareness to reduce their reactivity to their children in stressful parent–child interactions. Recognizing activation of child modes, they can pause to give themselves or their inner child compassion, instead of reacting automatically to their child. Recognizing activation of parent modes (punitive or demanding parent), they can pause, label the mode, and take a moment to decide whether they want to react to their child in this way.

GUIDELINES FOR SESSION 5

Box 9.1. Agenda Session 5

1. Sitting meditation including emotions (30 min) + inquiry (15 min)
2. Discuss home practice in pairs (20 min)
3. Reactive parenting and schema modes (50 min)
4. 3-min breathing space (5 min)
5. Break (15 min)
6. Walking meditation inside (15 min)
7. Holding your emotions (20 min)
8. Review home practice (10 min)

1. SITTING MEDITATION INCLUDING EMOTIONS

We invite the group for a sitting meditation focusing on the breath, body, sounds, and thoughts and add at the end the new element emotions (Box 9.2). As Martine Batchelor pointed out, we might feel uncomfortable if we notice no emotional state at all, a "neutral feeling tone" (p.c., March 2009). Particularly when parents come from a more emotionally intense place, such as when having had an emotionally intense youth, or an intense relationship, or an intense working environment or have a more intense personality, they may find it difficult to feel neural. We may avoid such a neutral feeling tone by looking for some excitement, positive or negative. For example, I often find myself, when in a neutral feeling tone, opening the mailbox, looking for exciting mail, like a nice invitation, a letter of acceptance of a paper, and exciting results from a new research project. More often I find something bringing me in a negative feeling tone, such as a rejection letter, disappointing or null results, or administrative tasks that I should be doing or should have done, but such a negative feeling tone is at least familiar, I feel so I'm alive! Allowing ourselves to spend more time resting in this neutral feeling tone can decrease our suffering.

Box 9.2. Sitting with Emotions

If you are ready for it, let go of the focus on thoughts . . . bringing awareness to emotions . . . noticing your emotions tone at this moment . . . the emotional tone can be somewhat negative . . . anxiety, irritation, a bit sad . . . more intensely negative . . . fear, anger, depressed . . . or somewhat positive . . . a bit excited, happy . . . or very positive . . . joyful, relieved, proud . . . but mostly, the feeling tone is neutral, not positive or negative. See if you can accept your present feeling tone, letting go of any attempt to change your emotional state, just noticing your emotional tone as it is in this moment and any changes in it from moment to moment.

You may find a neutral feeling tone a bit boring, or empty . . . but see if you can appreciate this neutral feeling tone, as a place to rest, a place to come home to, a nurturing state.

VOICES OF THE PARENTS

Eva, who has a very demanding management job, has an important deadline today. She decided to still go to the group, but during the sitting, thoughts are running through her mind constantly: "I don't have the time for this," "I'm too restless to meditate today," "Why is this practice taking so long," "When is this finished." While meditating, it was difficult for her to see her thoughts as just thoughts. The teacher asks her what the effect was of her thoughts on her body and mind. She answered that it made her more restless and unhappy, and that that made her perceive the time of the sitting as even longer. The teacher invited her to explore this "restless state" further, where could she feel it in the body? She described tension in her legs and arms, pressure in her head, a tendency to move. And what would she normally do when in such a restless state? She would walk back and forth, do things in a mindless or chaotic way, be impatient with her children or staff. And does this restless state help to get your work done more efficiently? No, she replied. How would it be to next time, when she recognizes this state "ah, restless state!," to sit with it for 5 or 10 min, observing in detail what is going on in her body and mind, without acting? And see what effect that would have on the efficiency of her work?

Jane came to the group because she had suffered from bipolar disorder, which had taken her away from taking care of her young son the first years of his life. She was struck by the experience of being okay with a neutral emotional state. She realized how she has not been used to being in neutral feeling tone, and how it used to make her feel uncomfortable, looking for anything to feel.

Mark reflected on his busy life as an architect working on competitions in a top firm. He said: "I'm almost addicted to working so hard, day and night, to make the dead-line and try to win the competition. I don't see my family for days at the final phase, but I feel highly excited, rushed, in control. After we've made it, it takes time to get used to feeling normal. It is as if I'm depressed, but I might simply be in this neutral feeling tone, which makes me feel not at ease. I avoid it by doing exciting things, such as rafting or climbing. Which means that I see my family also less than I would want to when I do have the time because the project is over." Mark plans to sit more often exploring his feeling tone, resting in a neutral feeling tone when it's there.

2. DISCUSSING HOME PRACTICE

In pairs (e.g., the .b pairs made last week), parents discuss their stressful parenting moments from the past week. Each participant reviews one stressful moment he/she recorded, preferably reading it aloud, and what effects a possible breathing space before, during, or afterwards had or could have had. The other participant practices mindful listening. Parents also share experiences in writing the short autobiography. There is no need to share the content of what they wrote down but the experience of writing about it, the experience of recognizing similarities or dissimi-larities in how they were raised and how they now raise their child, and how they felt afterwards, while doing a breathing space. Parents often like to exchange their experiences of practicing the 3-min breathing space with the .b sms. They may talk about how connected they felt to each other and how much easier it is to remind the other parent to do a breathing space by sending a .b (and then doing a 3-min breathing space) than reminding yourself to do one.

3. REACTIVE PARENTING AND SCHEMA MODES

We invite parents to notice automatic patterns or action tendencies in their interactions with their child and to investigate if they see similarities or connections with aspects of their relationship with their own parents. We ask parents to notice when their angry or vulnerable child modes are activated in interaction with their own children and when their punitive or demanding parent modes are activated. They are taught to label it, in the same way they have learned to label thoughts and feelings. "I'm in angry child mode" or "Punitive parent mode is here." Simply labeling the mode puts some distance between the experience and the parent, raising the possibility that the thoughts, feelings, and sensations the parent is experiencing may not be the "truth" and that he doesn't have to react to this experience. We also invite parents to notice when their punitive or demanding parent mode has been activated, either in relationship to their child or to themselves. In earlier sessions, we have asked parents to notice when they are being harsh and judgmental towards themselves. This judgmental "voice" can also be heard in the voice of the punitive or demanding parent. Labeling this voice as "punitive parent" is simply another way to help a person decenter from this voice, by seeing it as something separate from himself or herself.

The teacher announces that we are going to do an exercise to help become aware of and identify modes in parenting. First, the teacher writes on a flip chart or white board the three parental modes a parent may be in when interacting with the child:

1. Parent as self (or healthy adult)
2. Parent as child—for example, angry and vulnerable child mode
3. Parent as internalized parent—for example, demanding or punitive parent mode (see also Chapter 4 and Handout 9.2)

We explain that we think of ourselves as parents as being healthy adults, but that in emotionally challenging situation, we may shift into child and internalized parent modes. We may give a personal example based on our own parenting or partner experiences. We then write on a flipchart four columns:

	Reactive parenting		Child and internalized
Triggers	pattern	Background	parent modes

A group member is invited to describe a trigger (a typical parenting situation or behavior of the child—or partner—that causes stress) and asks what the parent's usual automatic reaction is. Make sure that a *dysfunctional* way of reacting gets identified. The third question concerns a possible background of this way of reacting, mostly from parent's own upbringing history in his or her own family of background, sometimes from the history with the child. In the fourth column, the parent searches to identify child or internalized parent modes. When a parent cannot come up with child or parent modes, group members can be invited to help with suggestions, as they may struggle with similar patterns. It is always the parent who decides whether he or she recognizes this suggestion or not, so the teacher only writes down the suggestions of group members when the person working recognizes the suggested mode. The exercise is led by the teacher in a light and curious way. We find that group members are very active in helping each other identify automatic ways of reacting and modes, as they often recognize themselves in other participants' reaction patterns (or in the opposite patterns) and modes.

VOICES OF THE PARENTS

Mary gives the following trigger example: The teacher talks to her about problems he has in class with her highly-gifted son (column 1). She recognizes that she panics on such occasions and that she has the tendency to react dependently: to rely on her husband for support (column 2). She remembers that her parents were very protective with her and solved things for her that she could have done herself as a child, being a single, highly intelligent but anxious temperament child (column 3). The child mode at work here is the vulnerable child (column 4). The healthy adult could help the vulnerable child by comforting her and saying that together they are capable of coping with difficulties.

Other parents in the group respond to Mary's pattern description with similar reaction patterns, or opposite ones, or different ones.

Karen, a foster mother, with two severely physically handicapped children, who is usually silent in the group, comes with the following pattern description. The trigger is that the house is a mess, and she is tired. Her automatic pattern of reacting is not asking for support from her husband or others, and working too hard. As a background of this pattern she recalls that she received little emotional support from her hard-working parents as a child, who expected her to function independently from a young age. She identifies an internalized parent mode: the demanding parent. The healthy adult could say to the demanding parent that she has done enough for today, that she is okay, and that she can rest now and ask her husband to help.

*Ann, recently divorced and mother of young twins who are in their "terrible threes"
adds the following pattern. Her trigger is that her children ask for things she does
not want to give them (e.g. sweets before dinner). She has the tendency to give in,
and then feel angry with them for making her give in. Asked about a possible background for her giving in, she mentions that she feels guilty towards the children
because she split up with their father, who suffers from addictions. As a child she
suffered from her parents' divorce. She identifies an angry child mode, her anger
about her parents divorcing, and her not being allowed to express that anger. The
healthy adult could tell her that she has the right to be angry about the divorce of
her parents, and feel compassion for herself that she had to go through this, just as
her children have the right to be angry about the divorce.*

Other mothers recognize the "giving in" and then feeling angry pattern.

*Judy says that she gives in to her adolescent daughter because she is afraid that they
would otherwise get so much into conflict that the daughter would not want to live
with her anymore and would go to live with the father. Kate "gives in" to her adolescent son who refuses to take his medication, because she is afraid to lose the
relationship.*

*Ted describes as a trigger his children crying while he is driving. He automatically
responds with ventilating his frustration. He sees a connection with his youth, his
father did not allow the children to cry, and would threaten: "I will give you something to cry about." He recognizes the mode of the punitive parent, his father pun-
ishing him for expressing emotions.*

*Jill's trigger is that her adolescent daughter is seeking autonomy and pushes her
away. Her first response is to block or freeze. She sees a relation with her parents not
really seeing her the way she was, and that she had to be independent from a young
age, solving things alone. She recognizes a vulnerable child mode, she felt vulnerable as a child as she did not get much support.*

*Maud's trigger is when her son is not performing well at school. She describes as her
a pattern a tendency to control him. The background Maud mentions is that as a
child, she changed schools often, and eventually did not finish, because of lack of
motivation. The mode she identifies is demanding parent, as her parents had high
expectations and were disappointed with her results.*

The sharing of automatic parenting patterns (or action tendencies),
recognizing similarities and differences, across parents of children of
very different age ranges, can be a nurturing experience.

The exercise can be ended with the question: Why are we doing this? Do we need to identify our reactive parenting patterns and schema modes in order to change them? Isn't it enough to simply recognize moments of stress and take a breathing space, in order to change our dysfunctional ways of parenting? Yes, that would be enough. Yes, if we would be able to recognize our stress moments and take a breathing space, even without insight in where our reactive patterns come from and what child or internalized parent modes are involved, we would create space, use the "high road" (our frontal brain), and be able to respond more wisely rather than react impulsively. But it is often hard to recognize our stress moments and respond with a breathing space, precisely because we find ourselves in a child mode or internalized parent mode, whereas it is our healthy adult mode that is able to recognize stress and take a breathing space. That is why recognizing the child and internalized parent modes can help to step back when under stress.

4. 3-MIN BREATHING SPACE

After an intense period of sharing such personal experiences and insights, in the spirit of mindfulness, we check in a moment using the breathing space.

5. BREAK

The group takes a short break.

6. WALKING MEDITATION INSIDE

Walking meditation is a deceptively simple practice. We walk, with full attention to the physical sensations of walking, with no other goal except to experience walking fully. Thus, we do not walk to arrive at a particular destination, and we don't need to hurry because we're not going anyplace. In a sense, walking meditation is a metaphor for being mindful in our lives, particularly as parents. We find ourselves on this path, yet the point is not where we are headed, or getting there. The point is, as Chodron (2000) says, "Bringing everything we encounter to the path. . . . The path is the goal." This sums up mindful walking—we are moving, we are on a path, but we attend to what we experience in each moment, each step, without regard for where we are going or where we have come from. "The path is uncharted. It comes into existence moment by moment and at the same time drops away behind us." As parents, we are always planning—planning our child's day, planning what to make for dinner, planning how we'll get our work done, and planning where our child will go to high school, then college. This is fine, and for practical reasons, we need to do all that. But walking meditation is an invitation to let go of our illusion of control and walk without plan, without purpose, and without goal.

What does it feel like to walk a step? What do I feel, literally, in the soles of my feet as I walk? In my legs, my back, my arms? Thich Nhat Hanh speaks the words, "I have arrived, I am home, in the here and in the now" in rhythm with his footsteps, as a reminder that where you are, right now, is the only place to be. For me, as a mother who is always rushing, always late for something, these words remind me to pay attention to where I am right now, in this moment, and that this is "home." When you take the goal out of walking, it's amazing what you see. Mindful walking can awaken the beginner's mind in you; you become alert to things which you normally pass by in your hurry to reach your destination. You may notice things which you have passed a thousand times, only this time you "see" them, really see them for the first time. This is especially true during walking meditation on outside, which we introduce in Session 6, when we find ourselves noticing small details of a flower, a blade of grass, a bud about to bloom, and the texture of a tree trunk. But walking meditation indoors can also open our beginner's mind, allowing us to see details in the room as if for the first time or experience the physical sensations of walking, as if for the first time. We may realize what a wonder it is indeed to be able to walk—what an achievement of coordination, balance, strength, and volition—all of which we do completely automatically, without thinking about it. When we walk mindfully, like a beginner, we are reminded of the child's first steps, full of wonder, and which required full attention to the act of walking. When I walk mindfully, I think of my mother, now paralyzed and unable to walk, and about what a wonder it is that I can walk, what a pleasure it is to simply will the body to walk and it does, and how lucky I am that my body can do this, with so little effort.

Mindful walking is also a useful practice for looking at our own impulsivity. When we meditate sitting down, there is a higher threshold for acting on our impulses, since we've committed ourselves to sitting down for a period of time. But when we are practicing walking meditation, an impulse to act may be more quickly translated to action, since we are already moving. Moving brings out our doing mode. For example, let's say I have the impulse to drink a cup of coffee. If I'm sitting, I would probably be able to inhibit that impulse and wait until the meditation is finished before getting up to get my coffee. But if I'm walking, I may find myself walking to the kitchen to make my coffee, before I've even realized I've made that decision. Another example is that participants report that when they do a walking meditation inside, they tend to pick up what's on the floor to clean up. So walking meditation is a practice which brings us closer to our everyday situation in the world, in which we may automatically follow our impulses rather than pausing to choose what is wisest. In walking meditation, we can practice letting our impulses rise up and becoming aware of them before acting on them in a way which is more challenging than sitting meditation (J. Teasdale, p.c., April 7–11, 2010).

In this session, we practice mindful walking inside (see Handout 9.4 for instructions). We begin by suggesting parents to walk more slowly than usual. This is just to help bring awareness to the act of walking. Later, parents can choose to experiment with walking more quickly or more slowly and how that affects their experience.

7. HOLDING YOUR EMOTIONS

We have been working with becoming aware of our child and parent modes this session. We now invite parents to bring an open, accepting and welcoming attitude to the angry or vulnerable child mode in themselves. This is the same as welcoming all emotions and letting them be there, as Rumi's poem *The Guest House* so beautifully illustrates (the poem can be found in Segal, Williams, & Teasdale, 2002). We start with holding your emotions as if it were your baby, by moving towards and embracing a strong emotion.

If parents feel comfortable, we invite them to literally welcome the angry or vulnerable child, by beginning a dialogue with him. This technique has been used in Young's (1994) schema therapy and also by noted meditation teacher Thich Nhat Hanh (2001). When parents are aware of the child modes, we then invite them to talk to them. After acknowledging the presence of the vulnerable child mode, the parent is invited to comfort the child. In this way, the healthy adult mode "talks" to the vulnerable child mode. This technique achieves the decentering which has been found to be so crucial to the mechanism for why mindfulness works for depressed individuals (Segal et al., 2002). The strong emotions, thoughts, and action tendencies of the angry child mode can be there, in this present moment, but they are held in awareness and held emotionally by our healthy adult mode, which can comfort the childlike part and which can remind us that this is just a transient experience which we don't have to act on.

The labeling also helps parents "talk back" to this voice or to replace the punitive parent voice with the healthy adult voice. The healthy adult voice can be kinder, more compassionate towards the person.

Nhat Hanh (2010) suggests the following dialogue when a person becomes aware of their inner child's deep emotions: "I see you and I am here for you. Your emotions are real, and I understand them. But we are grown up now, we are no longer a child. We can take care of ourselves. And the sun is shining, and the tea is delicious. Come take my hand and we will drink it together!" In this delicate balancing act, Thich Nhat Hanh illustrates how present moment awareness can hold the emotions from the past, compassion can comfort the child experiencing those emotions, and awareness can help make a bridge to bring the person into the present moment experience. There is no denial of the feelings nor does the person get lost in ruminating about the past. Past and present are held lightly, together, in the present moment.

Nhat Hanh also uses the metaphor of holding anger like your baby to deal with the angry child mode. He suggests: when you are angry, go to your baby. Your baby needs your attention. Just as a mother drops everything to attend to her crying baby, you too must attend to your baby (your anger). Hold your baby, comfort him, and take care of him. When we first read this, we felt it was a helpful practice, but didn't understand why it was helpful. Now we understand that Nhat Hanh's insight is that our strongest angry states usually are activations of child modes and that we need to respond with compassion to our child modes and that we need to respond with compassion to our child modes rather than responding with judgment or criticism.

Note to teachers: For some participants, this may become too intense. We suggest that parents choose a strong emotion but not too overwhelmingly strong. They are also free to focus on the specific body sensations if they want; this can lower the intensity of the emotion. You may want to read the practice of mindfulness of difficulties, described by Williams and Penham (2011) in *Mindfulness in a Frantic World*.

Box 9.3. Holding Your Emotions, Holding Your Inner Child

Sit comfortably and call to mind a recent experience where you felt strong emotions such as anger, sadness, fear, or other emotions. See if you can feel the emotions in your body, now. What sensations do you feel? If there are thoughts, noticing them. Just staying present with the emotions and noticing what you feel in your body. And now moving in closer to the emotions and body sensations. You don't need to try to fix it or solve it, or change the feeling in any way. Just see if you can be present with it. And now embracing this emotion—this anger, fear, sadness, etc.—as if it's your baby. Holding it gently and with compassion, attending to it, being there for it. Can you bring a little gentleness or kindness to yourself in this moment? And just holding the feeling for as long as you like.

If you become aware of a child mode, you can experiment with talking to it from your healthy adult mode. You can try giving your child mode a name such as "Little _____ or just talk to that part without a name. You can say, for example, "Little _____, I know you are there. I can feel you are very angry right now. It's okay for you to be here, and I'm here with you too. I'm here for you now. What do you need from me right now?" Or, if the vulnerable child mode has been activated, you can try giving comfort or compassion to that part of yourself. You can try using whatever words feel most comfortable to you.

8. REVIEW OF HOME PRACTICE

This week's mindful parenting practice (see Handout 9.1) concerns taking a 3-min breathing space when your child behaves in a way that is difficult for you. It is helpful to make a round and ask each parent to mention a behavior of the child that really annoys or triggers them, to use as a meditation bell for a 3-min breathing space the coming week. It should be something that happens regularly, such as child crying at night, child coming out of bed, child spilling food, adolescent throwing the jacket on the ground, eating with open mouth, being disrespectful, cursing, and siblings fighting. Parents are also invited to identify their schemas when under parenting stress, by filling in the record form, in a similar way as we did in the group today. The formal meditation practice is sitting meditation (including emotions) as well as walking meditation, on alternate days.

HANDOUT 9.1 Practice for the Week After Session 5

Reading

Read the handouts mindfully.

Mindful Parenting

Do a 3-min breathing space every time your child is behaving
_____ (your child's worst behavior being your meditation bell) and
if needed add extra self-compassion.
Fill in the parental stress calendar including identifying schemas (Handout 9.6).
Be aware of strong emotions during the week, which may signal your
angry or vulnerable child mode being activated or your critical or
demanding internalized parent mode. Try to hold them as if they were
your baby. Can you bring gentleness, kindness, and acceptance to yourself in this moment?

Formal Meditation

Sitting meditation including emotions, three times per week; see Handout 9.3. Walking meditation (inside), three times per week; see Handout
9.4.

HANDOUT 9.2 Reactive Parenting and Schema Modes

At the moment of giving birth to a child, is the mother separate from the child? You should study not only that you become a mother when your child is born, but also that you become a child.

                                    Dogen Zenji (edited by Tanahashi, 1985)

Our experiences being parented by our parents and others (teachers, caretakers) are re-experienced when we become parents ourselves to parent our children. Much of our knowledge and skills about parenting comes from our past parenting experiences. But we are not doomed to repeat the mistakes that our parents and caretakers have made with us (and of course, we will make new ones that we hope our children won't repeat when they become parents). However, when under stress, or when strong emotions are challenged in parent–child interactions, we tend to fall back on our earliest experiences: the way we have been raised. Schema modes refer to modes of thinking, feeling, and behaving in adults which reflect activation of child-like patterns. In these modes, the person can take on either the child role or the parent role, since what is internalized is the (perceived) relationship between parent and child. For example, a person may go into the angry or vulnerable child modes or the punitive or demanding parent mode.

The parent–child relationship appears to evoke such schema modes, especially in highly charged emotional interactions between parent and child. In these highly charged situations, parents' own early (maladaptive) schema modes may be triggered, out of their awareness. A parent may find himself or herself becoming enraged at his or her child, suggesting triggering of the angry child mode. Or a parent may feel rejected or powerless by a child's behavior, suggesting activation of the vulnerable child mode. In general, very strong emotional reactions or overreactions suggest the possibility of activation of early schemas. Early (internalized) parental schemas can also be activated in a parent's interaction with a child. For example, a parent may become overly harsh with a child (punitive parent mode) or may have unreasonably high expectations (demanding parent mode). In addition to the early child modes and parent modes (internalized based on the parent–child relational experiences), a parent has developed a healthy adult mode, which consists of wisdom about parenting, relationships, what works with this child, etc. In sum, three Parent modes are active when parenting: the self as parent (healthy adult), the self as child, and the self as internalized parent.

In emotionally charged parent–child situations, the modes can switch rapidly. For example, a mother may start in the healthy adult mode, but in the course of the interaction, she may feel provoked to

HANDOUT 9.2 Reactive Parenting and Schema Modes (continued)

anger by the child's behavior or words. This may trigger her angry child mode, so that instead of her anger being tempered by her healthy adult understanding of her child, she becomes enraged at her child. The angry child mode may then trigger her punitive parent mode, which she then directs at her child, becoming more harsh and punitive that she actually believes is appropriate for the situation. The child may react by becoming more angry and oppositional, saying things like "I hate you! You're the worst mother ever!" This may trigger the mother's vulnerable child mode, so that she feels hurt or abandoned by this statement, rather than her healthy adult mode understanding that her child is just expressing anger. Finally, the punitive parent mode may be reactivated but this time against the mother herself, as she berates herself "I really am a bad mother for yelling at my child like this; even she hates me!"

Notice when your angry or vulnerable child modes are activated in interaction with your child and your punitive or demanding parent modes. In general, when emotional reactions seem out of proportion to the situation, it's likely that the vulnerable or angry child has been activated. You may want to label it, in the same way you have learned to label thoughts and feelings. "Oh, I'm in angry child mode" or "Oh, there's my punitive parent mode." Simply labeling the mode puts some distance between the experience and you, raising the possibility that the thoughts, feelings, and sensations you are experiencing may not be the "truth" and that you don't have to react to this experience. This is similar to the decentering effect of watching thoughts or schema modes, noting that "thoughts are just thoughts" or "schema modes are just schema modes." Second, try to be open to the child mode, allowing it to be there, instead of pushing this part away, denying it, or criticizing it (with the punitive parent).

Many of us spend a lot of energy pushing away the child modes, and simply recognizing and allowing them to be there is a crucial step. When you are aware of the child mode, you can experiment with talking to it from your healthy adult mode. It may feel a little silly, but some parents have found this exercise helpful. You can try giving your child modes a name such as "Little _____" or just talk to that part without a name. You can say, for example, "Little _____, I know you are there. I can feel you are very angry (or afraid) right now. It's okay for you to be here and I'm here with you too. I'm here for you now. What do you need from me right now?" You can try giving comfort or compassion to your child mode.

Whether or not you talk to the child mode, when you recognize activation of parent or child modes, talking a 3-min breathing pause (or follow three breaths), is always the first step in not repeating old parenting. We have a choice!

HANDOUT 9.3 Sitting with Emotions

You can practice being with emotions either at the end of a formal sitting meditation on breath, body, sounds, and thoughts, and ending with a focus on emotions, or as a meditation on its own, starting with sitting, focusing on the breath, and then on emotions.

1. If you are ready for it, bringing awareness to emotions. Noticing your emotional tone at this very moment.
2. The emotional tone can be somewhat negative: you may notice a sense of anxiety, irritation, and a bit sad. Or it can be more intensely negative feelings of fear, anger, and sorrow. Or the emotional tone is somewhat positive: a bit excited and happy. Or very positive: joyful, relieved, and proud. But mostly, the feeling tone is neutral, not positive or negative.
3. See if you accept your present feeling tone, letting go of any attempt to change your emotional state, just noticing your emotional tone as it is in this moment, and any changes in it from moment to moment.
4. You may find a neutral feeling tone a bit boring, or empty. But see if you can appreciate this neutral feeling tone, as a place to rest, a place to come home to, and nurturing state.

HANDOUT 9.4 Holding Your Anger as If It Were Your Baby

Anger is like a howling baby, suffering and crying. The baby needs his mother to embrace him. You are the mother for your baby, your anger. The moment you begin to practice breathing mindfully in and out, you have the energy of a mother, to cradle and embrace the baby. Just embracing your anger, just breathing in and out, that is good enough. The baby will feel relief right away . . . embrace your anger with a lot of tenderness. Your anger is not your enemy, your anger is your baby.

Thich Nhat Hanh (2001), *Anger*

HANDOUT 9.5 Mindful Walking*

1. Find a place (indoors or outdoors) where you can walk back and forth in a lane, in a location that is protected enough so that you will not be preoccupied by a feeling that other people are watching you do something they (and even you at first) perceive as strange.

2. Stand at one end of your walking lane, with your feet parallel to each other, body width apart, and your knees "unlocked" so they can flex gently. Allow your arms to hang loosely by your sides of hold your hands loosely together in front of your body or behind it. Direct your gaze, softly, straight ahead.

3. Bring the focus of your awareness to the bottoms of your feet, getting a direct sense of the physical sensations of the contact of the feet with the ground and of the weight of your body transmitted through your legs and feet to the ground. You may find it helpful to flex your knees slightly a few times to get a clearer sense of the sensations in the feet and legs.

4. Allow the left heel to rise slowly from the ground, noticing the sensations in the calf muscles as you do so, and continue, allowing the whole of the left foot to lift gently as the weight is shifted entirely to the right leg. Bring awareness to the sensations in the left foot and leg as you carefully move it forward and allow the left heel to come in contact with the ground. A small, natural step is best. Allow the rest of the left foot to make contact with the ground, experiencing the weight of the body shifting forward onto the left leg and foot as the right heel comes off the ground.

5. With the weight fully transferred to the left leg, allow the rest of the right foot to lift and move it slowly forward, aware of the changing patterns of sensations in the foot and leg as you do so. Focus your attention on the right heel as it makes contact with the ground. Be aware of the weight now it shifted forward onto the whole of the right foot as it is placed gently on the ground and of the rising of the left heel again.

6. In this way, slowly move from one end of the walking lane to the other, aware in particular of the sensations in the bottom of the foot and the heel as they make contact with the ground and of the sensations in the muscles as each leg swings forward. You can also expand your awareness whenever you care to, if it seems appropriate, to include a sense of what the breath is doing in the various phases of the walking, when it is coming in and when it is going out, as well as the sensations of breathing. Your awareness can also include a sense

*From *The Mindful Way through Depression* by Williams, Teasdale, Segal, and Kabat-Zinn (2007), pp. 91–93. Copied with permission of Guilford Press.

HANDOUT 9.5 Mindful Walking (continued)

of the body as a whole walking and breathing, as well as the changing sensations in the feet and legs with each step.

7. When you come to the end of the lane, stop for a moment or two and just be aware of standing, then turn slowly around, aware of and appreciating the complex pattern of movements through which the body changes direction, then mindfully continue walking. You might also notice from time to time what the eyes are drinking in as your position changes and you receive whatever the view is that is in front of you.

8. Walk back and forth in this way, sustaining awareness as best you can of the full range of your experience of walking, moment by moment, including the sensations in the feet and legs, and of the contact of the feet with the ground. Keep your gaze directed softly ahead.

9. When you notice that the mind has wandered away from awareness of the experience of walking, gently escort the focus of attention back to whatever aspect of the walking you are attending to as your object of attention, using it as the anchor to bring your mind back to the body and to the walking. If the mind is very agitated, it is helpful to stop for a moment and just stand here, with feet a body width apart, in touch with the breath and the body as a whole standing, until both mind and body re-stabilize themselves. Then resume the mindful walking.

10. Continue to walk for 10–15 min or longer if you wish.

11. To begin with, walk at a pace that is slower than usual, to give yourself a better chance to be fully aware of the sensations of walking. Once you feel comfortable with walking slowly with awareness, you experiment with walking at faster speeds up to and beyond normal walking speed. If you are feeling particularly agitated, it may be helpful to begin walking fast, with awareness, and to slow down naturally as you settle.

12. Remember to take small steps in the walking. And you don't need to look at your feet. They know where they are. You can *feel* them.

As often as you can, bring the same kind of awareness that you are cultivating in walking meditation to your normal, everyday experiences of walking. Of course, if you are a runner, you can always bring a similar quality of attention to the step-by-step, moment-to-moment, breath-by-breath experience of running you have cultivated in the mindful walking.

HANDOUT 9.6 Parental Stress Calendar:
Schema Mode Recognition

Be aware of the activation of schema modes this week. In particular, see if you can notice vulnerable or angry child modes. Also see if you notice punitive or demanding parent modes. Try also to identify a pattern in your automatic reactions. If possible, take a breathing space at some point during the stressful event, or afterwards, or in anticipation of, and add self-compassion if needed. See what effect that has, if any. Write down your experiences at a later time using the table on the next page.

Describe the stressful situation	What is your automatic reaction pattern? Do you recognize a schema mode?	(Did you) take a breathing space or self-compassion?	(How) did that change the situation?
Example: My ex wants to have our daughter on her birthday, but she said she wants to be with me. I give in first to him, and then mail him about what she wants. He mails back that I set up our daughter against him but that she will be with me	Reaction: giving in too fast (to avoid fights) but then getting angry Modes: first vulnerable child, then healthy adult, then angry child	Not at the moment of giving in or of mailing him, but when I received his angry mail, I took a breathing space and gave myself compassion for having to deal with a difficult ex, extending to feeling compassion with all divorced parents who have to share their children on birthdays, with all children of divorced parents who cannot divide themselves in two	I could feel compassion for all of us and mailed him back to thank rather than responding with anger
My daughter asks if she can watch something on You Tube after dinner. I say no, but then she says, "But Daddy said I could." I say, "it's late and you've been really tired in the morning, I'd like you to get to bed early." My husband comes in and says, "I did say she could do it, it doesn't seem fair not to let her." I explain my reasoning, plus add that I don't want her to think she can get her father to approve of something after she's heard no from me. He gets angry, and in the end, I give in and say she can do it	Reaction: giving in, not taking a strong stand because I don't want my daughter and husband to be angry at me, but then I feel very angry Modes: Angry child—I felt furious Vulnerable child—I felt very impotent, like I had no power in the family and my child won't respect me Punitive parent—My daughter came downstairs and asked me something, and I bit her head off because I was so angry!	At the moment, no, because I was so angry. Later, when I was calmer, I took a self-compassion break, reminded myself of how difficult families can be, and forgave myself for lashing out at my child, reminding myself that other parents have lost their tempers. I gave compassion to my daughter for how she must have felt when I yelled at her, also for being a child who wants to have special privileges from her daddy, which all little girls would like! I gave compassion to my husband, who was not meaning to cause a fight but just wanted to connect with his daughter	After I was cooled down, it made me realize that my husband wasn't trying to undermine my authority and that he was just trying to spend some time with his daughter, that it was intended innocently

257

HANDOUT 9.7 Home Practice Record Form Week 5

Fill in the record form each time after you practice (mindful parenting, formal or informal meditation). Write down what comes up for you during the practice, so that we can discuss it in the next session.

Day/time	Practice (Yes/No)	Comments

HANDOUT 9.8 Notes Informal Practice
and Mindful Parenting Practice Week 5

You may want to use this sheet to make notes about your experiences during the informal meditation practice and the mindful parenting practice. Or to make notes during or about the group session.

CHAPTER 10

SESSION 6: CONFLICT AND PARENTING

"Life is stress, and so is evolution. . . . Fetuses must struggle with mothers who have lives of their own and might reproduce again; then the two must go through labor and delivery, the timing of which cannot be ideal for both. Parent-offspring conflict pervades this and later interactions; if the mother becomes pregnant again, the siblings are immediately in competition with each other. Siblicide in frogs, birds, and princes shows the extreme of this competition, as pedicide and abandonment show the extreme of parent-offspring competition."   Konner, 2010

I F YOU made a holiday card to send around this year, chances are you selected a photo of your children smiling and laughing or one of the whole family smiling, perhaps with arms around each other. Or perhaps you made a photo collection of your last holiday with images of smiling happy children and smiling happy parents.

But if our cards and collections were to reflect reality instead of fantasy, they would look a bit different. In addition to the lovely, happy, cooperative photos, we would also have to include pictures of family conflict: siblings fighting with each other, parents fighting with kids, parents fighting with each other, family members crying, and so on. In fact, family conflict is so ubiquitous that this second collection might be a more realistic portrayal of our family life than the first. Research has shown that siblings have a conflict on average once an hour, and on average, parents have a conflict with their adolescent child once a day (Feinberg, Solmeyer, & MacHale, 2012). And we only need to look at divorce rates to see that conflict between partners is the norm rather than the exception. In fact, from an evolutionary point of view, family conflict is ubiquitous since each member of the family often has divergent goals and needs which often conflict with those of other family members.

Yet somehow we persist in our fantasy that our home life should be smooth and conflict free. We become irritated when our children pick fights with each other, distressed when we argue with our partners, and upset when we fight with our children. We may feel guilty when we fight "in front of the children" or when we have a bad fight with one of our children.

When we get caught in a fantasy about ideal family life, we miss out on important opportunities for learning and growth in the family. Conflicts occur when people love each other, and conflicts are excellent opportunities for getting closer since issues can be resolved as a result of having a conflict. Siegel and Hartzell (2003) call this "rupture and repair." Conflicts are also good opportunities for parents to teach children important lessons about conflict: that conflicts can occur between people who love each other and that conflicts can be resolved. This last point is key, since more than two decades of research by Cummings (1994) and his group his demonstrated the deleterious effects of unresolved interparental conflict on children. While children respond with distress to any interparental conflict, when conflicts are resolved, children's distress levels return to their pre-conflict levels. Cummings suggests that children learn important cognitive, social, and interpersonal skills by observing parents resolve their conflicts. So the point is not to avoid conflict between parents or with children, but to learn how to have conflicts in nondestructive ways and to resolve conflicts. Mindfulness can help with both of these aspects. In earlier sessions, we invited parents to use mindfulness during "hot" or high-emotion situations which often involve a conflict with children or partners, to lessen reactive parenting. In Session 6, we address repairing the effects of conflict and resolving conflicts.

After a strong conflict in which family members may have "lost it" and reacted with anger, criticism, or yelling, or may have had their feelings hurt, it is important to go back and repair the relationship. After a conflict, a child may feel so angry or hurt that on an emotional level, he or she may experience a rupture in the parent–child bond. Siegel and Hartzell emphasize that this kind of rupture is completely normal and occurs in all parent–child relationships. However, they also note that parents rarely return to the child to discuss what happened and repair the emotional damage done to the relationship. As parents, we may feel guilty about our role and therefore hesitate to open Pandora's box and expose our mistakes. We might also fall into the trap of thinking that since it's over and done with, better to move on.

However, there is ample research on parent–child conflict to suggest the opposite: children and adolescents can often nurture old wounds, about unresolved conflicts, as well as harbor misrepresentations about the parents' motives or feelings. Children and adolescents are less likely to be able to approach parents in order to discuss painful conflicts, so their silence does not mean they are not upset or suffering (Diamond & Liddle, 1999). When parents are able to return to their child or adolescent to discuss what happened in an open, nonjudgmental and loving manner, the conflict can be transformative for the relationship as well as for the child. During adolescence, when teens are balancing their needs for autonomy and relatedness, resolving parent-child conflict constructively becomes even more important. Adolescents continue to need to be able to use the parent–youth attachment relationship as a "safe base" emotionally, that is, to be able to go back to parents when emotionally distressed. Unresolved parent-child conflict, either small "ruptures" or actual traumas, can disrupt the attachment relationship, leaving a child or adolescent on his or her own to deal with emotional difficulties. Repairing these ruptures or even more severe ruptures due to trauma or abandonment can reduce symptoms of depression and suicide in adolescents and can improve the parent–child relationship (Allen, Hauser, Bell, & O'Connor, 1994; Allen, Moore, Kuperminc, & Bell, 1998; Diamond & Siqueland, 1998; Diamond, Reis, Diamond, Siqueland, & Isaacs, 2002; Diamond et al., 2010).

Repair requires being able to understand the other person's feelings and desires, in other words, to see things from their perspective and to empathize with their feelings. Perspective taking requires the ability to understand a situation from the perspective of another person and the ability to imagine what other people think, feel, and want. It is a skill that children learn during development, in interaction with others. The parent–child interaction is very important in children's development of perspective taking. Parents who are able to see the world from the perspective of their child and are sensitive to their child's need facilitate their child's ability to place him or herself in other people's perspective and be sensitive to other people's needs (e.g., Duncan, Coatsworth, & Greenberg, 2009).

. But during intense conflict, it is difficult to see the perspective of the person we're in conflict with. This is something which is hardwired into our biological beings, so we don't have to feel so bad about it! When we perceive danger and are under stress, our *fight, flight, or freeze* system is activated via the fast route in the brain, with the accompanying *adrenaline* hormone being produced, allowing us to make a *fast* judgment and a fast response. This fast judgment makes it difficult for us to take the perspective of another person. Perspective taking takes time; is *slower*;

requires taking the longer brain route, involving the frontal brain; and is facilitated by the so-called attachment or affiliation hormones like *oxytocin*. Oxytocin is produced during breast feeding, love making, hugging, being comforted, and feeling connected and seems to help people empathize with and bond with others. Research shows that when animals lick each other, oxytocin is released. So while adrenaline makes us *turn away from* the other person, and rely on our own, fast, and often faulty or biased judgment, oxytocin makes us *turn towards* the other person, *opening up* to the perspective of the other person as well (Theodoridou et al., 2009).

To make it a bit more complex, based on evolutionary differences between men and women, females also have a different response under stress next to the fight-flight-freeze response: *tending* their children and *befriend* strangers (Taylor et al., 2000). As a result, mothers may, when in an intense conflict with their (ex)partner, turn towards their children to protect them, or respond with pleasing behavior towards an attacker, the latter simply because they don't have the physical strength to fight the attacker effectively.

To illustrate, I once got on a train on my way home after a long flight, with my money in a small backpack on my back. Suddenly I felt pulling on my backpack. When I turned, I saw a man with a knife trying to cut the handles of the bag. To my (later) surprise, I gave him a big smile. He smiled back, and he and his mates jumped out of the train. I still had my bag. I could not understand why I smiled at him and why I had not screamed, so that he and his mates could have been caught, until I read about this different evolutionary response in the face of danger in women.

Intense conflict with our children or partners can often trigger maladaptive childhood schemas or send us into angry or vulnerable child mode or punitive parent mode. We invite parents to notice which schema modes are triggered for them and whether they shift into child or parent schema modes. Noticing these modes can help parents to take some distance on the interaction or to decide to wait to come back to the interaction until they have had a time to sit with their strong emotions. They can use the 3-min breathing space and/or take a self-compassion break, or if a schema mode has been triggered, they can take a moment to recognize it and "talk" to their child mode.

Let's go back again to the example of the conflict with my daughter after the dentist, that was described in the introductions of Session 5 and 6. When my daughter jumped off the bike and walked home, she created a pause in the interaction, which helped me to become mindful of my bodily state of tension, my anger, fears, shame, and despair and all the thoughts that had run through my mind. Although still angry, my mindful awareness helped me realize that I was not yet ready to repair the relationship at that moment. Instead, I gave myself the time I needed to calm down. Once calm, I was able to see the situation from my daughter's point of view as well as my own. At this point, I was ready to go back to my daughter to "repair."

I came home and found her writing in her diary in her room. I invited her to sit down together on my bed and hugged her. I told her that I was very sorry about my outburst and that it was wrong what I said. She said that when I'm angry like that, she gets the feeling she is a bad child. I hugged her and expressed how much I love her. I told her how proud I was of her for undergoing the anesthesia and said that it must have been difficult for her to trust the dentist and get the injection. She nodded. She said that she was embarrassed about my scene as we were biking through the city. I agreed that it was embarrassing and promised her not to do that again. I said that she was right to shout at me to stop and that when I did not, was very wise to put her fingers in her ears and jump off of the bike when I was in that state, and that next time she could also tell me that my behavior is unacceptable. I explained to her that my outburst was related to my being worried about her teeth and to my being discouraged that all my attempts to make her brush better and more often had not produced the result I had hoped for. She said that she finds it difficult to remember to brush and that it is boring. We talked about how she could remember better to brush her teeth and we agreed that the idea of not receiving allowance when she had forgotten was a good one. She brainstormed about other solutions as well. I also told her about my embarrassment when she resists being treated at the dentist, and she smiled and said that next time she will behave braver, as she has now done it once. As we were both shocked from the difficult morning, I proposed to her that we would take the day off to rest.

As this example shows, it is important that the parent goes back to the child to reconnect. The primary goal of repair is to emotionally reconnect, not to teach your child a lesson, scold or set limits. The second point is that the parent starts the interaction by apologizing for her behavior. The parent takes full responsibility for her own actions and admits she was wrong. Only then does she attempt to discuss her two different perspectives. In this way, the child trusts that she won't be blamed and understands that her parent is open to hearing her perspective. Empathizing with the child's perspective makes the child feel emotionally understood, so that the child can allow the parent to comfort her. Finally, only at the end, when the emotional relationship has been repaired, the child's role in it is addressed too. At this point, the child is in a much better position to reflect on it, as she has felt understood and empathized with.

In Session 6, we invite parents to call to mind a recent conflict with their child, and through an imaginal exercise, we ask them to first focus on their own emotions, then on their child's. Mindfulness can help us create more space, so that we can take into account both our perspective and the perspective of our child. We also invite parents to try repairing a conflict with their child (or partner) during the following week.

GUIDELINES FOR SESSION 6

Box 10.1. Agenda Session 6

1. Sitting meditation, with choiceless awareness (20 minutes) + inquiry (15 minutes)
2. Review of home practice in pairs (10 minutes)
3. Group discussion of pattern and schema recognition home practice (20 minutes)
4. Walking meditation outside (25 minutes)
5. Break (15 minutes)
6. Perspective taking, repair (60 minutes)
7. Review home practice (10 minutes)
8. Read poem (5 minutes)

1. SITTING MEDITATION, WITH CHOICELESS AWARENESS

Meditating with no specific anchor, following the attention wherever it goes from moment to moment, is my favorite meditation, because of the free format and because it gives me the most insight into my condition at this moment. It can be very confronting when I find myself being restless, hurried, on edge, nervous, and exhausted, but when I allow myself to look at all that from a place of stillness, as Mark Williams (p.c., December 16, 2011) suggested, not wanting things to be different as they are right now, it brings me right in this moment, with some acceptance and clarity. On retreats of Martine Batchelor, I learned to use the "What is this?" question in this free-floating meditation, to help investigate any experience coming up with the beginner's mind. The poem of Asai Ryoi (translation by Lane, 1957), from about 1665, fits nicely with this meditation.

WHAT IS THE FLOATING WORD?

Living only for the moment, turning our attention to the pleasures of the moon, the cherry blossoms and the maples, singing songs, drinking wine, and diverting ourselves in just floating, floating, caring not a whit for the poverty staring us in the face, refusing to be disheartened, like a gourd floating along with the river current: this is what we call the floating world.

Box 10.2. Choiceless Awareness Meditation, What Is This?
(Inspired by M.Batchelor, p.c., January 27–31, 2011)

Settle into a sitting posture that reflects dignity, falling awake, presence. Taking your time to feel where the body touches the chair or cushion, anchoring yourself in this space, this moment. . . . Turning your attention to the breath for a few moments, following each breath going through your body as best as you can . . . this breath . . . and this one . . . every breath is a new opportunity to be fully present in this moment. . .

Then, when you are ready for it, let go of the focus on the breath . . . allowing your attention to just float, from moment to moment. It may go to physical sensations, thoughts, sound, emotions. See if you can follow your attention from a silent place behind it. . . . You can try to let this question drop from time to time: "What is this?" The "What is this?" question can help you investigate any experience with curiosity, open attention, beginner's mind. . . . "What is this?" . . . .

When you feel overwhelmed by the experiences, you can always go back to the breath or the body to re-anchor yourself in the present moment.

We continue with this free–floating awareness for about 10 minutes in silence.

INQUIRY

When asked how this meditation was for them, participants may talk about very different experiences, such as feeling chaotic as the attention was hopping around or feeling very serene when moments of nothingness were experienced. Whatever is coming up, welcome each experience, positive or negative, and bring parents' curiosity to the experience, asking about accompanying bodily feelings. We encourage acceptance of the "way things are," allowing things to be as they are right now, just noticing from a quieter space, without adding judgments and without trying to change them (Batchelor, 1997).

2. REVIEW OF HOME PRACTICE IN PAIRS

Parents share with each other their attempts at recognizing patterns of reacting under stress and doing a breathing space and see whether that gives new possibilities of responding. They also can share how using the worst behavior of your child as a your meditation bell to do a 3-min breathing space went, as well as the formal practice (sitting including emotions, walking meditation).

3. GROUP DISCUSSION OF HOME PRACTICE

In the entire group, we come back to questions about and experiences with pattern and schema mode recognition and about choices in ways of responding.

VOICES OF THE PARENTS

Mary had recorded in her diary a quarrel with her stepdaughter, in which she felt not seen and accused without reason. She could see her pattern from the past: the hurt child, who in response becomes an angry child, and a punitive parent. Mary saw that she said mean things to her stepdaughter after having taken a breathing space, she could come back to it from a different mind state.

Ted had told his son of 11 do his homework, which he refused. Ted became angry, and the conflict escalated, his son screaming at him, Ted about to hit his son, Ted was able to take a breathing space, and could recognize his pattern. He went to boarding school, where the teachers were quite harsh with the pupils. Ted included. He learned to be obedient, as otherwise he would receive physical punishment. Ted's fear that his son would be punished if he did not follow the rules, turned him into a punitive teacher! After the breathing space, Ted went to his son and offered to help him with his homework.

It is helpful to when parents realize that there are endless ways of responding, that we are not doomed to keep responding according to old patterns, and that meditation can help us recognize patterns and break the cycle of automatic responding. Children and partners can also help us to recognize stress and patterns. For example, my daughter had developed a little rhyme that she said in the morning when she saw me getting stressed because of running late for school. The rhyme was: "You not stressed, me not stressed, we work together, we get to school on time." She also once made me a little bag as a present when I was stressed because I could not get the television to work, with the following words: "NO STRESS" and a heart.

Experiences with the other home practice (your child as your meditation bell, the formal practice of sitting with emotions and walking meditation may be discussed as well.

Sue took as her personal meditation bell her daughter's coming out of bed again after Sue had finally put all the children to bed, and "her" evening would start. This happened almost every evening, and several times per evening. Sue used to respond the first time warm and friendly, but when her daughter would come out of bed a second and third time, become more angry and frustrated with her daughter, and also anxious about how to finish her own work and how her daughter would feel next morning. Taking a breathing space every time her daughter came out of bed, changed Sue's pattern of reacting. She was less warm and friendly the first time (if only as she first had to meditate) and less angry at later times. She also became aware of how worried she was about her daughter's sleeping problems, and the consequences for her daughter's and her own functioning. Then she realized that she had exactly the same sleeping problems at that age, would read long hours in bed, and would still be able to function well at school. As a result, over the week Sue became more accepting of her daughter's sleeping difficulties, and allowed her to read longer in her bed.

4. WALKING MEDITATION OUTSIDE

The walking meditation fits with the theme of today of rupture and repair, that is, after an intense conflict, one choice would be to take a long, mindful walk, or do a longer sitting, or even take a few days if needed, before coming back to the conflict. Walking meditations in nature, because of the strong sensory input, are for some the best way to step out of the repetitive angry thoughts that accompany conflicts and hinder conflict resolution. We first introduce the walking meditation outside (Box 10.3).

Box 10.3. Introduction Walking Meditation Outside

Last week, we practiced walking meditation inside. Today, we are going to practice the same but outside. Set out a path for yourself; it can be a circle, or a path going back and forth, or a longer walk that can be done in 10 min. The whole point of the walk is that there is no goal, no place to be reached. Simply experiencing, as best as you can, the sensation of walking, outside. You may want to start with paying attention to the movement of walking, step by step, as we did last week. This is helpful as all the sensory input can be a bit overwhelming: seeing, hearing, smelling, and feeling, outside. After paying attention to the movement of walking in the body, you may want to gradually shift your attention to other aspects of the walking: the sensation of the different surfaces on which you walk and the sensation of wind, humidity, temperature differences on parts of your body, the smells, seeing, and hearing.

Some participants may feel embarrassed to do a walking meditation outside. Give anybody the permission to do the walking meditation inside if they prefer that.

Before or after the walking meditation, you may want to read this poem of Emily Dickinson, from about 1864, copied with permission from Bartleby.com

I stepped from plank to plank
I stepped from plank to plank
So slow and cautiously;
The stars about my head I felt,
About my feet the sea.
I knew not but the next
Would be my final inch,--
This gave me that precarious gait
Some call experience.

5. BREAK

Take a short break.

6. PERSPECTIVE TAKING, REPAIR

The practice is introduced shortly, saying that intense conflicts, called ruptures, happen regularly when people love each other and live together such as in families and that the following practice focuses on exploring ways to resolve them.

Box 10.4. Imagination Exercise Rupture and Repair
                    (Inspired by Siegel & Hartzell, 2003)

Take a comfortable sitting position and pay attention to how the body feels in this position and where the body makes contact with the chair, cushion, and ground. Let a situation in which you were very angry with your child (or (ex) partner, or other intimate person) and in which you were not happy about your own behavior, for example, because you exploded or felt out of control, come to the surface. Imagine the conflict as vividly as you can, as if it is happening right now. Who were you with? What were you doing/saying? What were are other person(s) doing saying? What were you feeling? What did you notice in your body? What thoughts ran through your mind? What action tendencies did you feel?

When you have a vivid image of the conflict situation shift your attention to the here and now, what bodily sensations, feelings, and thoughts do you become aware of, right now? Can you be compassionate towards yourself? Say to yourself, whatever I feel, it is okay, let me feel it . . . welcoming any emotion coming up, whether it is fear, sadness, anger, pain . . .

Then, bringing your attention to your breath, the movement of the breath in your body . . . following three breaths with full awareness . . . widening the attention to your body as a whole, in this sitting position . . . aware of any tension . . .

And then, when you are ready for it, on the next outbreath, shift your attention as best as you can to your child (or partner, or other person,) how is the other person feeling, what emotions may the other person experience, what bodily sensations . . . thoughts . . . action tendencies . . . desires . . .? Can you not only allow yourself to feel what you are feeling . . . but also allow the other person to feel what he or she is feeling . . . can you allow him or her to feel angry . . . sad . . . hurt . . . or afraid . . . can you tell him or her, whatever it is he or she is feeling, it is okay . . .?

Can you understand the other person from his or her perspective? Can you feel compassion for the state the other person is in now?

What would you want to say to the other person from this understanding and compassion? Could you let go of your pride and—really from yourself—apologize for what you did wrong? Because, if you cannot do it, how can your child (or other person) do it?

Apologize in your imagination, and become aware how this is for you . . . and for the other person.

INQUIRY

Participants may share their surprise that, after having paid attention to their own anger, they could suddenly see the perspective of the other person much clearer. This may go together with guilt feelings about the outburst and negative judgments ("I'm a bad parent"). In such cases, the teacher can ask whether the parent could see this negative self–thoughts as thoughts and briefly explore what effect the negative thoughts had, that is, whether the participant noticed any changes in the body while feeling guilty, how it affected the mood state of the participant (usually negative), and the attention for the other person (usually negative). The teacher also asks whether the participant could let go of the thought or mind state and redirect attention to the other person's perspective, moving from guilt back to compassion. Participants may also be so angry that the shift in perspective did not occur. This is fine; in very intense emotional states, it may be enough to keep repeating the message: it is okay, let me feel it, holding the anger as if it is your baby. Taking care of yourself is very important when you are in a state of extreme anger.

After or during the inquiry of the perspective taking and repair practice, the teacher can put the experiences of the participants in a broader perspective of how conflicts are great opportunities for growth in the relationship, on the importance of solving conflicts between partners and with children, for the sake of the children and on the role of hormones in perspective taking. The teacher may want to put the two hormone systems on a white board with the accompanying cognitive and behavioral skills (see Introduction and Handout 10.2).

VOICES OF THE PARENTS

Jill went to pick up her son from scouting, and was in a hurry as she left her other child home. He was playing happily and did not listen when she told him to put on his shoes and jacket. She got angry, remembering all the times where she had to chase him to go home. When she placed herself in his position, she could see why he went on playing, and ignored the stressed and angry mother. In her imagination she could repair it by hugging him.

Irene described a severe conflict with her adolescent son about the time of coming home at night. She had been sending him text messages in the middle of the night, unable to sleep, and screamed at him when he finally came home. While paying attention to her own bodily sensations and emotions, she realized that she was not only worried, but also angry because she felt ignored by her son, and sad because she felt she was losing the relationship with him. When paying attention to his bodily signals and emotions, she could see him trembling (voice, hands) and could suddenly see his point of view: that she did not trust him and his choice of friends. Being able to see and hold all these emotions of herself and her son at the same time, helped her to feel the relationship between them: her son's trembling as a sign that he cares about what she thinks. From this understanding of her son's perspective, she could say in imagination to him that she does trust him, and that she was sorry for her screaming. Holding all these emotions also made her realize that rather than sending text messages in the middle of the night in an attempt to control the situation and her emotions, she could next time simply sit with whatever would come up if her son was out and she was awake. She smiled realizing now how many of those moments are yet to come.

Judy imagined a conflict situation with her partner. She had bought presents that the children could give her for her birthday, as her partner would usually forget. Since her son has been diagnosed with autism, it has become clear that also her partner has autistic traits. When he discovered the presents he got angry, and she too, blaming him for all the years he forgot her birthday, calling him her extra child. Seeing it from his perspective she could understand that he felt ignored, and could feel his pain too, of not having been able to do the things for her that would make her happy. This made her cry. She imagined sitting down with him and explaining him how she wanted her birthday to look like, and asking him if he needed any help from her to make that happen.

7. REVIEW OF HOME PRACTICE

This week's home practice (Handout 10.1) consists of further imple-mentation of the breathing space in difficult family interactions, by taking a breathing space and trying out the rupture and repair suggestions, and by asking your partner and child to remind you to take a breathing space when they feel you need one. Also, we ask parents to be aware of strong emotions during the week, trying to hold them as if they were your baby, while bringing gentleness, kindness, and acceptance to themselves (their vulnerable or angry child mode). To help parents prepare to establish their own daily meditation program for the following week. We also ask them to organize a mindfulness day at home or follow a mindfulness day between Sessions 6 and 7 at the institute.

8. READING A POEM: AUTOBIOGRAPHY IN FIVE CHAPTERS

You may want to read the poem of Portia Nelson (1977), called "Autobiography in five short chapters" to remind participants of the fact that changing patterns may take a lifetime and that we will fall back into them time and again but at the same time will slowly start to recog-nize our falling, and by recognizing that, we will eventually change our behavior.

HANDOUT 10.1 Practice for the Week After Session 6

Reading

Read the handouts attentively.

Mindful Parenting

If a conflict arises between you and your child, or you and your partner, or a conflict with another person, take a breathing space and try out the rupture and repair suggestions (Handout 10.3).

Ask you partner and child to remind you to take a breathing space when they feel you need one.

Formal Meditation

Make your own meditation program based on the meditations you have practiced during this course, of about 40 min a day. Make notes in your journal. Try also to practice without audio recording at least once. You may also want to try the choiceless awareness meditation once. Choiceless awareness meditation is not so easy, and therefore, it may be wise to do it for relatively short periods.

Organize your own mindfulness (half or whole) day at home (Handout 10.4). Alternatively, the institute where you follow this training may offer a silent (half or whole) day between Session 6 and 7. In that case, save your own mindfulness day for the next week.

HANDOUT 10.2 Stress and Perspective Taking

Perspective taking involves the ability to understand a situation from the perspective of another person and the ability to imagine what other people think, feel, and want. It is a skill that children learn during development, interaction with others. The parent–child interaction is enormously important in children's development of perspective taking. Parents who are able to see the world from the perspective of their child and are sensitive to their child's needs, facilitate their children's ability to place themselves in others people's perspective and be sensitive to other people's needs. One of the earliest forms of perspective taking that has been studied by developmental psychologists is called "joint attention," a process in which the baby points at an object that the parent is not yet seeing while looking at the parent, in order to draw the parent's attention. Then, they share the vision of the object; they both have the same perspective.

Stress enables us to take a fast route in the brain and use our fight-flight-freeze system, which is important in situations of real danger. Stress, however, negatively affects our ability for perspective taking. When the stress system becomes active, hormones such as adrenaline are released, and people rely on their own (fast) judgment and are not able to see other people's perspective. Adrenaline rushes can be sensed when almost falling from the stairs but also during a fight: watch how your heart beats and breathing pattern changes when you are having a fight with your partner! Hormones such as oxytocin, that help us to empathize with others and trust others, are released when people hug or caress each other, when breast feeding, and also during meditation. So when we are in a fight with our child, but also when we are under stress because our child is late for school, we have a diminished perspective-taking capacity. At such moments, we will probably not be able to understand our child, and we may not even be able to see or hear our child clearly. The more stressed we are, the less we can see our child's perspective.

Taking a breathing space in the middle of a stressful interaction, going for a mindful walk, meditation, taking a self-compassion break, or sitting with our child on our lap are all helpful ways to step out of our stress system and into our attachment system, to change our hormonal balance and be able to have a wider view of the interaction, and each person's perspective.

HANDOUT 10.3 Rupture and Repair

Conflict is a part of all close relationships and will invariably occur at times in our interactions with our children (and partners), especially when there is stress. These conflicts can sometimes feel like small "ruptures" in the relationship. However, it is useful to remember that *conflicts are important opportunities for learning and growth in the relationship between parent and child.* When you feel a conflict with your child arising, the first step is always: breathe. Take a breathing space, however small. Notice what happens in your body, and say to yourself, "it's okay, let me feel it." Even if the conflict has already escalated, you can stay in the moment and slow down your further reactions by simply staying with your breathing.

It is important to remember that after a rupture occurs, *we can always repair it.* You may need to take time to prepare yourself, by taking a breathing space or a sitting meditation. Take the time to feel the conflict situation again. See if you can go back to what happened between you and your child. Can you see what your role was in it? What patterns do you recognize from your child. Can you see what your role was in it? What patterns do you recognize from your own relationship with your parents or from the history you and your child have built up together? We tend to fall into conditioned reaction patterns with the people whom we are closed to—children and partners. Can you understand what made your child so angry? Can you let go of your pride? Can you go back to your child with an open and compassionate heart?

It's important to wait to come back to your child until you are emotionally ready for it, when your anger has subsided, and you are able to look at your own role in the conflict. If taking a breathing space is not enough, you can try doing a walking meditation or a longer sitting meditation.

When you're ready, come back to the rupture with a "repair conversation." See if you can create a feeling of spaciousness large enough to hold your own and your child's experiences and an attitude of compassion and forgiveness for yourself and your child. See if you can find the space in your heart to accept what you may have done in this conflict, to forgive yourself for it, and to acknowledge it to your child. This is a wonderful way to model for your children how to make responsibility for their own role in a conflict. On an emotional level, you are teaching your child that conflicts are solvable and can even lead to feeling closer to each other once they are resolved.

HANDOUT 10.4 Mindfulness Day at Home

Being mindful for a full day, as best as you can, in the midst of your family, is a practice that helps you to generalize the learned mindfulness practices and skills to daily life. It is also a nurturing practice that may have surprising effect on you and your family. Choose a day in which you are around your family, but can be without obligations or appointments, for example, a Saturday or a Sunday. Explain your partner that you are going to have a mindfulness day, and describe briefly how you are planning this day and what you need from your partner and the family.

On your mindfulness day, detach yourself from external input such as television, music from recorded sources (playing music yourself or listening to music of family members is okay), newspaper, e-mail, Internet, phone, and mail. Make sure that there is no computer, TV, or music on, or phones. Avoid also reading and the work that you usually do in your office.

Do whatever you are doing mindfully. When you are doing housework, or other chores, do it like a monk, fully dedicated to the chores (washing dishes, peeling potatoes) without rushing to reach a goal, to have it finished. The work you have decided to do on your mindfulness day, you fully commit yourself to, without asking yourself why some other family member is not doing it.

Make a program for the day, that consists of periods of meditation and yoga, mindful eating and drinking, work meditation (non-stressful, repetitive work such as cleaning, gardening, ironing), and doing mindful activities with the kids or being mindfully with the kids and with the partner. For example:

7:00 AM Morning sitting meditation.
7:45 AM Making breakfast mindfully
8:00 AM Drinking a cup of tea mindfully before waking up the other family members.
8:15 AM Waking up family members mindfully (take a moment to watch how they sleep before waking them up).
8:30 AM Mindful eating of breakfast, mindful speaking, and mindful listening, during breakfast.
9:30 AM Going for a 1 hour hike, alone, or with any family member that chooses to join you; in that case, practice mindful speaking and listening and also periods of silence during the walk.
10:30 AM Mindful playing, being, or talking with children.
11:00 AM Mindful working in the garden.
12:30 PM Mindful coffee drinking.

12:45 PM Preparing lunch mindfully.

HANDOUT 10.4 Mindfulness Day at Home (continued)

1:15 PM Mindful lunch.
2:15 PM Sleeping or resting.
3:00 PM Mindful playing, being, or talking with the kids.
3:30 PM Mindful yoga or some other physical activity that feels good for the body, for example, swimming.
4:15 PM Mindful reading of a spiritual book or mindful drawing, etc.
5:30 PM Prepare dinner mindfully, and give family members mindfully task that you want them to do around dinner.
6:30 PM Dinner, eat mindfully, speak mindfully, and listen mindfully.
8:00 PM Mindful walking, or mindful reading, or playing a game with the family.
9:00 PM Bringing the children to bed mindfully (or asking your partner to do that).
9:30 PM Meditation.
10:15 PM To bed.

HANDOUT 10.5 Home Practice Record Form Week 6

Fill in the record form each time after you practice (mindful parenting, formal or informal meditation). Write down what comes up for you during the practice, so that we can discuss it in the next session.

Day/time	Practice (Yes/No)	Comments

HANDOUT 10.6 Notes Informal Practice and
Mindful Parenting Practice Week 6

You may want to use this sheet to make notes about your experiences during the informal meditation practice and the mindful parenting practice. Or to make notes during or about the group session.

CHAPTER 11

SESSION 7: LOVE AND LIMITS: CULTIVATING COMPASSION AND SETTING LIMITS

Even poor or suffering people raise their children with deep love. Their hearts cannot be understood by others. This can be known only when you become a father or a mother. They do not care whether they themselves are poor or rich; their only concern is that their children will grow up. They pay no attention to whether they themselves are cold or hot, but cover their children to protect them from the cold or shield them from the hot sun. This is extreme kindness. Only those who have aroused this mind can know it, and only those who practice this mind can understand it.

Dogen Zenji (edited by Tanahashi, 1995)

D O YOU recall how you felt the first time you laid eyes on your newborn baby? Or how you feel gazing at your child as he lies sleeping? This is the mind of loving-kindness: wide open, boundless love and kindness. As parents, we are already intimately familiar with the mind of loving-kindness. With mindfulness, we learn to *practice* this mind.

Buddhist psychology teaches that we can cultivate compassion and love for ourselves, our children, and others by intentionally practicing kind and compassionate mind states. When we practice the mind of kindness, we cultivate a kinder mind; when we practice the mind of anger, we cultivate an angry mind. Whichever type of mind we choose to practice will determine the kind of mind we experience, which will in turn determine the kind of actions we undertake. Nhat Hanh (2009) uses the metaphor of "watering the flowers": We all have seeds of love and compassion within us, as well as seeds of hatred and anger. The more we water the seeds of love and compassion, the more love and compassion we cultivate for ourselves and for others.

There is a wonderful Native American folk legend which illustrates this simply. An old man wishes to teach his grandson his wisdom. He says: "Grandson, I feel like I have two wolves fighting inside of me—an angry wolf and a peaceful wolf." The grandson asks, "Which one will win, grandfather?" The grandfather replies, "The one I feed."

Practicing the mind of kindness is an antidote to the mind of anger, hurt, fear, and judgment. It's not that we want to get rid of negative emotional states. On the contrary, mindfulness helps us to tolerate different emotional states without rejecting, avoiding, or denying them. But when those difficult emotions arise in a mind which has practiced kindness, their effect is diluted. When we cultivate a mind of love and compassion, we cultivate a larger, more open, and spacious mind. Such a mind can more easily hold our negative states with love and kindness.

There is now evidence from current psychological research to support these ideas (Neff, 2011). For example, in contrast to the idea that venting angry feelings helps diminish them, expressing and thinking about anger has been shown to increase angry feelings. On the other hand, practicing self-compassion has been found to increase compassion for others.

Kindness is at the very heart of mindfulness; indeed, we could say that kindness *is* the heart of mindfulness. That is, the underlying attitude of mindfulness is open-hearted kindness, compassion, and love for oneself and for others. From the first class, we embody this attitude, and we invite participants to do the same. Interestingly, William Kuyken and his colleagues (2010) recently found that mindfulness training (MBCT) increased participants' self-compassion, even when no specific practices to develop compassion or kindness were taught.

There are also specific practices within the various mindfulness traditions which have been developed to cultivate kindness, compassion, and love. These practices are generally referred to as "loving-kindness" and compassion practices. We have found it useful to introduce these specific practices in the context of mindful parenting. The Buddha often used the metaphor of a mother's love for her only child to describe the basic attitude of mindfulness; within the Christian tradition, the Madonna and child is perhaps the most powerful image of love and compassion. While Mindful Parenting is a secular program, we feel it is helpful to acknowledge that the love of a parent for a child is universally seen as profoundly powerful. From an evolutionary perspective, we have seen how the mother-child bond probably led to the evolution of compassion, making us understand why this relationship has come to symbolize the deepest expression of love in many cultures. We want to highlight this for parents, especially parents who are struggling with their own difficulties or their children's difficulties. It is a simple reminder to parents: *You already have what it takes to be a loving parent, no matter what the difficulties are.*

We have found that many parents seem to benefit from the practice of loving-kindness meditation. Parents report a kind of softening towards themselves, as well as towards their children, when they practice loving-kindness meditation. Loving-kindness practice also helps parents get in touch with their own *lack* of compassion for themselves. For example, when we teach loving-kindness meditation, some parents easily experience loving feelings for their child but have difficulty experiencing love for themselves. For some parents, loving-kindness practice elicits painful feelings of what they have missed from their own parents. Getting in touch with these painful feelings can be an important step towards healing themselves.

Loving-kindness practice is powerful because it capitalizes on parents' inherent capacity to love as a means to intentionally cultivate love and compassion for themselves and their children. Many of the parents in our groups suffer from shamed-based disorders such as depression and anxiety, feel inadequate as parents due to their children's difficulties, or have had difficult or traumatic backgrounds. Yet no matter how stressed, frustrated, or inadequate they may feel at times, how difficult the relationship with their child, or how traumatic a past they had, they have all experienced at one moment or another the intense, boundless love for their child. It is common for parents to describe this by saying "Until I had a child, I never knew I could love someone this much." It doesn't matter that they don't feel that way all the time or that they may often feel strong negative emotions towards their children. When parents can connect with the largeness of their love for their children, they recognize their own inherent capacity to love, to care for their children, and ultimately to heal themselves.

MINDFULNESS: WISDOM AND COMPASSION

In Buddhist psychology, the word for mind (*chitta*) is best translated as "mind and heart." Mindfulness is better understood as "mind- and heart-fulness" (J. Teasdale and C. Feldman, p.c., April 7–11, 2010). In other words, mindfulness comprises both wisdom and compassion. We can think of mindfulness and compassion as two sides of the same coin, complementary to each other, and both essential. This was perhaps the essential insight of the Buddha: we cannot face reality as it is, with all its inherent dissatisfaction and suffering, without the solace of compassion (Batchelor, 2001; Germer, 2009). Mindfulness helps us become aware of what there is in the present moment, including painful sensations and emotions. Compassion helps us to deal with the pain of suffering—our own, or others—helping us to acknowledge rather than deny it, by bringing the balm of kindness and understanding to suffering. When we feel pain – physical pain or the pain of anxiety or depression or loss—we use mindfulness to bring present moment awareness to the experience, but we need compassion to hold the experience and comfort ourselves. Just as a mother comforts her baby in distress, just as a hand reaches down to caress an injured limb, just as a friend consoles us in a time of loss, we can comfort, console, and soothe ourselves in difficult times and through difficult emotions.

But many of us feel uncomfortable with the idea of comforting ourselves when we are struggling or feel that it is self-indulgent to deliberately bring an attitude of self-compassion to ourselves. In fact, many of us feel more comfortable being judgmental and self-critical of ourselves when we feel we have made a mistake or "failed" at parenting. However, compassion for ourselves is the basis of compassion for others: in order to be able to empathize with the suffering of others, we need to be able to empathize with our own suffering. Rather than leading to selfishness or self-absorption, true compassion for ourselves and others connects us with others in the most profound way (Batchelor, 2001; Neff, 2011). As parents, having self-compassion for our own suffering is important for us to be able to tune in to our child's suffering (Siegel & Hartzell, 2003).

WHAT IS COMPASSION?

Goetz, Keltner, and Simon-Thomas (2010) offer this definition of compassion: " . . . the feeling that arises when witnessing another's suffering and that motivates a subsequent desire to help." So, it is an emotional state we experience when we are aware of another's suffering, and most importantly, it motivates us to take action, to alleviate the suffering. Compassion can be differentiated from empathy, which is "the vicarious experience of another's emotions," and also empathic distress, which occurs when we become distressed by the suffering of another. In order to feel true compassion, we have to understand that we are separate from the one who is suffering and that his misfortune is not our own. When we don't understand this distinction, we are likely to feel empathic distress—distress in the face of another's suffering—rather than true compassion. This is important, because research has shown that when we feel distressed, we respond in ways to diminish our distress, such as avoiding rather than helping. But when we feel compassion, we tend to approach others in order to alleviate their suffering. This differentiation helps explain "compassion contagion" which can occur in helpers such as therapists or rescue workers who experience empathic distress instead of compassion when they are unable to emotionally separate the experience of the sufferer from their own experience (Goetz et al., 2010).

Matthieu Ricard, a French monk who has volunteered to participate in many studies of meditation and compassion, describes how he was asked to empathize with the world's suffering, while his brain was being scanned. He described how by the end of the period, he felt in agony, as if he were personally suffering along with the people he was empathizing with. He was then asked to practice compassion. Immediately, he felt calm and relief, and he was able to practice the compassion meditation for a long time without experiencing any distress. This seems to be an excellent description of the phenomenology of compassion compared to empathic distress. This distinction is particularly relevant for parents, as we can sometimes lose sight of the fact that our children are not ourselves. Unfortunately, when this happens, we become empathically distressed—sad, anxious, scared, or mad—and our response is likely to be less effective or include avoidant rather than approach strategies. When we teach compassion practices to parents, we can help them understand this subtle, but crucial difference and help them recognize when their own emotional distress is being triggered by their child's suffering. When we recognize this, we can pause, look at it clearly, and let it go. We can remind ourselves, *This is her experience, not mine*; we can orient towards our child, see clearly what she is needing, and move towards her rather than away from her, as we consider what kind of compassionate action is needed.

This distinction has helped me tremendously as a parent. Picking up my children on the school yard has been a major trigger for social insecurities which I have not experienced since childhood. For example, when one of my kids would come out of school looking a little dejected, and I would notice other children making playdates and my child was not, I would start to feel very bad. Without realizing it, seeing my child looking dejected was triggering my own experiences of feeling dejected on the schoolyard, and I would slip into a feeling of empathic distress. Then the emotions related to my childhood social insecurities would get mixed up in my child's situation. The more distressed I would feel, the less I could actually attend to the real child in front of me, who was perhaps just a little tired and maybe not suffering the rejection I was imagining. Once I realized what was happening, I could recognize and even embrace this part of myself, give myself some compassion, and then deliberately orient myself to my child to see clearly what he was needing in that moment.

LOVING-KINDNESS OR METTA PRACTICE

"Loving-kindness" or metta is a specific practice to help cultivate the attitude of open, unconditional friendliness. With metta, we cultivate unconditional friendliness towards ourselves, towards loved ones and friends, towards people we find difficult, towards strangers, and finally, towards all living beings. Metta practice breeds spaciousness: we begin small, and we end up directing our loving-kindness out to infinity. Metta practice waters the seeds of compassion and kindness.

Although loving-kindness is mentioned in many discourses by the Buddha, the formal practice of loving-kindness meditation was established several centuries after the Buddha lived. The story goes that a group of monks were sent into the woods to meditate, but they returned, frightened. Their teacher sent them back to the woods with the loving-kindness practice to help them with their fear. This story reminds us that those monks, separated from us in time, space, culture, and lifestyle, also struggled with the same basic anxiety that we still struggle with today.

The essential purpose of loving-kindness meditation is to cultivate an attitude of openhearted friendliness towards all beings. As human beings, we tend to go around with all sorts of judgments and categories about who is lovable and not. We may find our children, loved ones, and friends inherently deserving of our love and compassion, whereas strangers, people who are different from us, or political opponents may seem less deserving of our love and compassion. People who are difficult for us may seem entirely undeserving of compassion and love, and we may feel justified in disliking or hating them.

It is exactly these arbitrary divisions that the practice of loving-kindness seeks to dissolve. The formal practice follows a standard structure of sending kind, compassionate, or loving intentions to several different categories of individuals: (1) oneself, (2) a cherished person or "mentor," (3) a friend, (4) a neutral person or stranger, (5) an "enemy" or difficult person, and (6) all living beings (Salzberg, 2006). The practice works precisely because it builds on our natural tendency to express love and compassion easily to those close to us and to have more difficulty expressing love and compassion to those at a distance or enemies. The emotional "break-through" in this practice comes when we suddenly feel that there is no difference in being compassionate towards our children than towards a stranger's child, towards a close friend, or towards our enemy himself. The depths of our hearts are such that we can feel compassion for all humans, indeed, all living beings, once we open to that. In these moments of compassion, the distinctions are truly dissolved.

Sending friendly wishes to neutral people and our enemies also helps with perspective taking and empathy, which we discussed in Session 6. It's easy to have empathy for people close to us but more difficult to have empathy with the difficult people in our lives, or for strangers, from whom we can expect nothing in return. Metta practice helps us take a wide perspective in which we recognize our kinship with all creatures, including people we normally categorize as "enemies" or as different from us. In metta we make a deliberate intention to be friendly, despite our other feelings or despite the lack of personal gain.

However, metta is not about pretending to feel friendly when you are angry or forcing yourself to feel friendly when you feel otherwise. Metta is about setting an *intention* for openhearted, unconditional friendliness, rather than about *feeling* friendly or loving. That is what makes it powerful, since while wishing your friend well is easy, it takes real commitment and practice to wish your enemy well! We cannot dictate how we feel; we can only set up the conditions which may open our mind to a friendly attitude. The goal of metta is not to feel a particular way but to incline the mind towards openhearted friendliness towards ourselves and others (M. Williams, p.c., December, 16, 2011). What's important is our intention to cultivate this attitude, on the one hand, and our intention to be mindful of what we are experiencing in the moment, whatever the feelings. There is a kind of paradox here: the goal of metta is not to increase our feelings of love and kindness; however, that may sometimes happen.

Sometimes, metta can lead to a different relationship to difficult people or "enemies." When we feel anger or hatred towards another person, we enlarge them in our minds. In fact, we invite them to take up residence in our mind, where they grow larger and scarier, increasing our suffering. Practicing metta can transform this relationship.

I recall an experience I had with loving-kindness meditation when I was first learning the practice. I was preparing for a meeting with a supervisor who was often critical. In the past, I had prepared for these meetings by making a list of all the things I had accomplished, in order to defend myself. This time, I decided to do a brief loving-kindness meditation. After recognizing my own anxiety and suffering and sending myself friendly wishes, I contemplated the suffering of my supervisor, first personally and then in terms of his interaction with me. I thought about how difficult it must have been for him to have this strained relationship with me and how he must have also been suffering, anticipating my angry reaction. The whole meditation couldn't have lasted more than 5 min. When I went into the meeting, I felt softened towards my supervisor, and I even noticed a maternal feeling towards him. He seemed more vulnerable than I had realized before. The result was that he shrunk down to normal size. In my fear, he had become larger than life, more powerful than he really was. With this focus on his suffering, he became just another human being, struggling to get through his day with some semblance of self-esteem still intact.

Traditionally, metta practice begins by wishing ourselves well. It was assumed that loving oneself was the easiest way to open the floodgates of compassion. However, in the West, we often encounter the reverse: many people express discomfort in wishing themselves well. There are accounts of depressed or traumatized individuals suffering from an upsurge of very strong negative feelings about themselves, *in reaction* to directing loving-kindness towards oneself, precisely because they do not feel worthy of love. Christopher Germer refers to this as "backdraft." In Western culture, an attitude of self-criticism may be considered normal and even necessary to accomplish life's goals, and many individuals suffer from feelings of worthlessness, shame, or doubt about their inherent lovability. In a well-known anecdote, Jon Kabat-Zinn recounts a meeting with the Dalai Lama in which a psychologist used the term "low self-esteem." The Dalai Lama struggled to understand what the term meant. When he understood it finally, he was saddened to realize that so many people in the West feel such self-loathing and inadequacy.

We have been greatly helped by Christopher Germer and Paul Gilbert's experiences in working gently and compassionately with these kinds of feeling states which can arise during loving-kindness practice: feelings of being unworthy, unlovable, or deep shame. As Paul Gilbert explains, loving-kindness practice opens us up to our deep attachment and affiliation needs. When these needs have not been fulfilled, or when there has been trauma, these feelings will come up: "For some people it starts a profound grief process because it opens them to the desire for connectedness and to feel loved" (Gilbert, June 23, 2012).

Christopher Germer likewise sees the negative feelings which come up for some people during loving-kindness as an essential part of the healing process: "When we give ourselves unconditional love, we discover the conditions under which we didn't receive much love as children. And then we repair that old relational pain with a compassionate response to ourselves simply *because* we're struggling. The main question of self-compassion training is 'What do I need?' especially when we experience backdraft, and then we learn to give ourselves what we truly need. Mindfulness says, 'Open to suffering with spacious awareness and it will change'. Self-compassion says, 'Give yourself kindness when you're suffering and it will change'" (C. Germer, p.c., June 1, 2012).

When participants feel unable to send themselves friendly wishes because of negative feelings about themselves, we sometimes invite them to get in touch with themselves as a child, at a moment when they were feeling vulnerable, as we described in Session 5. For example, we can invite a participant who feels undeserving of love to call to mind how she looked as a child and to talk to that child gently, asking her "What do you need from me now?" What's amazing about this practice is that very often out inner child will give us an answer, loud and clear. We often find that parents who insist they are not deserving of love soften and can feel love towards this childlike part of themselves, with little effort. In this way, we use our grown-up, healthy adult part of ourselves to comfort and heal the childlike part of ourselves who is still hurting. This is really just another way of giving kindness to ourselves when we are suffering.

We have also found it helpful to stress intention over feelings, as Mark Williams and Martine Batchelor recommend (M. Batchelor, p.c., March, 2009; M. Williams, p.c., December 16, 2011). This takes some of the pressure off when people don't feel friendly towards themselves or others. We emphasize the mindful awareness aspect of loving-kindness, by inviting participants to notice their reaction to the phrases and to be curious about whatever bubbles up. Mark Williams describes this approach as follows: "When you say the phrases, imagine you are dropping them into a well; then listen for whatever response comes back up" (M. Williams, p.c., December 16, 2011). When participants notice thoughts like "I don't deserve kindness" or feelings of sadness, we can invite them to be curious about this reaction, instead of identifying with it or assuming it is true.

We also warn parents that some people may feel uncomfortable sending loving-kindness to themselves, but we suggest that they try it anyway. In this way, we normalize any negative reactions. In cases where a parent feels strong love for their child, but feels undeserving of love themselves, we highlight this contradiction. When we invite these parents to begin the loving-kindness meditation with their child, this can sometimes open up a well of feeling in them which makes it possible to then direct friendly feelings to themselves. However, it's important to keep in mind that *whatever* feelings arise are okay, loving or not. We don't want to unintentionally convey the idea that we should always feel loving towards our children or that we should feel positive emotions when we do loving-kindness meditation.

ACCEPTANCE AND PARENTING

From the first session, we invite parents to bring an accepting and nonjudgmental stance towards themselves: acceptance of what there is, here and now, even if we don't like it. Acceptance is letting go of wanting things to be different than they are, either by avoiding pain or grasping at pleasure. It is also letting go of judgmental and critical thinking, letting go of categorizing things as good or bad, black, or white. Acceptance can start very small: just *being* with the grasping, the avoiding, the judging, and accepting these states of mind is enough.

Acceptance also means tolerating difficult body sensations, thoughts, and feelings. Christopher Germer describes acceptance as a kind of letting go of the aversion to painful emotions and learning to "befriend" rather than resist them. He describes a patient with anxiety symptoms who learned to say "Don't fight it" to himself when he noticed his anxiety symptoms, rather than criticizing himself. Similarly, Joy, a mother in one of our groups who had spent a long time pushing away feelings of anger and sadness, used to repeat "let me feel it" to herself as a way to open to those feelings rather than resist them. The goal for both these participants was to open to accept uncomfortable feelings rather than resist them (C. Germer, p.c., September 12–13, 2012).

In Mindful Parenting, we also emphasize tolerating and holding the strong emotions of our child and ourselves. Thich Nhat Hanh's (2001) lovely metaphor to "embrace anger as your baby" conveys this stance of being able to hold ourselves and our children, whatever the emotions, with compassion and acceptance.

In addition to accepting our emotions, we can also talk about accepting ourselves and our child. In their Mindful Parenting program, Duncan, Coatsworth, and Greenberg (2009) highlight the importance of nonjudgmental acceptance of self and child. Acceptance of ourselves and our children means nonjudgmental awareness of ourselves as we are, here and now, with all our imperfections, and of our children as they are, here and now, with all their imperfections. It doesn't mean that we have to *like* everything about ourselves or our children or even tolerate certain actions. As Jon and Myla Kabat-Zinn(1997) put it, "Acceptance is a door that, if we choose to open it, leads to seeing in new ways and finding new possibilities. . . . Viewing our children's difficult behaviors in a more non-judging, compassionate and open manner allows us to remain their ally and keep a heartfelt connection with them even when we don't like how they are acting."

Mindful acceptance is based upon seeing ourselves as we really are, free from our concepts about ourselves as being good or bad, success or failure. When we give up these inherently judgmental categories, we are able to see and acknowledge what is there in this particular moment, and we don't need to push it away to preserve our positive self-feeling or grasp at some idealized view of ourselves. The Buddha understood this when he taught that clinging to a fixed view of oneself was a cause of suffering. Once we become attached to a particular view of ourselves or our child, we are set up for inevitable disappointment and suffering when the reality doesn't fit this view. Attachment to a particular view of ourselves also prevent us from seeing things as they really are.

For example, when I became a mother, I vowed that I would be more emotionally expressive than my own parents had been. Without fully realizing it, I became quite attached to the idea of myself as a warm and loving mother. Certainly, I have my moments of being warm and loving. But sometimes my need to see myself as *only* warm and loving has made me blind to the times when my children have experienced me as distracted, not interested, or angry. Acknowledging these moments would mean that perhaps I wasn't the warm loving *Mother* I had vowed to be. Fortunately, my children are usually pretty good at letting me know how they are experiencing me, even if it doesn't fit my idealized version. In this way, our children can really help us, by holding up a mirror for us to see ourselves more clearly. Letting go of the need to see ourselves in a particular way opens up the space for us to see things from their perspective, to acknowledge it with compassion for ourselves and for our children, and to deal with it realistically. Not only can we learn and grow from this experience, but we also validate and accept our children's experience.

Accepting our children as they are is not always easy for us as parents. We all have fantasies of how special our baby is, how precocious our 2-year-old is, and how talented our 4-year-old is. This is probably one of the most natural impulses we have as parents, and it has some benefits (like making our 8-year-old stick with piano lessons as we imagine our little Beethoven playing at Carnegie Hall). But it has its downsides too. We may feel disappointed when our actual child doesn't live up to our imagined child. One afternoon a couple years ago, I was watching my son's swimming lesson. At one point, I looked over at him and saw he was swimming freestyle across the pool. The light was streaming into the hall, making the water sparkle with white light. In that moment, it was as if he were a part of the water itself, flowing seamlessly across the pool. I felt a sense of relief and ease. I had been feeling worried about him, but in that moment, I felt he would be fine. A moment later, however, I found myself imagining him as a champion swimmer, as I thought to myself, "Maybe we should sign him up for the swim team." My son had recently quit the soccer team after a frustrating year. To my surprise, I realized that I felt disappointed: I wanted him to be a good athlete. Somehow I turned my moment of enjoying him into a story about how I wanted him to be—a great swimmer—instead of just accepting the moment, and him, as it was.

In our Mindful Parenting groups, parents often struggle with intense feelings of disappointment that their child is different from other children, "not normal," or in some cases, may not be able to have the kind of life they had imagined. Parents also struggle with feelings of guilt ("What did I do wrong to cause this?"), anger ("How come I have such a difficult child?"), fear ("What will become of her?"), and hopelessness ("There's nothing I can do to help him"). Accepting our children, as they are, and accepting ourselves, as we are, are not always easy. Here we work with acceptance in its smallest form—just noticing the feeling of disappointment in your child, in yourself. Can you acknowledge the fantasy and remember that all parents dream of their infant's noble future? Can you notice the thoughts "I am a failure," "It's all my fault," "It's my partner's fault," and so on and allow them to be there without getting too attached to them or taking them too seriously. And after this, can you look at your child, really look at her before you, and notice what is there? And can you bring a little kindness, compassion, and forgiveness to yourself for those moments when you wish things were different?

LIMITS AND LIMIT SETTING

It may seem strange to find limit setting in the same session as acceptance and compassion. But we understand limit setting as something which grows out of acceptance and compassion. We view limit setting as a kind of ruthless compassion which is needed in raising a child: out of our strong love for our child comes our intention to set limits and weather the storms which can follow.

When parents are able to acknowledge and accept their present moment experience in their bodies and minds, they can also recognize their own limits, which is the first step in setting limits with children. We deliberately wait until the end of the course to address limit setting, because we want parents to have a solid foundation in their own mindfulness practice before approaching the challenging task of setting limits. We want parents to approach limit setting from the "inside-out" as Siegel and Hartzell put it, that is, from a connection with their own bodily and emotional limits which they have been getting to know during the various mindfulness practices. We also want them to be able to bring an attitude of kindness and self-compassion to themselves when they experience the inevitable difficulties with limit setting.

Many parents struggle with setting effective limits, particularly those we see in mental health settings, either because of the challenges of children with diagnoses such as ADHD, oppositional, or other developmental disorders; because of parents' own difficulties with depression, anxiety, inattention, or stress; because of circumstances such as marital difficulties, divorce, and single parenting; or because of past histories including trauma and harsh limit setting. In Mindful Parenting, we are interested in helping parents explore their own reactions to limit setting which may interfere with their ability to effectively set limits. Our approach is different from behavioral parent training, in which parents learn specific limit-setting techniques. We don't teach any specific discipline techniques. This kind of approach may be useful for parents who simply lack information about more effective parenting tactics. In our experience, many parents who have taken such courses know intellectually how to set limits, but they still have difficulty with setting limits. Many of the parents we see have difficulty setting limits due to their own emotional reactions to limit setting, sometimes due to their experience as children with their own parents. For these parents, parent training alone may not be sufficient, and Mindful Parenting is recommended. Furthermore, parents with their own emotional or behavioral difficulties, such as ADHD, tend to do more poorly in behavioral parent training courses (Sonuga-Barke, Daley, & Thompson, 2002). By bringing mindful awareness to the feelings, thoughts, and sensations that arise during limit-setting situations, parents can learn to slow down their automatic, impulsive reactions and understand their own experience better, including understanding the obstacles which make setting limits difficult for them.

And it's helpful to acknowledge that some children are more difficult to set limits on than others. Children with obsessive rituals may become extremely upset when told to stop. Other children may respond to limit setting by threatening violence, destroying things in the house, or with self-mutilation. Many parents feel intimidated by these reactions, and some have given up on setting limits. But even in these extreme-sounding examples, there may be more room for parents to set limits than they realize. Being mindfully aware of what happens during these difficult interactions can be a first step for parents to begin to look at this anew. We assume that parents first need to become aware of their own boundaries and limits, as they experience them in their body, in order to be effective in setting limits with their children. As parents become more aware of their own limits, they also become more accepting of them, and they learn to use this awareness as a kind of barometer. When we struggle to set limits, we often miss or ignore the cues that tell us that our child is crossing our boundaries, until they cross it in an extreme way. When we listen to our body, we notice these boundary violations earlier, and we can act earlier to help our child settle down, before he has gotten more out of control.

In addition, we have seen how we may automatically repeat patterns from our upbringing in our relationship with our child. Some of us may repeat the limit-setting pattern of our parents, consciously or unconsciously, while others of us actively reject our parents' form of limit setting. When we become aware of our reactions to limit setting, we can replace automatic responding with conscious choice, based upon their own values and beliefs. Finally, setting limits can evoke strong emotions in our children and ourselves, so the practice of tolerating and holding strong emotions in ourselves and our children helps prepare parents for limit setting.

We emphasize that limit setting with children has two essential functions: to structure the child and to enable parents to take care of themselves. We use the metaphor of the oxygen masks on airplanes which drop down in case of emergency: *Remember the wisdom of the airline stewardess: Put on your own oxygen mask first, before you put on your child's.* In order for our child to survive, we must survive; therefore, as parents, we need to protect ourselves and set limits on what we can and cannot do. For example, when we set a bedtime for our child, it helps structure him and give him the sleep he needs, and it also helps us to take care of our own needs, such as spending time with our partner, taking care of things, or just relaxing. When parents recognize and accept their own limits and boundaries, they can more clearly set boundaries for their children.

AWARENESS OF OUR OWN LIMITS

It is not uncommon for parents suffering from stress, burnout, depression, or anxiety to report that they have not paid enough attention to their own boundaries or limits, for example, by giving too much to friends or relatives, putting in too many extra hours at work, or allowing others to infringe on their boundaries. Often parents are not aware that their own personal boundaries are being crossed until it's too late—they have chronic pain or fatigue, psychological symptoms, or they need to take a leave of absence from work. Raising children and running a household are areas where it can be easy to ignore one's own limits and boundaries, since it may feel that "everything is high priority" when it comes to one's family and children. Mindfulness training helps parents become aware of the bodily and emotional signals arising when their personal boundary is being crossed.

During the initial practice of the body scan, parents may become aware of fatigue and bodily aches, which they may spontaneously connect to not taking good enough care of themselves, for example, by not sleeping enough, working too late, not taking enough time-out for themselves, or simply not paying attention to their bodies. This is a first step in recognizing that they have gone over their own limit. In the yoga practice introduced in Session 3, parents have begun to explore their own physical limits, approaching them, testing them out, and finding out what happens as they get closer or when they go over them.

This has a direct analogy in daily life, especially daily life with children. How often do we ignore our own bodies, push ourselves past our own limits, and automatically take care of children and chores without regard to our body's reactions? It's as if we say, "Not now, Body, I don't have time to listen to you because I've got to get dinner on the table, get the kids to bed, and finish the laundry. I'll listen to you later, I promise." Our bodies put up with this for a while, but eventually they may revolt and decide to go on strike, refusing to go on further.

When parents routinely neglect their own personal limits, it can have negative consequences for children. A typical pattern seen in ineffective or abusive parenting occurs when parents ignore their own reactions to small limits being crossed by their children. Eventually, as more limits are crossed, and more rules ignored, the child's behavior becomes increasingly disruptive, and parents may find themselves reacting suddenly with aggression towards the child. Ironically, often abusive behavior towards children begins with parents not recognizing their own limits, being too permissive, and setting the limit too late.

RECOGNIZING OUR HERITAGE FROM OUR PARENTS

Setting limits with children is also a good practice to help parents deal with unresolved issues leftover from their own childhood. Limit setting can be a highly charged interaction between parent and child; it involves saying "no" as well as the consequent emotions from the child and the parent. In stressful situations, parents are likely to automatically repeat old patterns of limit setting, often without being aware of it. At the same time, parents' unresolved feelings and reactions to how their parents set limits are also likely to get stirred up in stressful interactions with children. This can lead to contradictory behavior on the part of the parent. For example, a parent who experienced harsh limit setting as a child and who has not fully resolved her feelings about this may avoid limit setting, due to her identification with the child part of herself who still feels wounded. However, by avoiding limit setting, she may then be faced with more difficult behavior from her child. As her child's behavior escalates and her emotions run high, she may revert back to the patterns she experienced and react more harshly to her child than she intended. By bringing her awareness to her own experience while setting limits, which may include discomfort, thoughts that she is harming her child, fears that her child will suffer, and ultimately, unresolved pain or anger about how she was treated as a child, she can begin to find a place for these emotions and make space to see what is needed in the present moment with her child.

HERE AND NOW AWARENESS DURING LIMIT SETTING

We emphasize the importance of *feeling* the limits in our own bodies—to recognize the bodily signals when we've allowed our child to go over our limit. We invite parents to open to these sensations which they so often automatically ignore, to be curious and ask, "What is my body trying to say to me now?" or "Am I listening to my body now?" Listening to the body, and accepting its wisdom, goes counter to many habits we have learned as parents, so it is a good everyday informal practice for parents to use.

HOLDING OUR OWN EXPERIENCE, HOLDING OUR CHILD'S EXPERIENCE

Setting limits often elicits anger from children, and tolerating this anger can be difficult for some parents. They may feel guilty or feel that they are being too harsh, or they may feel angry in return. For other parents, it may feel like a break in the relationship if the child is angry at them. Perhaps they have unrealistic fantasies that their child should always feel happy or never be angry at them. Or they may fear that their adolescent will leave them or behave in out-of-control ways. Avoiding limit setting is one way to avoid these uncomfortable feelings. As parents, we need to be able to tolerate and hold our own emotions, while also holding the emotions of our children. Just being with our children's and our own emotions is an important form of practice which can help with this.

FEELINGS VERSUS BEHAVIOR

As child psychologist Ginott (1965) pointed out, it is important to distinguish between feelings and behavior: we can accept a child's feelings unconditionally, but it doesn't mean we have to accept her behavior unconditionally. Mindful Parenting does not mean unconditional acceptance of your child's behavior, no matter what! Rather, a parent brings mindful awareness to the situation, to her own reactions, and then to her child's feelings and needs in the situation. Ginott suggests that parents set limits clearly but at the same time verbalize the child's feelings. A parent can also verbalize her own feelings in a calm way.

Bringing mindfulness to bear on limit setting gives parents the opportunity to reflect on what is really important to them as parents, what they want to teach their children—in other words, the values they want to instill in their children. Mindfulness can help parents examine their own values, and distinguish them from the values of their own parents, or the values of their friends and community.

Children need limits as well as love to grow. In fact, limit setting, when done intentionally, is a loving act because it is a form of attention the parent gives to the child, because he knows it will help her grow and develop. When the limit setting comes from a clear vision of what parents value and want for their children, rather than an automatic replication of what they experienced as children, it is more consonant with their own intentions and may help parents weather the storms which may follow. For each parent, the discovery will be different, but the journey is the same: from awareness of the sensations, thoughts, and feelings which are triggered during their interaction with their child, recognition of childhood patterns, and awareness of their child's emotional reaction, and holding all of this in mindful awareness.

To sum up, the two central themes in Session 7 are cultivating compassion and loving-kindness and setting limits. We begin with the formal loving-kindness practice. We discuss parents' experiences repairing a difficult conflict with their child. We also pay attention to how parents can take care of themselves, using a "what do I need" meditation. In the second half of the session, we address limit setting through an imaginal exercise and a role-play. Finally, we end with the story of the two wolves to remind us that loving-kindness is something that we can practice.

GUIDELINES FOR SESSION 7

Box 11.1. Agenda Session 7

1. Loving-kindness meditation + inquiry (45 min)
2. Home practice review in pairs (10 min)
3. Review of rupture and repair home practice in the group (10 min)
4. Discussion of the mindfulness day at home or at the center, in pairs or group discussion (20 min)
5. What do I need? (15 min)
6. Break (15 min)
7. Limits: imagination exercise + discussion in pairs/trios (20 min)
8. Limits: role-play in pairs/trios (30 min)
9. Review home practice for next time (10 min)
10. Read story of the two wolves (5 min)

1. LOVING-KINDNESS MEDITATION

We introduce loving-kindness meditation briefly. Because this is a group of parents, we like to begin by explaining the Buddha's injunction to practice kindness and compassion "like a mother protecting her only child." The deep kindness and love that parents feel for their children is already there; we are just cultivating that mind-state. We like to inspire parents feel a sense of wonder and respect for the kindness and love they have for their children.

Kindness is the attitude underlying all meditation (J. Teasdale and C. Feldman, p.c., April 7–11, 2010). We do this practice to further cultivate the mind of kindness and compassion. We emphasize that in this practice, we are forming the *intention* to be kind, compassionate, and loving to all beings, including ourselves, but that we may not *feel* that way, and that's perfectly okay. If you wholeheartedly commit to this intention, that is enough. We are also making the commitment to practice kindness and compassion in our actions towards ourselves and others, since a mind of kindness leads to kind actions. There is an altruistic message to loving-kindness—we are trying to relieve suffering. Since this practice is about the intention to practice loving-kindness, it helps to sit or lie in a very comfortable, easy position, so that you are embodying kindness towards yourself. You can also experiment with breathing in and out of the heart region or placing two hands on your heart to stay connected with your heart.

In previous sessions, we have already been practicing self-kindness, and we can also practice sending kind wishes to others. This meditation begins with sending ourselves friendly wishes and then sending a beloved person, then a friend, a stranger, a difficult person, the group, and finally all living creatures. We observe that sometimes people find it awkward or difficult to wish themselves well; some people feel they don't deserve to wish themselves well. We invite parents to simply notice any thoughts or feelings when they arise and also to notice what whether these reactions change at all during the meditation. Some metaphors that are helpful are "Plant a phrase as if you are planting a seed—pause—then listen for response that comes up." Or "Drop the phrases into a well, and then listen for the response which comes up" (M. Williams, p.c., December 6, 2011).

Box 11.2. Loving-Kindness Meditation

Sit or lie comfortably, closing your eyes. Become aware of your body sitting or lying in this room here and now, breathing. Bringing your attention to yourself. Not focusing on what you may like or not like about yourself, but bringing attention to the fact that you are a human being, who is alive . . . who is breathing . . . who suffers. Remembering that all human beings long to be happy and free from suffering. We wish ourselves well:

May I be happy.
May I be at peace.
May I be free from suffering.

Letting the phrases drop, and noticing any reaction. . . . You can repeat this phrase, or any other, to yourself for a bit . . .

For parents who feel they cannot send themselves kind wishes first:
Sit or lie comfortably, closing your eyes. Become aware of your body sitting or lying in this room here and now, breathing. Bring your attention to your child (or a pet, hero figure), to the fact that he or she is a human being, who is alive . . . who is breathing . . . who is suffering. Remembering that all human beings long to be happy and free from suffering. And wish him/her well:

May you be happy.
May you be at peace.
May you be free from suffering.

Letting the phrases drop, and noticing any reactions. . . . You can repeat this phrase, or any other, to your child for a bit . . .
And now, calling to mind a beloved person—a mentor, teacher, someone who has been there for you. It can also be someone who has inspired you. And bringing your attention to this person. Not focusing on what you may like or not like about him or her, but bringing attention to the fact that he or she is a human being, who is alive . . . who is breathing . . . who suffers. Remembering that all human beings long to be happy and free from suffering. We wish him well:

May you be happy.
May you be at peace.
May you be free from suffering.

And repeating this to yourself for a few moments, noticing any reactions . . .
And now, calling to mind a friend (or relative, child, etc.). And bringing your attention to this person. Not focusing on what you may like or not like about him or her, but bringing attention to the fact that he or she is a human being, who is alive . . . who is breathing . . . who suffers. Remembering that all human beings long to be happy and free from suffering. We wish her well:

May you be happy.
May you be at peace.
May you be free from suffering.

Repeating this to yourself for a few moments, noticing what bubbles up . . .

And now, calling to mind a stranger or neutral person. Someone you've seen but don't know personally—it could be a clerk at a store, a bank teller, a parent at your child's school that you don't know, someone you've seen in the elevator at work . . . and bringing your attention to this person. Not focusing on what you may like or not like about him or her, but bringing attention to the fact that he or she is a human being, who is alive . . . who is breathing . . . who suffers. Remembering that all human beings long to be happy and free from suffering. We wish him well:

May you be happy.
May you be at peace.
May you be free from suffering.

Repeating this to yourself for a few moments, noticing what comes up . . .

Now calling to mind a difficult person, an "enemy." Someone who has been difficult for you, for example, because of conflict in the relationship. It can be a difficult co-worker or boss, a partner or ex-partner, family member, your child, a friend, or neighbor. Once again, bringing your attention to this person. Not focusing on what you may like or not like about him or her, but bringing attention to the fact that he or she is a human being, who is alive . . . who is breathing . . . who suffers. We wish him well:

May you be happy.
May you be at peace.
May you be free from suffering.

Repeating this to yourself for a few moments, being aware of what comes up . . .

And now, becoming aware that we are sitting here in this

room, breathing together. We breathe out, and that becomes the inbreath of our neighbor. Bringing our awareness to all of us sitting here, all of us parents, who are alive . . . who are breathing . . . who suffer. Remembering that all of us long to be happy and free from suffering. We wish all of us well:

May we be happy.
May we be at peace.
May we be free from suffering.

Repeating this to yourself for a few moments, being aware of what comes up . . .

And now, becoming aware of all living creatures. Realizing we are all breathing the same air, we are all sharing the same earth, we are all connected to each other. All of these creatures, who are alive . . . who are breathing . . . who suffer. Remembering that all creatures long to be happy and free from suffering. We wish them well:

May all creatures be happy.
May all creatures be at peace.
May all creatures be free from suffering.

Repeating this to yourself, noticing what comes up . . .

In a few moments, you'll hear the bell ring and you can slowly open your eyes.

For alternatives, see Handout 11.3.

INQUIRY

We begin by asking open-ended question such as "Would anyone care to share their experience?" We listen openly to all responses, asking questions to help participates elaborate on their experience.

There are several areas of experience to consider: the experience of repeating the phrases, what thoughts and feelings and body sensations arise after saying the phrases, and any changes that occur over the course of sending loving-kindness wishes to the different persons. We discussed earlier some of the difficulties which may arise—parents who may feel awkward or even unworthy when directing loving-kindness to themselves or experience of strong negative thoughts and feelings about the self. If participants only discuss pleasant or positive experiences with the meditation, we might ask: "Did anyone find this difficult?" or "Did anyone notice difficult thoughts and feelings coming up?" If no one responds, the teacher can mention that sometimes painful feelings can arise during this practice, so that participants are prepared in case they have this experience at home. If no one shares a difficult experience with this practice, it can be very helpful for the teacher to share a personal experience with this practice, for example, having difficulty feeling deserving of loving-kindness, feeling "nothing" after doing the practice, feeling angry at children or partners, or feeling bored or unmotivated. As teachers, it is important that we have sufficient experience doing loving-kindness practice, so that we can understand some of the potential reactions from our own experience.

For example, I make use of targeted self-disclosure to help embody the mindful stance of accepting all feelings which come up in loving-kindness. I often mention that certain of my dearly beloved's—my husband, my children, my mother, my sister and brother—often rotate through my loving-kindness practice, in a parade of musical chairs, sometimes occupying the enemy chair, other times the friend or mentor chair. Initially I found myself feeling guilty when my husband or one of my children ended up in the enemy chair, but I have come to accept this and now find it interesting to notice where the different characters in my life are sitting in my loving-kindness practice. I share this with the group to make the point in as personal a way as possible that loving-kindness practice does not mean we have to feel loving, even towards our loved ones! To the contrary, we often harbor all sorts of strong negative feelings towards the people we love, and isn't that interesting to notice?

If any of the participants choose to first send loving-kindness to their child, we can ask about their experience. For example, after sending loving-kindness to others, did anything change, or was the parent able to direct loving-kindness towards themselves? If any participants choose to send loving-kindness to their vulnerable or angry child, how was that?

VOICES OF THE PARENTS

Frederica described how difficult it was to feel unconditional love for herself, or from someone else to her. She felt awkward, and as she stayed with the awkwardness, she became aware of a feeling that she was not deserving of love. At the same time, she felt her heart brimming with love for her two young children. We focused on this moment of holding the paradox of loving her children so fully, and not feeling she could love herself. As she sat with this discrepancy, tears came into her eyes. The group could feel compassion for this woman who was so hard on herself. . The teacher asked gently "Who is it who is doing the loving?" The teacher was inviting her to feel that this love, which came from her, was the same love whether it was directed towards herself or her child..

For some parents, connecting with their love for their child may help them recognize that they can also be loving towards themselves. They may realize that they are deserving of compassion, not because they are good mothers or fathers, but simply because they are a human being, who is flawed and who suffers. They may also come to realize that there is no need to be perfect to be loved, as, after all, also their children are not perfect but deserve their love no matter what.

Other parents come face to face with old emotional wounds during this practice.

For example, one mother describes how loving-kindness practices brought up old painful feelings of hers which she had spent her life struggling to overcome:

When we did our first loving kindness meditation, we had to bring someone to mind who loves you unconditionally. It was my second mother, the woman who raised me. While seeing this image, again sadness comes up, tears stream over my cheeks, and my throat became tight . . . as soon as I go to this image, the wave of sorrow comes back with full intensity. I know what it is, that sadness, that fear. Someone who loves you unconditionally, I find deep inside really scary. The first one who did that with me died. In this way—with gentle attention—I come directly to my "old sadness." That is a step in the right direction—I know.

I had tried to process my old sorrow: I've talked a lot about it, I read, I analyzed, I went into psychotherapy, and came some way. But the basis was unreachable. No psychologist, no new mother, no patient husband, could solve it for me., could give me what my mother was not able to give me when I was young: unconditional love. The only one who can do that, is me. Only when I can be my "own" mother, I can be a mother for my children. I have learned how I can be my "own" mother.

In this moving account of her experience, Esther describes clearly how loving-kindness practice brought her in touch with deep feelings of loss, grief, and unworthiness related to her wishes for unconditional love from her mother, who had died. She also describes how this practice brought her closer to healing than the other things she had tried, because she finally was able to realize that she could "mother" herself—give herself the love, kindness, and compassion to deal with the part of herself that still suffered from her old pain. This illustrates so clearly how loving-kindness opens up the desire for connection and love and the pain when we have missed that connection and love. She illustrates how bringing self-compassion to her suffering—by becoming her own mother—helped her in the process of healing. Mindfulness helped her to realize that she had what was needed to heal herself—that she herself could be the mother she needed to heal the pain of her youth. In schema terms, Hannah realized that her healthy adult mode was capable of mothering and healing her vulnerable child mode.

This practice can also bring up ambivalent or negative feelings for children. Some parents may feel angry towards their child or guilty that they don't feel loving towards their child. Some parents may never have felt a sense of lover for their child, and this may be very painful, especially if they hear other parents expressing loving feelings for their child. It is important to be very sensitive and open to this experience, although it does not come up often. As discussed in Chapter 2, when mothers (or fathers) lack the social support that is so needed in raising children, their commitment to them will be affected. This is an important point to make, especially during a session where we are focusing on loving feelings for children.

To sum up, we invite participants to be aware of any and all reactions, to be accepting of all reactions, and to normalize this phenomenon of backdraft by explaining that we live in a culture which emphasizes self-criticism over self-compassion. We emphasize that you do not have to feel anything special during this practice. Sometimes, parents become aware of their pain and sadness about having missed that unconditional love. Responding compassionately to these painful feelings can initiate a healing process for some, as we saw with Esther.

As with all practices, as teachers, we use our own experience with loving-kindness practice and our own clinical skills to guide the inquiry and to support parents when difficult feelings come up. If a teacher feels concerned about a participant's strong negative reaction, she can invite the participant to speak privately after the class, to find out how upset he feels, how much distance he can take on his reaction, whether he anticipates feeling upset when he goes home, what kind of support he has (e.g., from a therapist, friend, or partner) if needed.

2. REVIEW OF HOME PRACTICE IN PAIRS

Participants share their experience with the home practice, especially any rupture and repair experiences. If time allows, parents discuss other home practice, such as holding your emotion as if it were your baby and how the daily mindfulness practice went. After 5 min, the teacher rings the bell, and the participants switch. The group then comes back together as a whole to discuss the home practice.

3. REVIEW OF RUPTURE AND REPAIR HOME PRACTICE

We ask participants to describe any experiences "repairing" a conflict with a child or partner. The teacher might ask if parents experienced any difficulties. It can be helpful to outline on the whiteboard the different steps of the repair practice as a parent describes it: (1) taking a 3-min or self-compassion break; (2) becoming aware of body sensations, feelings, thoughts, and action tendencies, noticing any schema modes (Angry or Vulnerable child, punitive or demanding parent); (3) viewing the conflict from your child's perspective and empathizing with his feelings; (4) returning to your child when ready and inviting him to talk about it; (5) telling your child you want to make up; (6) saying any regrets you have (e.g., "I'm sorry I made you feel bad") or apologizing for your actions ("I shouldn't have yelled at you like that—I see how it hurt you"); (7) empathizing out loud with your child's experience and invite your child to share his side; and (8) explaining briefly your experience.

The point of the repair conversation is to restore the emotional bond between parent and child (or partners). These steps don't have to be followed exactly, but the teacher should listen for whether the parent was able to express empathy with the child, apologize if necessary, and reconnect emotionally with the child. One common trap can be to get back into the conflicting interaction or for the parent to go on too long about the child's misbehavior. For this reason, we recommend parents wait until after the emotional bond feels restored to bring up the child's role in the conflict.

4. REVIEW OF MINDFULNESS DAY

We discuss how parents experienced the mindfulness day at home or at the center, either as a whole group or in small groups of two or three.

Jo was looking forward to this nice day for herself, but her partner was ill that day, needed care and could not take care of the children. She felt angry and disappointed. We suggested "mindful taking care of the ill patient" as part of a mindfulness day.

Sue announced to her partner that she planned to have a mindfulness day, but he reacted by saying "And when do I get my mindfulness day?" They agreed that he could have it on the following day. She noticed that "working like a monk"—doing the dishes with full awareness, preparing dinner attentively, and so on, made her more peaceful with the work of running a family of four children. When she announced she would go for a walk, her son reacted with surprise: "You never do that," and asked if he could join. As they walked together Sue practiced mindful talking and listening, and walking in silence. At the end of the day, her son said to her in surprise: "What a nice day was it today!" Sue was shocked, as she thought that the tension in the family resulted from her partner's stress, not from hers!

Milena noticed that a mindfulness day looks like a "pajamas day" that she has several times a year with her daughter.

Some parents ask the children to join them for a day of no computer, TV, electronic games, or mobile phones during their mindfulness day. They are often surprised by the positive effect this has on their family life.

5. WHAT DO I NEED?

The Buddha wrote, "If one going down into a river, swollen and swiftly flowing, is carried away by the current—how can one help others across?

We do a brief meditation on what we need to take care of ourselves as parents and individuals. The teacher rings the bell, and we sit for a few minutes. At the end of the outbreath, we let the question "What do I need?" drop into the space between the outbreath and the next arising inbreath; sometimes "What do I need as a parent?" sometimes "What do I need as an individual?" or "What have I learned about what I need, as a parent, and as an individual?" We listen for what comes up. After the meditation, the parents fill out the "What do I need?" form (Handout 11.5).

For many parents, the course and the group has become a way to nurture themselves, and we want to encourage parents to bring this kind of nurturing into their lives. Lack of social support is one important reason why parenting is stressful, as was pointed out in Chapter 2. Therefore, we pay in the "what do I need" exercise attention to the social support that parents need, to fulfill their parenting tasks as best as they can, and to handle more wisely parenting stress.

6. BREAK

Take a short break.

7. LIMITS

We begin this practice by explaining that all children need love and limits. Limits are a form of "ruthless compassion"—something we do out of love for our children, which may at times be difficult for them and us.

We start by connecting the theme of setting limits with our children to experiencing our own bodily limits, as we have been doing in the yoga practice, the body scan, and by bringing awareness to stressful interactions. Setting limits with our children starts with our being mindfully aware of our body, sensing when we feel a limit is being crossed with us.

We discuss how often we know the right thing to do with our children, but as we've seen in the course, our own stress, emotional reactions, and past experiences can sometimes interfere with carrying out what we already know. This is also true for limit setting. Setting limits mindfully means becoming aware of what we value, what is important for us to teach our children, and how we can effectively convey that. It also means becoming aware of our own experience with limits growing up in our families of origin. How were limits handled? How did we feel about them? How do we feel about our parents' style of limit setting? As we have seen, we sometimes find ourselves automatically repeating patterns we have learned from childhood, instead of choosing, with full awareness, how we want to respond to our child. When we are aware of these automatic tendencies as they come up, as well as our feelings about how limit setting was handled when we were children, we can make space for identifying our own values and choosing when and how to set limits. The teacher can give a personal example to illustrate this.

Box 11.3. Imagination Exercise: Limits

Call to mind an interaction with your child which was difficult, and where you felt your limits were crossed, or a particular behavior of your child which you feel you need to set more effective limits on (e.g., temper tantrums, stealing, hitting, or not cleaning up). See if you can imagine it as vividly as possible: Who is there? What is happening? Who is saying or doing what?

Now, see if you can remember how your body felt, your feelings and thoughts, what you felt like saying or doing. Did you notice a mind state (of anger, sadness, fear, etc.)? Were you aware of a childlike part of yourself that was triggered by this interaction? Angry or vulnerable child? Punitive or demanding parent? Notice also what you experience now. What comes up for you in your body, your thoughts, and your feelings, and what action tendencies do you notice?

And now, let go of the situation, and take a 3-min breathing space (*the teacher guides group in a 3-min breathing space*). See if you can also give yourself some self-compassion for your suffering. If you like, you can imagine saying kind words to yourself, put both hands on your heart, or stroke yourself, give yourself a little hug, or simply feel compassion for yourself as parent. If you feel the presence of your vulnerable or angry child, you can comfort him or her . . .

Did you recognize your own limits before or after your child went over them? What is it like for you when you try to set a limit? What would you avoid by not setting a limit? What do you want to do now?

Now open your eyes. Discuss in pairs or trios what you experienced.

VOICES OF THE PARENTS

Annie, mother of 6-year-old Lily, reported "I never feel it in my body when Lily crosses my boundaries." The practice for her was to tune into her body during interactions with her child, especially stressful ones, looking for any signals—tensing or tightening of shoulder or neck muscles, butterflies in her stomach, muscle cramps, etc.—which would tell her that a limit was being crossed.

Maya, the mother of a 7-year-old girl, observed: "I notice that by the time I realize there's a problem with my daughter going over my limits, it's too late—it's gone too far without my giving her the signal that it's not allowed, so she keeps going on doing what she's doing. I need to recognize it sooner, and say something sooner."

Many parents have even more difficulty saying "no" at home to their children or partners than at work. To give a personal example: after my divorce, I felt I had to devote all of my time to my children when they were with me, as they lived halftime with their father. At one point, I noticed how one of my children's teachers would routinely put up a Stop sign, which meant that for 1 hour, the children were not to disturb her and instead should consult each other if they had questions. I talked to my children (3 and 5 years at the time) and explained that I needed an hour of time on Saturday morning to read the newspaper undisturbed and that during this hour, they could play by themselves and help each other. Much to my surprise, they did not feel neglected by this and instead took this hour very seriously. They were careful not to disturb me, including telling people who called on the telephone that their mother was having her morning newspaper time and could not be disturbed! They helped each other with going to the toilet, using scissors wisely, etc. In this way, setting a limit to protect my own needs also helped the children develop important skills, such as recognizing that their mother has needs as well, developing concern, and being able to entertain themselves more independently.

Natalie, the mother of a teenage girl, found that she could use mindfulness to help her delay saying "No" long enough to give her daughter the feeling that she was being heard. Her daughter would ask "Can't you just hear me out and listen to my side of it, before you say No?" Natalie reflected on how she has changed her approach: "So now I bite my lip, I just listen, even if I'm thinking, 'Oh my god, what do we have here? How am I going to tell her no?' Then after I've listened, I say 'Wow, that is a great idea and I understand why you want to do it, but for this and that reason I can't let you'. And I find she accepts it better after she feels I've heard her. And sometimes, that waiting time gives me time to reconsider my initial impulse to say 'No', and I realize that I don't have to say No automatically, I can maybe say yes in this situation. So it gives me time as well and saves me from automatically responding."

Natalie would also acknowledge her daughter's feelings as well as her own when setting limits. When her daughter would begin to curse at her, which Natalie found unacceptable, she would say, "I am feeling angry that you are cursing at me. I understand you're disappointed and angry, and you can tell me that, but I don't want to be cursed at." In this way, Natalie set a clear limit, acknowledged her daughter's feelings, and also acknowledged her own anger. This helped her daughter recognize the effect of her action, as well as understand exactly why her mother was angry—she didn't like to be cursed at, instead of interpreting it in a more global, personal way ("I'm a bad child").

Wendy had been physically abused as a child, and had difficulty disciplining her 4-year-old son, because she felt he would experience it as a rejection. Her son was an active and impulsive boy, and was having problems at school, and Wendy recognized that he needed firmer limits from her. She was able to get in touch first with her own feelings of fear and helplessness as a child when her father, an alcoholic, would beat her, and she recognized the same feeling of fear coming up in situations where she needed to be firm with her son. In the following week, she was encouraged to experiment with setting a limit on her son's hitting his younger sister. The task was to set the limit, which she chose ahead of time, and while setting the limit, bring mindful awareness to her experience and reaction to her child. When she set the limit, which was to bring him to a time-out chair, she focused on her breath and body sensations, thoughts and feelings. When her son screamed and had a temper tantrum, she was able to stay connected with feelings of fear and anger, tension in her belly, and thoughts that she was a terrible and cruel mother. She was also able to bring her own wisdom to bear on the situation, by reminding herself that she knew he needed help in controlling his behavior. She also gave herself compassion for her feeling distressed at her son's crying. To her surprise, his temper tantrum was short-lived, and he sat through the time out. When he came out of it, he was calmer, and did not seem upset. This new experience—seeing that she could be firm, and seeing that it helped her son—gave her a new perspective on limit-setting, and enabled her to see herself in a new light—as a competent and firm parent who did not always give in to her son.

8. ROLE-PLAY: LIMITS

In pairs or trio's, parents role-play the same situation that they practiced within the imagination exercise (Box 11.3), using what they've learned from the exercise to guide them. The parent explains to the partner(s) in the role-play the situation shortly. If time permits, parents may want to try both positions: playing the parent who sets the limit and playing the child who receives the limit. It is helpful to first let your "child" role-play the difficult behavior, and be mindful of the effect that has on you, maybe also practicing an inner smile, and take your time before you set the limit. Set the limit mindfully, aware of yourself, and your child, in contact.

VOICES OF THE PARENTS

Mary imagined the following situation: She was ironing in the living room when she heard her two children playing in the bath together, splashing water on the bathroom floor which she had just cleaned. From the living room, she screamed at them that they must stop splashing and not make a mess in the bathroom. When she finally went in to the bathroom and saw the mess, she exploded at the children. Imagining this situation in the group, she became aware of how tired she was, and how she was trying to do two things at the same time. She also recognized her demanding parent mode—needing to do so much at the same time, as well as her angry child mode—that others did not take her into account.

During the role play, when two participants played the children having fun in the bath, she put down her ironing and went to the children, stopped a moment to notice how much fun her children were having together, but still set the limit that they could not make such a big mess.

Miriam, mother of an autistic son, had difficulty setting limits on her son when he would scream intensely. She noticed how upset she felt by his screaming, which she experienced as a kind of clenching in her belly and chest. She also felt an urge to scream back and hit him, and recognized her angry child and punitive parent modes. When she discussed her experience with her role—play partner, the partner suggested that she try holding her son firmly, with love. She tried both positions: the mother holding the child and the son being held. In both positions, she felt herself calming down.

Sue had difficulty setting limits on her two children, who often fought intensely. Imagining the fighting children, she became aware of the intense arousal in her when her children would fight, which she experienced as a tightening in her chest and throat, difficulty breathing, and a headache pressing on her forehead. She remembered how fighting between siblings was forbidden in her family of origin, whereas her parents would fight constantly. She identified her vulnerable child: feeling vulnerable because her parents were fighting, and tried to give that child compassion. She also recognized her punitive parent mode which told her "Your children should never fight!" During the role play, she found she was able to relax seeing her partners role-play her fighting children, and was able to assert a limit firmly but non-punitively, from a position of strength rather than vulnerability.

9. REVIEW OF HOME PRACTICE

In the home practice for this week, we ask parents to continue their own 40-min formal practice each day. We also invite them to try out loving-kindness meditation, and suggest just before falling asleep as one possible time, but they are free to choose another time. We also ask them to pay attention to limit setting with their child as it is happening. Finally, we ask them to bring in an object, poem, song, or narrative description of their process during the past 8 weeks, to share with the others in the group in the last session.

10. THE TWO WOLVES

We tell the story of the two wolves to illustrate why we practice loving-kindness meditation (see Handout 11.7).

HANDOUT 11.1 Practice for the Week After Session 7

Reading

Read the handouts mindfully.

Mindful Parenting

Try paying attention to how you set limits this week. Notice what it feels like when you have reached your own personal limits (with children, partners, colleagues, work). Notice when you feel you want to set a limit with your child. Notice any body sensations, thoughts, feelings, and impulses to act. Set the limit, as best you can, and notice how that feels, including noticing your child's reaction and your reaction to his reaction. Remember it doesn't always feel good to set a limit, yet it is one of the most important things to do for your child and yourself. As best as you can, bring kindness to yourself and to your child when it feels difficult.

Formal Practice

Continue you own formal practice program of about 40 min a day. If you have not done it last week, investigate your obstacles, take care of them as best as you can, and try with new intention this week. You may want to follow this daily meditation program after the course ends. You can use the journal to make notes.

Try one or more loving-kindness meditations. Choose a restful or relaxing time (e.g., when you go sleep at night) and do a brief loving-kindness meditation. Make yourself comfortable, and practice bringing an attitude of unconditional friendliness to yourself (see Handouts 11.2 and 11.3 for instructions). Notice your reactions to the meditation.

Your Personal Journey

Bring in something to next week's session which symbolizes your personal learning process or journey. It may be an object, music, art, a poem, or anything else. Write a description of your personal process during the past 8 weeks of taking the Mindful Parenting course (see Handout 11.6). As you reflect on your journey in the past 8 weeks, think about how you want to continue this journey after the courses ends.

Optional: Books

If there are any books that you have read that have helped you particularly with mindful parenting, you may want to bring them to show the group next week.

HANDOUT 11.2 Loving-Kindness Meditation:
Basic Instructions*

You can do this meditation any time you like, for as short or as long as you like. It can be nice to do before falling asleep at night.

Sit or lie comfortably, closing your eyes. Become aware of your body sitting or lying in this room here and now, breathing. Bringing your attention to yourself. Not focusing on what you may like or not like about yourself, but bringing attention to the fact that you are a human being, who is alive . . . who is breathing . . . who suffers. We wish ourselves well:

May I be happy.
May I be at peace.
May I be free from suffering.

Letting the phrases drop, and noticing any reactions . . . . You can repeat this phrase, or any other, to yourself for a bit . . .

If you find it difficult to send yourself kind wishes first, here are two suggestions:

1. Send kind wishes to yourself as a vulnerable child. If it helps, you can call yourself "Little [your name]."
2. Send kind wishes first to your child, a beloved pet or friend, a mentor or other cherished person, or an inspiring figure.

We repeat the above phrases for the following individuals:

1. Yourself (or your child or your inner child)
2. Beloved person or mentor or inspirational figure or pet
3. Friend
4. Neutral person (stranger)
5. Enemy or difficult person
6. Your neighbors or community
7. All living beings

Don't worry if you don't have time to get through the whole list. Sharon Saltzberg, the guru of loving-kindness meditation in the West, describes how she spent months just sending herself loving-kindness wishes!

Have fun playing around with the order of the individuals, and notice how you react.

*Adapted from Martine Batchelor, p.c., March 2009.

HANDOUT 11.2 Loving-Kindness Meditation:
Basic Instructions (continued)

Finally, keep in mind that loving-kindness practice is also mindfulness practice. See if you can notice with curiosity and kindness your own reactions to repeating the phrases—irritation, frustration, doubting yourself, feeling inadequate—any and all feelings may come up, and that's okay! You don't have to feel loving when you practice loving-kindness meditation!

HANDOUT 11.3 Variations of Loving-kindness Meditation

You can think of loving-kindness phrases as recipes that can be borrowed, swapped, and adapted as needed. When we cook, we like to combine a few recipes until we get something we like. You can also do the same with loving-kindness phrases!

Here are some that you might like to try. Of course, feel free to make up your own!

Sylvia Boortein's version:

> May I feel happy.
> May I feel safe.
> May I feel strong.
> May I live with ease.

John Teasdale's version:

> May I be safe and protected.
> May I be peaceful.
> May I live with ease and kindness.

Christopher Germer's version:

> May I be safe.
> May I be peaceful.
> May I be kind to myself.
> May I love myself as I am.

One of my versions:

> May I be happy.
> May I accept myself as I am.
> May I love myself for who I am.

For your child:

> May [name of child] be happy.
> May I accept [name of child] as he/she is.
> May I love [name of child] as he/she is.

Your own version:

> May I . . . .?

HANDOUT 11.4 The Mind of Love

At the moment of giving birth to a child, is the mother separate from the child? You should study not only that you become a mother when your child is born, but also that you become a child.

> Dogen Zenji (edited by Tanahashi, 1995)

Even poor or suffering people raise their children with deep love. Their hearts cannot be understood by others. This can be known only when you become a father or a mother. They do not care whether they themselves are poor or rich; their only concern is that their children will grow up. They pay no attention to whether they themselves are cold or hot, but cover their children to protect them from the cold or shield them from the hot sun. This is extreme kindness. Only those who have aroused this mind can know it, and only those who practice this mind can understand it.

> Dogen Zenji (edited by Tanahashi, 1995)

After I had a child I realized that all the love I had experienced in the past—especially with partners—was selfish. I was constantly thinking, what's in this relationship for me? And if my expectations weren't met any good feeling would dry up altogether. My daughter has taken me to hell and back but there's nothing she can do to make me stop loving her.

> Mother quoted by Napthali (2003) in *Buddhism for Mothers*

I teach my children how to behave from a base of love and unconditional acceptance. I'm now learning to do the same for myself.

> Mother quoted by Napthali (2003) in *Buddhism for Mothers*

Being with Strong Emotions

We re-visit the raw emotions of our own childhood when we have a child. We feel intense love, undiluted hate and anger, as well as extreme anxiety and fear, and can swing from one extreme emotion to another.   Figes and Zimmerman (1998), *Life After Birth:*
> *What Even Your Friends Won't Tell You About Motherhood*

What makes [metta] such a different approach is that we are not trying to solve a problem. We are not striving to make pain go away or to become a better person. In fact, we are giving up control altogether and letting concepts and ideals fall apart.

> Chodron (2000), *When Things Fall Apart*

HANDOUT 11.5 What Do I Need?*

You only have to let the soft animal of your body love what it loves.
                    Mary Oliver, "Wild Geese"—in Segal, Williams,
                                              and Teasdale (2002)

Stopping to ask the question, "What do I need, as a parent.. and as an individual?" is the first step towards self-compassion in daily parenting life.

How can I take care of or parent myself (physically, mentally, emotionally, relationally, spiritually)?
How do I already care for myself (as an individual and parent)?
Are there new ways to care for myself?

What care do I need from others to feel supported as a parent (my children, my (ex) partner, other caregivers, school, my parents, friends, etc.) [remember you don't always get the care you want, but most important is that you become aware of and express what care you would want—and deserve—even if you will never get it from that person]?

How do they already care for me (as an individual and parent)?
Are there new ways I would want them to care for me?

*Adapted from Chris Germer, p.c., June 2012.

HANDOUT 11.6 Acceptance and Limits

Feelings, no matter how strong, can be unconditionally accepted. Validating the feelings of our children helps them to become aware of their feelings and for them to be accepting of their own feelings. Just as we are learning to accept own feelings, we can also welcome and allow all of the feelings of our children to be there. We accept the feelings; however, we don't have to accept all *behaviors* in reaction to feelings.

As parents, it is important that we become aware of our own limits, rules, and values and that we make these clear to our children. To become aware of your own limits, particularly at times when you feel you have allowed your child to go over that limit, you can use your body as a barometer to help sense when a line has been crossed for you. It may be a particular behavior or pattern of behaviors that you have allowed while feeling uncomfortable with it. Have you been clear with your child about this? Can you bring creative awareness to the situation, to help your child to be able to respect your rules and limits? For example, during a calm moment, enlisting your child's help in making a list of family rules.

Keep in mind that limit setting has two functions: it provides children with the structure they need, and just as importantly, it allows parents to take care of their own needs, which is necessary for them to be able to take care of others. *Remember the wisdom of the airline stewardess: Put your own oxygen mask on first, before you put on your child's. If you don't take care of yourself, how can you possibly take care of anyone else?* For example, when you set a bedtime for your child, you not only provide him with structure and help him get the sleep he needs, but you also give yourself time to take care of yourself, for example, by spending time with your partner or friends or just relaxing and recharging your battery.

Sometimes our own childhood experiences can make it difficult for us to set limits. For example, if we have experienced abuse or neglect growing up, we may feel uncomfortable setting any kind of limit, even appropriate limits, because we worry that we may be too punitive with our child. We may feel guilty about setting limits or have difficulty when our children become angry with us. If these were issues in your own upbringing, you may find yourself giving in to your child at times rather than setting appropriate limits. On the other hand, we may automatically repeat the limit-setting techniques our parents used and may become overly punitive or rigid in limit setting because we are not aware of what we are doing.

Our current situation or stress may also make it difficult to set limits effectively. If we are going through a personal crisis or divorce, we may feel so guilty that we have trouble saying no to our children, or we

HANDOUT 11.6 Acceptance and Limits (continued)

may feel we have to give them all our time and attention when we are with them.

The way some children respond to limit setting may make limit setting particularly difficult and even frightening for parents. Some children may panic when their routines or rituals are interrupted. Some children may become threatening or physically aggressive when confronted with limit setting. For example, a young child holding his breath, an adolescent threatening to leave the house, or an adolescent who threatens to break something or hurt the parent, a sibling, himself. Taking a moment to be mindfully aware can help calm you down and give you a chance to assess the situation. Sometimes what our child or adolescent is doing feels terrible but, in fact, poses no danger to himself of others. So you might decide to let your child hold his breath, or let your adolescent storm out of the house, once you realize there is actually no danger. In situations where a child or adolescent is acting aggressively or out of control, pausing mindfully is just as important so that you can assess the situation realistically and keep yourself and your child safe. One mother of an autistic teen described how he broke the door to his room when she told him he had to turn off his computer game. This mother was convinced that her limit was correct, and she felt it was important to set the limit, despite his reaction. She did make sure that she and her other children stayed out of the way, so that everyone was safe. If a child physically threatens a parent or a sibling, then it's important to make sure you feel safe. One mother's daughter would come up very close to her and scream at her. The mother felt afraid to set a limit, until she realized that she could walk away from her daughter.

If you find yourself experiencing any of these difficulties, or other difficulties not mentioned here, the first step is to be aware of the stress, feel it in your body, and be present with it. See if you can bring compassion to yourself for the difficulty you are experiencing with limit setting and recognize that other parents have also struggled in similar situations. Give yourself a moment to be aware of the body sensations, feelings, and thoughts, without having to react immediately. See if you can open to your own inner source of wisdom—What do I need in this situation? What does my child need? What would I tell my best friend to do in this situation? And finally, recognizing that you don't have to be perfect to raise your child, it's okay not to know what to do.

HANDOUT 11.7 Two Wolves

Native American folk legend recounts the story of an old man who wishes to teach his grandson his wisdom.

> *The grandfather says: "Grandson, I feel like I have two wolves fighting inside of me—an angry wolf and a peaceful wolf."*
> *The grandson asks, "Which one will win, grandfather?"*
> *The grandfather replies, "The one I feed."*

HANDOUT 11.8 Personal Learning Process

Describe your personal learning process during this 8-week Mindful Parenting training. If you want, you can read it aloud next week in the group.

HANDOUT 11.9 Home Practice Record Form Week 7

Fill in the record form each time after you practice (mindful parenting, formal or informal meditation). Write down what comes up for you during the practice, so that we can discuss it in the next session.

Day/time	Practice (Yes/No)	Comments

HANDOUT 11.10 Notes Informal Practice and Mindful Parenting Practice Week 7

You may want to use this sheet to make notes about your experiences during the informal meditation practice and the mindful parenting practice. Or to make notes during or about the group session.

CHAPTER 12

SESSION 8: ARE WE THERE YET? A MINDFUL PATH THROUGH PARENTING

Mindfulness is neither difficult nor complex; remembering to be mindful is the great challenge.

Feldman (2004)

*A*RE WE *there yet?* How many times have we heard that question coming from the back of the car? "We'll be there soon, just another 5 minutes," we might respond. But what does it mean for us to "get there?" Will we ever get there, and if we did get there, what would it look like? Once I had the good fortune to be seated next to Myla Kabat-Zinn during a presentation on mindful parenting, and she observed that it is natural for parents to want to feel that if they work at it hard enough, they will someday become a "mindful parent." Shaking her head with some humor, she reflected on how there is n o such thing as a "mindful parent" or a "mindful child" for that matter. There is no "there" to get to! Mindful parenting is a *process* that continues your whole lifetime, as you grow with your children. Feeling both embarrassed and relieved by her comments. I realized I was one of those parents, waiting for the day that I would be pronounced, finally, a "mindful parent" (by whom—my children?), finally feeling that I had arrived, had figured it all out. What a relief to find out that Myla Kabat-Zinn, like everybody else who cares about mindful parenting, has to practice working with whatever arises. It is the journey that is critical. There is no final destination, and we will never "figure it all out." I often think back to that conversation when I am feeling critical of myself, frustrated with my "lack of progress," or when I'm having a rough day with my kids and all my mindfulness goes out the window. It's helpful to remember that it's the path that's important, not the end point.

Nonetheless, many of us persist in wanting to finally get there, arrive, and succeed at this thing called mindfulness. It's part of our nature that we strive to achieve something, put another feather in our cap, or cross another thing off our to-do list. The Buddha is said to have left home to wander in the forest, and he frequently used the metaphor of a path to describe the process of becoming awakened. For some of us, it's hard to resist the temptation of wanting to arrive at the end of that path. As if our navigator could pronounce, in that crisp British voice, "You have reached your destination." The Buddha said, "The path is lovely in the beginning, lovely in the middle, and lovely in the end." Meditation teacher Christina Feldman invites us to ask ourselves, "What would I have to let go of to make the path more lovely for me?" (C. Feldman, p.c., April 7–11, 2010).

Raising children brings this so poignantly home to us. Where else is it so clear that it is the path, the journey, and the process, which takes precedent over the end goal? Yes, of course we want our children to grow up to be happy, fulfilled, and moral citizens of the world, but if we are in too much of a hurry to get to that goal, we risk missing out on our children growing up.

In the eight session of Mindful Parenting, we take a moment to reflect on this process: what has this experience been like for us, what have we learned in these 8 weeks, and what if anything has changed. Secondly, we invite participants to ask how they can take care of themselves and continue this process of learning for the next 8 weeks in the absence of the group.

This is often a very moving session. Parents have struggled to find the time to do the exercises, have dealt with frustration and lack of progress, and have sat with difficult emotions. Some have also had moments of insight and made changes in their lives or their perspective on their lives and children. The children may have also been affected by this process. We return to the body scan to bring the circle round, but the emotional core of this session is the object that parents bring in to symbolize their process, and their describing this to the group.

GUIDELINES FOR SESSION 8

Box 12.1. Agenda Session 8

1. Body scan and review (30 min)
2. Review of home practice in pairs (15 min)

3. Gratitude practice (15 min)
4. Meditation on what have we learned (5 min)
5. Meditation plan for the next 8 weeks (15 min)
6. Break, including review of books and websites (15 min)
7. Process descriptions with objects (70 min)
8. Reading: Some suggestions for everyday mindful parenting (5 min)
9. Announcement of follow-up meeting (5 min)
10. *Metta meditation* (5 min)

1. BODY SCAN + INQUIRY

The group is led into a guided body scan, in order to make the circle round, as this is where we began our journey. The teacher speaks less and allows more silence than in the beginning of the course.

INQUIRY

The group discussion of the body scan may focus on how this body scan is different or similar to the first body scan done in the group. For example, group members may notice how tired they were in the beginning of the course or how they fell asleep during the body scan, and how that is different now (or not); or how their patience has grown with doing the body scan; or the nurturing feeling they sensed now when the teacher announced the body scan. Or they may have sensed resistance with the idea of doing again a body scan. Whatever is brought up, the inquiry focuses on experiences, including bodily experiences, and if only positive experiences are discussed, the teacher should ask about negative ones as well, in order to continue bringing the message that negative feelings are just as important and welcome as positive ones.

2. REVIEW OF HOME PRACTICE

Participants share the experience of settling on their own meditation practice in pairs. Also, they share the limit setting practice they have tried out and the metta meditation that they have practiced.

Based on the time schedule (with a large group, there is less time than with a smaller group today because of the object practice), there may be more or less time to come back to the home practice in the full group. Participants may have felt resistance when doing the metta at home, or did not like the phrases, which can be explored if time allows. It is however important to note that this way of practicing loving-kindness is just one way; other ways may speak to some participants better, such as the hand-on-heart meditation that we have practiced. Or, metta can be practiced in real life, for example, by doing a random act of kindness. That is, do something kind, unconditionally, to someone you don't know, and be aware what that does to you.

The limit practice can bring up new insights. For example, Desy became aware of her tendency to do too much for her son, who is developmentally delayed, when he said "My book is still upstairs" just before they needed to leave. She recognized her usual tendency to get it for him in order to be on time. Instead, she now said, "okay, go pick it up, I'll wait for you!" and took a breathing space, which made a difference for her day and for her relationship with her son.

3. GRATITUDE PRACTICE

Simply saying what you feel grateful for in your life improves your subjective experience of happiness (Emmons, 2007). This corrects our tendency to focus on the negative and cultivates an attitude of savoring and appreciating our lives here and now.

Participants are invited to sit in small groups, for example, groups of three, and close their eyes. The teacher asks, "What are three things you feel grateful for in your life?" and suggests to see what comes up spontaneously. Parents are then asked to go around in their small group, each one saying aloud one thing they feel grateful for, for three rounds. Next, if time allows, the group sits again in a big circle, making one round in which each one says aloud one thing they feel grateful for. This is an excellent practice to recommend doing first thing in the morning.

4. MEDITATION ON WHAT HAS BEEN LEARNED

After having settled in the sitting posture, with eyes closed, the teacher rings the bell and invites the participants to go back to the beginning of this course, 8 weeks ago.

Box 12.2. Meditation on What We Have Learned

Go back to how it was before you started the Mindful Parenting course, about 8 weeks ago.

How was your situation back then? What were your concerns, symptoms, and sufferings? How was your family doing, how did you feel about your child and your parenting? What were your expectations of the course? Which hopes did you have? . . .

And what has changed? In you, your child(ren), your relationship(s), your family, and your work? Not only in behavioral changes but also in changes in insight, experience, emotions, and thinking . . .

What did it cost you? What price have you paid? What did you have to let go of?

How do you want to continue with what you have learned? To begin with, what is your intention for the next 8 weeks in terms of daily (or weekly) meditation, formal and informal? What is your intention in terms of mindful parenting?

5. MEDITATION PLAN FOR THE NEXT 8 WEEKS

After the bell, the teacher asks participants to write down their meditation plan for the next 8 weeks in their workbook form (see Handout 12.2). It is important to warn not to be overambitious and then feel guilty if they cannot follow the plan but develop a realistic plan that can be carried out. It is helpful to be very concrete in when and how to practice and how to remind yourself of the plan (e.g., write it in your agenda, your phone, put a photo or text on the wall, ask your partner to remind you, meditate with others). Having written it up, volunteers can read aloud their plan in the group.

It can be helpful to end with an intention meditation on this plan (J. Dumas, p.c., 2002). The teacher asks the group to settle in their sitting position. Imagine yourself 4 weeks from now. Imagine yourself in your busy family and working life. Imagine how you are carrying out little bits of your plan during the week. . . . Imagine how you are going to find the time to withdraw a moment from your busy day, how you will announce to your children and partner you are going to meditate . . . where and when and what you will be practicing, make a picture of the place, the moment, how you feel, and how you return to your busy life after the practice. . . . Imagining ourselves doing the practice, bringing intention to it, helps to actually do it!

6. BREAK AND BOOKS

Group members may have brought their own mindfulness books that they want to share with others, and teachers have brought their favorite mindfulness books, particularly those related to parenting and children. Either one can put the books somewhere in the room and have people go by or those who have brought books tell shortly why they appreciated this book so much. During the 8-week course, we don't encourage further reading aside from the handouts because it may take time away from what is most important during the 8 weeks: the personal practice. Also, too much reading in the beginning may get participants in a more intellectual rather than experiential mode, and the goal of the course is to experience the effects of meditation practice on our daily life. Also, websites can be exchanged, which have information on retreats, further courses, etc.

7. PROCESS DESCRIPTION WITH OBJECTS

The group sits in a circle. We explain that during the next hour everyone gets a chance to show the object they brought, put it in the middle, tell something about the object, and read aloud the description of their process during the 8-week course or tell about it. Based on the number of group members, it is wise to calculate in advance how much time there is per group member and explain this in advance. Each person can choose his or her own moment when he or she wants to speak. Between the descriptions, there may be short silences until the next person starts to speak, with no group discussion.

VOICES OF THE PARENTS

John brought music of Leonard Cohen. He explained that he had not been very convinced that meditation could help him (he suffered from chronic depression), although he practiced daily, until he heard that Leonard Cohen, of whom he is a big fan, meditates daily. He played the following song, with tears in his (and our) eyes:

"Anthem" of Leonard Cohen
The birds they sang
at the break of day

Start again
I heard them say
Don't dwell on what
has passed away
or what is yet to be.
Ah the wars they will
be fought again
The holy dove
She will be caught again
bought and sold
and bought again
the dove is never free.
Ring the bells that still can ring
Forget your perfect offering
There is a crack in everything
That's how the light gets in.

Patricia has brought a painting of a mountain that she painted herself, when she still lived in Peru. The mountain stood for peace, strength, finding her base, the painting of the mountain for full attention in the moment. She read aloud the following description:

I'm seated in a little bay hearing how the water rhythmically slaps the rocks of the shore.

I hear the singing of birds now and then, the sounds of a train passing, a car.

At the other side of the shore there is a line of trees of different sizes and types in grayish green shades.

It's a misty midday. Everything looks as if it's seen through a moistened piece of glass.

The sun starts reflecting silver sparks on the water.

One more train passes by.

I had left my house this morning before my kid wakes up.

It's Sunday. I have decided to take some time, just for myself.

Maybe my kid will miss me or maybe not.

I feel a bit guilty.

He'll be fine, I tell to myself.

I realize that that's the kind of moments that makes me a happier person, therefore a better, a much better mother.

I feel so lucky of having been able to attend this course, together with this caring and open-hearted group of women.

*It has taught me so many things, confirmed others, gave me strength and what is
    more important:*
It filled myself with a sense of self-confidence and possibility.

I stay with a few keywords:
Stopping.
Not judging.
Believing in myself as a source of solutions and new ways of looking at daily events.
*Perseverance. The realization of the fact that nothing comes by itself with no effort
    or attention involved.*
Wonderment of seeing how unlimited human capacities are.
*Brotherhood for finding people who are willing to put their time and energy in order
    to develop a healthier relation with the others and themselves.*
Peace, the best counselor we can get.

All my thanks to you all.
*I hope you find the strength in your heart and plant the seed of mindfulness in every
    person you have around.*

Patricia Vega

*Sue brought a piece of red silk. She explained that the red color expressed emotion
and the feeling of the silk softness. She read aloud: "I had totally pushed myself
away by the divorce and gave myself no space as a result- not in my house, not in my
new relationship, and not in parenting. The most important is that I allow myself
to feel my emotions again. These were so far away that I had lost them."*

*Peter, a musician, diagnosed with autistic-spectrum disorder after his daughter had
received that diagnosis, brought his saxophone. He explained that learning meditation was like learning to play a music instrument, first enthusiasm, then avoidance,
frustration, disappointment with the slow learning process, not being able to hear
the sound of it anymore, asking yourself why you ever started it, and telling yourself
you just have to do it, you don't have to like it. He read aloud: "Meditation and
yoga were totally new for me, and I really did not have much room in my life for
them. It took a lot of effort for me to give it a place in my life. I felt much resistance
and resentment towards the daily practice. At the same time, I notice that I am
thinking about it more recently, and about the subject of "feelings." I'm still very
rational, but it is a start. . . . I've noticed that I am very stressed and tired. . . . The
texts on the CD give me the feeling that although I don't practice regularly, I can
start again every day without guilt feelings. I'm planning to do the whole course
again on my own during the 8 week follow-up period"*

*Irene, a single mother of two, quietly laid a beautiful handmade quilt in the center
of the circle of parents. "This quilt was made for me by my mother, when I was preg-*

nant with my first son. It represents the fact that I've learned that I need to take care of myself, that I need to put myself in the chain of caretaking, from my mother, to myself, to my boys. Raising my boys alone has been really challenging. Sometimes I have been really exhausted from the effort. At the same time, it has felt like the most important thing I needed to do. I guess they have needed so much from me, that I forgot about myself. I forgot that I have to also think of my own needs, what I need to feel happy and fulfilled. This group has helped me to see this; that in addition to taking care of them, I can take care of myself. I can wrap myself in this quilt when I need to. It has also made me think about the fact that I don't have a relationship now, and I think I might like to make room for that in my life. Up until now, it hasn't seemed possible. I'm not sure I'm ready for it yet, but I am ready to think about it, which for me is new. I also would like to thank the group for being there for me."

Hannah announced that her object was too large to bring in. It is a large, red exercise ball. It symbolizes the enormity of her feelings when she started the group. Often she would feel like the ball was inside her, growing larger and larger when she became angry or frustrated at her children, her husband or her situation, until finally it (or she) exploded. At times, it felt like her rage was bigger than her, filling her home, out of her control. Mindfulness has helped her with this big red ball. She still feels the feelings, but she feels she can observe the ball, getting bigger and smaller, and she doesn't feel that she is carried away by it anymore. The ball no longer controls her. This has affected her relationship with her children and her husband. In the past, when she felt frustrated or angry, she would often explode at them. Mindfulness has helped her become aware of feelings of anger and frustration as they begin to build, before they have become so large and explosive. Her children have also changed. . . . Partly they have changed in her perception of them . . .

8. READING SOME SUGGESTIONS FOR EVERYDAY MINDFUL PARENTING

The group is asked to settle again in the sitting posture to listen to reading. After the bell, the teacher reads aloud the suggestions (Handout 12.1)

9. ANNOUNCEMENTS

The date and time for the follow-up meeting is announced as well as the goals of the follow-up meeting: to share experiences with the continued practice in the absence of the group and to share the longer-term effects of the course on parenting and the functioning of the child and family. A follow-up meeting may help participants to keep the mindful parenting alive and may help not to fall back in old patterns. Also, we will do some meditation practice.

10. CLOSING MEDITATION

The teacher chooses a brief meditation to end the group, whatever fits best with the particular group and teacher.

HANDOUT 12.1 Some Suggestions for Everyday Mindful Parenting

1. Remember the wisdom of the airline stewardess: put your own oxygen mask on first, before you put on your child's. If you don't take care of yourself, how can you possibly take care of anyone else? If you feel too guilty to take care of your own needs for yourself, then do it for your child.
2. Do a loving-kindness meditation every night before bed. It's okay if you fall asleep in the middle of it.
3. Chose your own personal meditation bell—the telephone ringing, a new e-mail coming in, your children fighting, your child screaming, a fight with your partner, and a difficulty with the colleague. Use the situation to take one or more mindful breaths; to investigate your body, mood, and thoughts; and to slow down.
4. Take three mindful breaths when you first wake up, before getting out of bed.
5. Once a day, observe you child mindfully, with a "beginner's mind." Do this at a regular time each day so you don't forget, for example, when your child comes out of school, goes to bed, wakes up, and eats a meal. See if you can stay present with the wonder of your child for just one moment.
6. In stressful interactions with your child or others, take a mindful breath each time the speaker changes.
7. Listen mindfully to your child or others.
8. Speak mindfully to your child or others.
9. Remind yourself that your child is your personal Zen master, sent down to you from a higher authority to teach you everything you need to know about yourself, your child, and the world. Remind yourself of this especially when your child is driving you crazy.
10. Take a mindful moment as you walk (or run, in our case) to pick up your child from school or daycare. Pay attention to your breathing, body sensations, thoughts, and feelings. What do you feel in your body? What thoughts and feelings are swimming around your head? Are you ready to be present for this moment of greeting your child again?
11. Try asking yourself "What is this?" as you enter a new situation with your child, as a way to open to the moment and what your child may be needing.
12. When you feel overwhelmed by stress and strong emotions, go into your body—what do you feel, where? This will bring you back to your experience in this moment.
13. Pay attention to your breathing when waiting . . . in traffic, in line at the supermarket or anywhere else, or on the train. See if you can

HANDOUT 12.1 Some Suggestions for Everyday
Mindful Parenting (continued)

transform your irritation at having to wait into an opportunity to slow down and bring your awareness to the moment.

14. Practice mindful housework, mindful tooth-brushing, mindful showering, mindful eating, mindful feeding your child, mindful picking your child up from school, etc., throughout the day. See if you can create more and more of these mindful moments each day.

15. Wake up _____ minutes early to practice (read Jon Kabat-Zinn's (1994) piece "Early Morning," for inspiration).

16. Read a book that inspires you.

17. Find a meditation community or create one yourself.

18. Make a list of the ways mindfulness practice has benefited you. Ask your children, your partner, your friends, or family to tell you what changes they have noticed in you in the last 8 weeks and write that on the list. Put the list in a drawer next to your bed, and when you feel your motivation is lagging, take it out and read it to yourself. Read it every day if you need to!

19. Make mindfulness part of your daily routine, something you do whether you feel like it or not, like brushing your teeth, showering, and eating. It doesn't matter whether it's 1 min or 1 h; just build in the routine.

20. Reflect on whether mindful practice is something you do for yourself, because of your intention and the benefits it brings, or if it feels like a "should." If it feels like a "should," how can you transform it into your own intentional choice?

21. Remember it is never too late to renew your intention to cultivate the path of mindfulness, no matter how little you may have practiced. The very next breath is always waiting for you . . .

HANDOUT 12.2 Personal Meditation Plan
for the Next 8 Weeks, Until We Meet Again

Think about any formal and informal practice you want to continue and mindful parenting practice. Make a plan that is concrete (where and when, and in what frequency, are you planning to practice), that is doable in your life in the next 8 weeks, and that you feel like doing.

HANDOUT 12.3 Evaluation of the Mindful Parenting Course and Personal Change*

1. Do you feel you got something of lasting value of importance as a result of taking the training?

   Yes   no

2. Have you made any changes in your lifestyle, in dealing with your child or family, or in your child-rearing practices as a result of the training?

   Yes   no

3. Did you become more "conscious" in parenting as a result of the training? Did this change something in relation to your thoughts, your feelings, and your reaction on your thoughts and feelings as a parent?

   Yes   no

4. Is it your intention to keep on practicing the formal exercises, i.e. the body scan, sitting mediation, 3-min breathing space, walking meditation, laying and standing yoga?

   Yes   no

5. Is it your intention to keep on practicing to be conscious in daily parenting life?

   Yes   no

6. Has the training been sufficient to move on with your life as a parent?

   Yes   no

7. How many times a week, on average, did you practice the meditation exercises during the 8-week training?

   Never   1–2 times   3–4 times   5–7 times

8. How many times a week, on average, did you practice meditation exercises during the 8-week follow-up?

   Never   1–2 times   3–4 times   5–7 times

9. How many times do you pay attention to your child in moments you are together, compared to before the training?

   Less than   As much as   More than   Much more than
   before   before   before   before

---

*Adapted from the evaluation form developed at the Center for Mindfulness of the University of Massachusetts Medical School.

HANDOUT 12.3 Evaluation of the Mindful Parenting Course and Personal Change (continued)

Did, as a result of the Mindful Parenting training, something change on the following issues?

1.	Knowing to take better care of myself	Negative change	No change	Some positive change	Positive change
2.	Actually taking better care of myself	Negative change	No change	Some positive change	Positive change
3.	Periods of parental stress or frustration	Negative change	No change	Some positive change	Positive change
4.	Intensity of parental stress or frustration	Negative change	No change	Some positive change	Positive change
5.	Believing that I can improve the relationship with my child and family	Negative change	No change	Some positive change	Positive change
6.	Feeling self-confident as a parent	Negative change	No change	Some positive change	Positive change
7.	Feeling hopeful as a parent	Negative change	No change	Some positive change	Positive change
8.	Dealing with emotions (anger, sadness, fear) in parenting	Negative change	No change	Some positive change	Positive change
9.	Awareness of what is stressful in my life	Negative change	No change	Some positive change	Positive change
10.	Awareness of stressful parenting situations at the time they are happening	Negative change	No change	Some positive change	Positive change
11.	Ability to handle stressful parenting situations appropriately	Negative change	No Change	Some positive change	Positive Change
12.	Do you want further training or treatment with respect to your parenting, own problems, your child's problems, partner relation problems, family problems?				

Parenting:	No	Maybe	Yes
Own problems:	No	Maybe	Yes
Child's problems	No	Maybe	Yes
Partner relation problems	No	Maybe	Yes
Family problems	No	Maybe	Yes

HANDOUT 12.3 Evaluation of the Mindful Parenting Course and Personal Change (continued)

Evaluations of parts of the Mindful Parenting training (1 = not important at all, 10 = extremely important)

1.	How important has the training been for you?	1	2	3	4	5	6	7	8	9	10
2.	Sitting meditation in the group	1	2	3	4	5	6	7	8	9	10
3.	Sitting meditation at home	1	2	3	4	5	6	7	8	9	10
4.	Walking meditation in the group	1	2	3	4	5	6	7	8	9	10
5.	Walking meditation at home	1	2	3	4	5	6	7	8	9	10
6.	Body scan in the group	1	2	3	4	5	6	7	8	9	10
7.	Body scan at home	1	2	3	4	5	6	7	8	9	10
8.	Yoga in the group	1	2	3	4	5	6	7	8	9	10
9.	Yoga at home	1	2	3	4	5	6	7	8	9	10
10.	3-min breathing space	1	2	3	4	5	6	7	8	9	10
11.	Awareness in daily parenting	1	2	3	4	5	6	7	8	9	10
12.	Awareness of parenting patterns and schemes	1	2	3	4	5	6	7	8	9	10
13.	Self-compassion and metta	1	2	3	4	5	6	7	8	9	10
14.	Group discussions and education	1	2	3	4	5	6	7	8	9	10
15.	The diaries	1	2	3	4	5	6	7	8	9	10
16.	The texts in the workbook	1	2	3	4	5	6	7	8	9	10

CHAPTER 13

FOLLOW-UP SESSION: EACH TIME, BEGINNING ANEW

[Mindfulness] is something that evolves gradually, patiently, over time. How long does this process take? I would say it takes the rest of our lives.

Chordon (2000)

HOW DO we remember to be mindful as parents and persons, and go on with some regular formal or informal meditation practice, after the course has finished? After the 8th session of the course, an intense period of mindfulness practice has come to an end. Parents may have felt relieved, as participating in the Mindful Parenting course may have been a challenge in their busy lives. On the other hand, the weekly group meetings may have functioned as a reminder to practice, formally and informally, and the sharing of home practice in the group may have provided the social pressure needed to keep on practicing. The course itself may have become a main reason to practice.

So where do we find the motivation to keep on practicing once the course has come to an end? One of the functions of the follow-up session is to give participants one more reason to continue practicing during the follow-up period, as they can share once more their experiences of home practice with the group. The fact that there is one more session to come after Session 8 may help them remember some of the practices they have learned in the course, such as checking in regularly, taking a breathing space when under parenting stress, and sitting on their cushion or chair to meditate. A second function of the follow-up session is to boost the skills and attitudes they have learned. In the follow-up session, we repeat some of the practices, we address any questions about the practice that have come up in the meantime, we discuss how to continue practicing without the support of the group, and hear suggestions from other group members about how to continue practicing and to remember to be mind-

341

ful. We introduce a new mindfulness exercise—the mountain meditation for parents—to give participants experience with a different meditation practices, this one using visualization.

Another reason why a follow-up session is helpful is that the farewells are postponed to that session, so that the 8th session's primary theme can be to look back at what has been learned and on how to continue practicing. Saying goodbye is an important theme in any therapy and group. We include two practices that support ending he course and saying farewell—the "wishing well," in which we wish each other well, and the stone meditation, in which the teacher gives a stone as a present to each participant to meditate on.

We had started to organize follow-up sessions initially for research purposes, as we wanted to evaluate whether the effects of the course would be maintained in the absence of the course. But even without formal research taking place, teachers want to know how participants are doing in the longer term and whether what they have learned in the course continues to have an effect on their lives after the course is over. Such formal and informal assessment can be done in a follow-up session.

In mental health settings, participants have come to the course because they have a problem with their child or with parenting. After the 8-week follow-up period, we evaluate with parents whether the Mindful Parenting course has been sufficient in helping them with this problem, as it may take time for the skills learned to affect the parenting and child problems. We can also assess at this time whether they want additional help.

GUIDELINES FOR THE FOLLOW-UP SESSION

Box 13.1. Agenda Follow-up Session
1. Sitting meditation (40 min)
2. In pairs: sharing experiences of the last 8 weeks (10 min)
3. In group: discussing experience of the last 8 weeks practice (20 min)
4. Mountain meditation for parents (10 min)
5. Stone meditation (10 min)
6. Wishing well (10 min)
7. Announcements (silent days, research, etc.) (5 min)
8. Individual evaluation of how group members are doing and further help requests (about 5–10 min per person, depending on group size)

1. SITTING MEDITATION

The group is guided in a regular sitting meditation of about 40 min, including awareness of breath, body, sounds, thoughts, emotions, and choiceless awareness, allowing more silence.

2. SHARING OF EXPERIENCE OF LAST 8 WEEKS (IN PAIRS)

In pairs, group members are invited to share experiences with their practice during the past 8 weeks, in terms of formal and informal meditations and mindful parenting. They can also share how things are going with their children, their families, or themselves. The person speaking may want to start reading aloud the plan as formulated 8 weeks ago. The listener holds back any advice but simply listens. After 5 min, the bell rings and speaker and listener change.

3. GROUP SHARING OF LAST 8 WEEKS

Several themes typically come up during the group sharing. First, some participants may say, full of guilt, that they have not managed to practice at all, but their family life has become much more fulfilling and less stressful. It is important to explore this in more detail. For example, they may do a lot of informal mindfulness and mindful parenting without realizing it. They may notice and enjoy the sky when going to work, be with their children in more attentive ways, be less reactive as parent or partner, etc. Once, a follow-up session was planned after summer holidays. Many group members hardly did any formal meditation, because during summer holidays, families went away, travelling and camping. But one mother did notice that where she normally needed at least a week to get out of her stress and into the holiday, this now occurred almost immediately. A father said that he was much more present with the family than on previous summer holidays, where his focus was to rest outside of the family, whereas now he rested inside of the family. Another mother described how she would get up every morning before the kids would wake up, to take a walk on the beach on her own, and how that helped her be more centered and present with the family the rest of the day. So even if none of the planned meditations have been carried out, participants may discover how they practice mindfulness in their everyday lives, which is all that counts.

For those who have not practiced, it is helpful to explore with an open mind about how that has been for them. For example, have they noticed any effects of not meditating? What attitude do they notice towards themselves about not having done formal practice—one of open curiosity, or judging themselves harshly? The teacher helps participants explore this, with no other agenda in mind than to help participants clarify their own experience and intentions. It is important to remain open to all possibilities, including that a participant may decide for now not to practice. Sometimes it can be helpful to share our own struggles with keeping a regular practice or to note that this is often difficult for many people. In any case, bringing an attitude of kindness, compassion, and acceptance to whatever the participant is experiencing will give the most space for exploration.

Some participants struggle to integrate mindfulness into their daily lives. It may be helpful to build in brief meditations into natural breaks in the day. Also, making the meditations very short may help (sitting on the cushion to follow three breaths), since, as Mark Williams pointed out, making the transition from a busy life to the cushion is more important than the length of practice. It can also help to tune in to what can motivate us to continue practice and to invite participants to make a personal list with reasons to practice, based, for example, on experiences of how they have benefited from the practice.

Life continues, and with each breath, we have another chance to practice mindfulness. It is never too late.

4. MOUNTAIN MEDITATION FOR PARENTS

The mountain meditation can be a helpful meditation for parents in the midst of their busy lives, being critical about what they don't do well as a parent, to realize that all they have to be is a mountain for their family. The mountain reminds us that we can remain stable and balanced in the face of the storms of our family lives and that that is what our children need from us.

Box 13.2. Mountain Meditation for Parents
(This Meditation Is a for Parents Modified Version of the Mountain Meditation a Developed by Jon Kabat-Zinn, 1994)

Take your time to drop into this sitting position, into your body, aware of your breath . . .

When you are ready imagine a mountain . . . . It may be a mountain you have seen in real or on a picture that made a particular impression on you, or a mountain you may have climbed, or a fantasy mountain. . . . What shape does your mountain have, tall, broad, square or pointy . . . imagine how the mountain is firmly grounded in the earth . . . and how it rises towards the sky, high above everything else, strong and steady . . .

Imagine that you are that mountain, your legs and bottom being the foot of the mountain, your arms as the sloping sides of the mountain, your head being the peak, standing firm, the whole body majestic and magnificent, as mountains tend to be.

Imagine the different landscapes on the mountain. For example, at the bottom, the grassy part, then the oak trees, higher up the mountain the pine trees, and even higher only rock. . . . You can also imagine the seasons on the mountain. . . . For example, depending on where your mountain is, winter, with ice and snow. . . . Imagine the skiers coming down from the slopes, animals finding shelter in holes. . . . Spring, the snow melting and coming down in waterfalls and little streams, first green leaves and flowers, rain falling down, animals coming out of their holes, farmers sowing seeds. . . . Summer, the top of your mountain may or may not be white, with people climbing the mountain until the top, further downhill everything is green, full of flowers, it is warm, people are resting in the grass, or picking fruit from the trees, animals are grazing the land. Autumn, leaves turni ng orange and red, falling down, fruits being harvested, thunderstorms and lightening . . .

Whatever season, the mountain is always grounded, rooted in the earth, stands firm, unmoved by storms, rain, and ice. . . . While animals and people are climbing the mountain . . . the mountain stands firm. . . . It has stood there for centuries and will, for centuries . . .

Imagine that you are a mountain in the midst of your busy family life, family members coming to lay down and rest with you, to ask your support, your shelter, to compete or fight with you, to be fed by you . . . and you, standing firm. Knowing that all you need to be a mountain in the family, steady and erect, the mountain that is always there, day and night, summer and winter. . . . Reminding yourself of this mountain when you are home with your family, also in the midst of a family crisis. . . . You can always be that mountain.

5. STONE MEDITATION

The teacher brings stones for all group members (bought in a shop, or, more personal, selected during a mindful walk, make sure there are more than the number of participants, to allow all participants to choose a stone that fits with them, and make sure the stones are washed). The plate with stones goes around the group so that each participant can select a personal stone. Participants are asked to bring full awareness to the process of choosing this personal stone, this stone that is there especially for them. What characteristics make you choose this very stone? Then, a meditation is carried out focusing on the stone, led by the teacher, as we did with the raisin at the start of this course.

Box 13.3. Stone Meditation

Take the stone in your hand to explore it. . . . Look at the stone . . . shape, colors, curves, depths, shiny or matte surfaces. . . . Feel the stone (maybe close your eyes to feel even better); is it hard, soft; what is the shape, size, temperature; are there hard and round surfaces; what happens when you squeeze it in your hands?

You can also bring the stone to your nose to smell it; how does it smell . . . and notice what effect that may have in your body. . . . Now, bring the object to your mouth . . . touch it with your lips . . . if you want, lick it . . . what do you taste? Noticing what happens in your body . . . . What happens to the color where you lick it or make it wet with your hand . . .

Dwell a moment on the thought of where this stone comes from. Imagine that this stone may have been thousands of years on earth, imagine where it came from, how it traveled, to finally arrive here . . And imagine how the stone will continue to exist, long after you have died . . . imagine where it may go . . .

This stone, this personal stone that you selected for yourself, can function as a reminder of what we have practiced, to be mindful persons and mindful parents. Put it on a place where you will see it regularly, to remind you of this course and your process, your path.

6. WISHING WELL

There are many ways to say goodbye. One way that we found helpful is to invite participants to formulate a wish for themselves. We then make a round and the person whose turn it is says aloud a wish for himself or herself. For example, participants may wish to take care of themselves, to accept themselves as they are, to accept their children as they are, to be able to love and receive love, and to continue practicing. When a group member has formulated his or her wish, the rest of the group sends this wish in silence to that group member, wishing him or her well. The teacher may or may not repeat the wish aloud to send it to the participant. For example, a group member says: "I wish to myself that I can enjoy life more," and the teacher looks at him or her and says "I wish to you that you can enjoy life more."

7. INDIVIDUAL EVALUATION

The last hour of the follow-up session can be used for individual evaluations with each of the parents or parent couples. These individual evaluations have three functions: (1) parents may have questions or remarks that they want to share with the teacher personally; (2) an assessment of how the parent is doing himself or herself, how the problem of or with the child (or children) for which the parent came to follow the course has evolved, and how the family is doing may be needed in mental health care contexts to decide whether additional care is needed or not; and (3) individual feedback is given about the results from any assessments that are taken pre- and post-course and at the 8-week follow-up, to inform the participant on the changes as reached according to these assessments.

We ask participants to fill in an evaluation form, modeled after the post-program assessment of the stress reduction program of the Center for Mindfulness of the University of Massachusetts Medical School (Handout 12.3) before the follow-up session. They mail the evaluation form to us well before the follow-up meeting so that we can read it to prepare for the individual evaluation. The teacher also studies the results of the objective assessments, particularly the pattern of change from pre- and posttest and follow-up (see Chapter 3 for examples of measures to be used), in order to be able to inform the parent about his or her progress. An example of a series of graphs of a mother, age 46, of two children, showing changes from pretest to follow-up, is given in Box 13.4.

Box 13.4. Series of Graphs about Changes from Pretest to Follow-up

If this short evaluation gives an indication that further intervention (for parent, child, couple, or family) may be helpful, a longer appointment can be made. Instead of a short individual evaluation, individual appointments can be made with all participants after the follow-up meeting, or only with those who would like to have an individual evaluation.

CHAPTER 14

VOICES OF THE PARENTS: LIFE AFTER THE MINDFUL PARENTING COURSE

"I can set my boundaries better, in a calm manner, I hardly ever blow up! Instead of anger there is much more love and collaboration now. I also see this between the children. It is the harvest of two years' regularly meditating." *(Mother of two children)*

W E OFTEN wonder how participants who have taken a Mindful Parenting course are doing. Do they still meditate, formally or informally, with or without the support of a meditation community or yoga course? Do they remember from time to time things they have learned during the course, such as how to take care of themselves and how to be less reactive in their parenting? And how do they cope with new transitions and challenges in their family life, such as restarting a job, children going to high school, children becoming adolescents fighting authority, their parent dying, a divorce, a new love relationship that the children are ambivalent about? Have they sought further treatment for themselves or their child or not? Some of the parents we see again on one of our mindfulness days that our treatment center *UvA minds* organizes several times a year and which are open for all parents who have taken a Mindful Parenting course. But as these days are in silence, we don't talk with them and don't get verbal feedback. Some of the parents we still see because their children are in therapy at our treatment center or they themselves receive further parent training or support. And on rare occasion, we bump into a parent on an unexpected moment in a completely different context and may have a chat if they initiate it. However, most of the participants of our courses we never see again after the 8-week follow-up.

In order to get an idea about whether parents still do mindfulness practices, we contacted all parents who had finished their Mindful Parenting course 1 year ago (*n* = 41), of whom 35 answered. All but one reported still doing mindfulness-related practices such as body scan, sitting meditation, yoga, or breathing space. They reported practicing daily (14), weekly (13), monthly (6), or once every 3 months (1). The average duration of their meditation practice was 15–30 min (20), shorter than 15 min (9), or longer than 30 min (6). Thus, most parents continue with mindfulness practices long after the course has finished.

When we finished this book, we contacted all participants who had previously taken a Mindful Parenting course at *UvA minds* to ask them to send us a short report about how they were doing, and what they felt were the long-term effects of the Mindful Parenting course on their lives, if any. For some, the Mindful Parenting course had ended only months ago, but for most it was a year or several years ago. Here is a summary of their stories.

MOTHER OF TWO CHILDREN:

Mindfulness has especially taught me that everything is allowed to be there: thus also anger, rage. In the Buddhist monasteries where I once attended retreats, I sensed pressure that these feelings weren't allowed. But I came to the Mindful Parenting course because I sometimes burst out in anger towards my children in times of stress, and sometimes completely lost my temper. Because I learned to just observe this, there was room for my anger, it was allowed to be there, I got the tools to get started. Mindfulness brought me acceptance of the anger in myself, I don't condemn myself anymore. Therefore the eruptions become less frequent.

Meanwhile, after the Mindful Parenting course had ended, I've had therapy and I've discovered the cause of my anger. I processed an old trauma, and because of this the stress has reduced.

I walk mindfully on a daily basis, and meditate every month during the so called "city lights evenings," an organized group event. Mindfulness especially brought me the acceptance of my own anger, and my own imperfections. Maybe this doesn't make me a better parent, but it makes me a more humane one.

MOTHER WHO TOOK THE COURSE ALONG WITH FATHER; THEY HAVE TWO CHILDREN:

I thought the Mindful Parenting was a good course because I got more understanding of why it often goes wrong at our home. The four of us (father, mother, two adolescent sons, now 13 and 15) tend to react to every action of another family member. *Because of the course I've learned to not always react. To never do this anymore is impossible because it is in our personalities, apparently. Count till ten, or walk away to calm yourself first. This is quite difficult for my husband and myself.*

The first year I've been able to sustain meditating almost every morning when the kids went to school, and then doing yoga for about 15 to 20 minutes. The past year it crept in that I only did this one to two times a week. I did join a yoga center where I went two times a week. Now I've started up again meditating in the morning and do yoga afterwards. Mindfulness didn't really change our behavior, but we are more aware of things. We have more understanding of how our behavior influences the behavior of the children. But mainly it was very nice to do this course together.

MOTHER OF TWO CHILDREN:

For me, mindfulness is a new way of living. Meditation has made me more balanced and for me this is often a good beginning of the day.

I try to judge and condemn less quickly and I have a greater openness towards things that happen. I take the losses and am grateful for the gifts. Because of this I feel that I'm on the right track. Once in a few weeks three of us who participated in the Mindful Parenting course come together; we meditate and exchange experiences. It is a diverse group, but we recognize each other's dilemmas and we all experience the value of meditating and being in the here and now.

I'm very grateful for having been able to do this course. It expanded and enriched my world. It had a definite impact on my children and the atmosphere in our house.

FATHER OF TWO CHILDREN:

Mindful parenting has completely changed the way I look at myself, my parenthood, my work and my life. The greatest good is that I realize that my thoughts, feelings and perceptions of a situation are only MY experience of reality, and that these thoughts, feelings and perceptions are not the truth.

For example, my child gets a low grade at school, she is watching television and I say something about this, then she gets angry. My automatic response is to connect the events, low grade, television, rude. What I see is a lazy, disinterested, rude child. Previously I would respond much quicker to this idea, in an angry manner. But I also know that my child has trouble concentrating, the hormones are running through her body and that she is trying her best to "survive." I react differently to this situation when I look at her in this way.

Reacting automatically comes down to reacting angrily in the afternoon to a child who only becomes more and more contrary and sad. At night I'm sorry because I haven't seen the other side.

Because of mindfulness I see the automatisms in myself and others much better and I learned to deal with them. Actually it is the "Pietje Bell" method [Note: A famous Dutch child novel about a naughty, wild boy]; when you want to hit somebody, first count till 10.

I still meditate on a daily basis, I can see my own shortcomings and the shortcomings of others with much more kindness and sometimes I can just let things be.

Thank you very much for organizing all this.

MOTHER OF TWO CHILDREN:

On your request I'm sending you an impression of my experiences with mindfulness, how mindfulness improved the quality of my life and how mindfulness improved my family.

Two years ago I signed up for the course Mindful Parenting because I wanted to learn how to deal with stress better. I constantly felt hounded up. I set the bar very high and had difficulties with planning and structuring my life. Frustrations and anxieties were always there. I was quickly agitated and often lost my temper, at my children and husband. I exploded. I thought that was awful. In particular that my behavior was so capricious and so unpredictable towards my children. This was the main reason for me to search for help. A friend of mine and my yoga teacher told me about mindfulness, and I suspected that this actually could be a breakthrough. And it was.

I can easier "grasp" undermining thoughts and the feelings that belong to them and put these thoughts and feelings beside me, instead of running away with them and falling into automatic reaction patterns. What a lightness arises then, I feel calmer and begin to sail more on my own compass. This changed attitude towards myself I see reflected in my attitude towards my children. I feel more space to adjust to their needs and where they come from. I can set my boundaries better, in a calm manner, I hardly ever blow up! Instead of anger there is much more love and collaboration now. I also see this between the children. It is the harvest of two years regularly meditating; sitting mediation, the three minute breathing space, many informal exercises, and in particular the body scan.

MOTHER OF ONE CHILD:

The most important gift I received from the course Mindful Parenting in 2009, was to realize that there was no need to get angry with what I think as parent that my kid "should" be doing or behaving like. To accept things as they are, as hard as sometimes it can be. Knowing everything is a process and it will take the time it takes. No need to belittle yourself for not being the parent you wish you were.

What I have found is that there are no recipes for parenting. That's why being open to what goes on and hopefully keeping ourselves calm, are very useful tools to establish harmony in our relationships, specially at home.

What I find amazing is that kids are like sponges. They are so sensitive, that they reflect our changes whether they are positive or negative.

My life has proven that even if I carried a heavy load due to my past, I can raise healthy kids when I have consciousness of what's happening.

I have more confidence in myself and enjoy my life more than ever. I am very proud of my son and myself so far.

And even now that my son is almost an adult, I see how my improvements continue affecting his life for good, and his wellbeing comes back to me and spreads around.

MOTHER OF TWO CHILDREN:

At the beginning, there was a feeling of doubt whether this course would help me or not. But then, after joining the first meeting I liked the idea of going "inside" when we did meditation because it is the same as what I believe in, my faith. I am a Muslim and according to my religion I believe that to be peaceful we have to go inside. So, this course reminds me regularly to go inside, to make my mind zero and to try to do everything in 'being mode'.

Actually, I had heard this idea many years ago, but it's difficult to do after living in the Netherlands especially after I had many problems that related to culture shock and joblessness issues. I gave up my career as a medical doctor in my homeland, and I couldn't work here, in the Netherlands as a GP. When my children were toddlers, I was very busy with them so it didn't create many problems, but after they went to primary school, became more independent and didn't need me very often anymore, the problem started. I was stressed, became angry very easily, and argued a lot with my children. The course reminded me again to seek happiness and peaceful feelings from inside. I did the meditation and combined it with the way I meditate in my religion. It worked very well as I could reduce my anger and became calmer. My relationship and communication with my children also became better. Sometimes I still do the meditation, although the way I do it is not exactly the same as at the course because to be honest, I forgot. So I do it as my faith suggests, but I think the main point is still the same: to try to go "inside" every day even if it's only three minutes a day. I think the way we use it doesn't really matter, as long as we keep going "inside" and sometimes make our mind zero, then we will get the same benefit.

We would like to end with one mother's process description soon after the course ended. She had brought as her object to the 8th session a picture of herself as an infant, with her mother, who died when she was very young.

DOING INSTEAD OF KNOWING

Immediately in the first lesson my "first lesson" is clear. This is about training and not knowledge. First meditating, instead of the standard introduction round. And not a list of books with theory: no, even more so, you get that only after the training. Otherwise you might go read instead of practice, is the message. Well, that is true for me, I'm a "head on a stick" and fond of knowledge. But that is not the focus now, that becomes clear right away. I tell myself to practice well. The intention is there.

NOW INSTEAD OF LATER

I can practice at many moments. Make time, preferably now rather than later, because before I know the day is over.

FEELING INSTEAD OF THINKING

As said, I'm a head on a stick. I dwell on everything. But two weeks of almost daily doing the body scan, for the rest of the day made me—if I wanted it or not—aware of my body. Of how I feel, I see myself being busy and think: "Aha, this is how others see me." I see it, I feel it, but I cannot change gears.

TAKING CARE OF MYSELF, LISTENING TO MY BODY

Suddenly it went automatically. I had worked all night on a deadline, with a headache that took possession of my entire head, but I had to go on. At 6 in the morning it was done, I switched off the computer. My daughter came out of her bed, I went in. In the past I would have gone straight to bed, but now I took a shower first. I stood under the shower for a quarter of an hour with full attention, I felt the water on my head, felt how little by little the pain washed away.

THAT UNCONDITIONALLY LOVING MYSELF DOES NOT WORK (YET)

It happened in one of the first lessons. The practice was: take one of your children in mind and think about three things you are really grateful for, that you savor.

Well, that was easy: initiating, social, kind. And now think about three things you are grateful for in yourself. Nothing came, not a single thought. And from nothing it came up and I could not suppress it; tears, sadness, a tight throat. Well, that was clear. I found nothing to be grateful for in myself. Yes, if I thought longer, but that came from far. Sadness from a far past, I knew that, but that it would be brought up like this I had not expected. Yes, I knew that it gets "triggered" at impossible moments and tries to break through barriers, mostly with the consequence that I become angry.

A few weeks later we did our first loving kindness meditation. I had to take someone in mind who loves me unconditionally. It was my second mother, the woman who raised me. Last Christmas I went angrily from the dinner table when the room was full of visitors. I cannot recall the precise reason, but I did not think of that. I thought about how she came to me and held me, stroked my hair, without saying anything, and listened. While seeing this image, again sadness came up, tears streamed over my cheeks, and my throat became tight. I thought: "I want a handkerchief," and the sadness disappeared. But as soon as I go to this image, the wave of sorrow comes back in all intensity. I know what it is, that sadness, that fear. Someone who loves me unconditionally, this I find really scary, deep inside. The first one who meant that to me, died. In this way—with gentle attention—I came directly to my "old sadness." That is a step in the right direction—I know.

BEING MY OWN MOTHER FIRST

In a way I knew that the problems that I had with my eldest daughter were caused by her "triggering" me. The parent training that I took previously, "Listening to children" was helpful, but I could not bring it into practice. I had tried to process my old sorrow: I've talked a lot about it, I read, I analyzed, I went into psychotherapy, and came some way. But the basis was unreachable. No psychologist, no new mother, no patient husband, could solve it for me, could give me what my mother was not able to give me when I was young: unconditional love. The only one who can do that, is me. Only when I can be my own mother, I can be a mother for my children. I have learned in the Mindful Parenting course how I can be my own mother.

Six months later, she wrote about her longer-term process:

I can proceed with the tools I have now. The progress I made in the 8 weeks of the course is not continuing at the same pace. Old habits fight back hard. But I know that I have the key in my hands and that it is an issue of doing. I don't meditate daily but about three times a week, I am still looking for something to help me continue meditating.

Four months after the follow-up meeting I went to my first "silent day" [our note: at UvA minds we invite all parents who once attended a Mindful Parenting course to join a mindfulness day twice a year], led by Joke Hellemans. I came back superbly rested. And, I realized only the day after, this immediately had an effect on my environment. My eldest daughter crawled nicely into my arms, while she usually keeps some distance. "Yes, that is also caused by you," my husband confirmed. This is another reason to restart practicing more intensively and to simply do more often that, what I learned in Mindful Parenting.

—Esther Deerenberg, mother of two children

REFERENCES

Abidin, R. R. (1983). *Parenting stress index manual.* Charlottesville: Pediatric Psychology Press. Dutch translation: De Brock, A., Vermulst, A. A., Gerris, J. R. M., & Abidin, R. R. (1992). *Nijmeegse Ouderlijke Stress Index. Handleiding experimentele versie.* Lisse: Swets & Zeitlinger.

Achenbach, T. M., & Rescorla, L.A. (2001). *Manual for the ASEBA School-Age Forms & Profiles.* Burlington: University of Vermont, Research Center for Children, Youth, and Families.

Achenbach, T. M., & Rescorla, L. A. (2003). *Manual for the ASEBA Adult Forms & Profiles.* Burlington: University of Vermont, Research Center for Children, Youth, and Families.

Allen, J. P., Hauser, S. T., Bell, K. L., & O'Connor, T. G. (1994). Longitudinal assessment of autonomy and relatedness in adolescent-family interactions as predictors of adolescent ego development and self-esteem. *Child Development, 65,* 179–194.

Allen, J. P., Moore, C., Kuperminc, G., & Bell, K. (1998). Attachment and adolescent psychosocial functioning. *Child Development, 69,* 1406–1419.

Arnold, D. S., O'Leary, S. G., Wolff, L. S., & Acker, M. M. (1993). The parenting scale: A measure of dysfunctional parenting in discipline situations. *Psychological Assessments, 5,* 137–144.

Baer, R. A., Smith, G. T., Hopkins, J., Krietemeyer, J., & Toney, L. (2006). Using self-report assessment methods of explore facets of mindfulness. *Assessment, 13,* 27–45.

Baer, R. A., Smith G. T., Lykins, E., Button, D., Krietemeyer, J., Sauer, S., et al. (2008). Construct validity of the five facet mindfulness questionnaire in meditating and nonmeditating samples. *Assessment, 15,* 329–342.

Bailey, K. G., & Wood, H. E. (1998). Evolutionary kinship therapy: Basic principles and treatment implications. *British Journal of Medical Psychology, 71,* 509–523.

Bardacke, N. (2012). *Mindful birthing: Training the mind, body and heart for childbirth and beyond.* New York: Harper Collins.

Barnhofer, T., Chittka, T., Nightingale, H., Visser, C., & Crane, C. (2010). State effects of two forms of meditation on prefrontal EEG Asymmetry in previously depressed individuals. *Mindfulness, 1,* 21–27.

Batchelor, M., p.c., March, 2009.

Batchelor, S. (1997). *Buddhism without beliefs. A contemporary guide to awakening.* London: Bloomsbury.

Batchelor, M. (2001). *Meditation for life.* Somerville, MA: Wisdom Publications.

Batchelor, M. (2007). *Let go: A buddhist guide to breaking free of habits.* Somerville: Wisdom publications.

Beck, A., Freeman, A., & Davis, D. D. (2004). *Cognitive therapy of personality disorders.* New York: Guilford.

Belsky, J. (1984). The determinants of parenting: a process model. *Child Development, 55*, 83–96.

Belsky, J. (1999). Interactional and contextual determinants of attachment security. In J. S. P. R. Cassidy (Ed.), *Handbook of attachment: Theory, research, and clinical applications.* New York: Guilford.

Blackmore, S. (2009). *Ten Zen questions.* Oxford: One World Publications.

Bly, R. (1971). *The Kabir book.* Boston: Beacon Press.

Bodden, H. M., Bögels, S. M., Nauta, M. H., De Haan, E., Ringrose, J., Appelboom, C., et al. (2008). Child versus family cognitive-behavioral therapy in clinically anxious youth: An efficacy and partial effectiveness study. *Journal of the American Academy of Child & Adolescent Psychiatry, 47*, 1384–1394.

Bögels, S. M. (2006). Task concentration training versus applied relaxation for social phobic patients with fear of blushing, trembling and sweating. *behavior Research and Therapy, 44*, 1199–1210.

Bögels, S. M., & Brechman-Toussaint, M. (2006). Family factors in the etiology and maintenance of childhood anxiety: Attachment, family functioning, rearing, and parental cognitive biases. *Clinical Psychology Review, 26*, 834–856.

Bögels, S. M., Hellemans, J., Van Deursen, S., Römer, M., & Van der Meulen, R. (2013). Mindful Parenting in mental health care: effects on parental and child psychopathology, parental stress, parenting, co-parenting and marital functioning. *Mindfulness*, doi:1007/s12671-013-0209-7.

Bögels, S. M., Hoogstad, B., van Dun, L., de Schutter, S., & Restifo, K. (2008). Mindfulness training for adolescents with behavior disorders and their parents. *Behavioral and Cognitive Psychotherapy, 36*, 193–209.

Bögels, S. M., Lehtonen, A., & Restifo, K. (2010). Mindful parenting in mental health care. *Mindfulness, 1*, 107–120.

Bögels, S. M., & Mansell, W. (2006). Attention processes in the maintenance and treatment of social phobia: Hypervigilance, avoidance and self-focused attention. *Clinical Psychology Review, 24*, 827–856.

Bögels, S. M., Mulkens, S., & De Jong, P. J. (1997). Task-concentration training and fear of blushing. *Clinical Psychology and Psychotherapy, 4*, 251–258.

Bögels, S. M., & Perotti, E. C. (2011). Do fathers know best? A formal model of the paternal influence on childhood social anxiety. *Journal of Child and Family Studies, 20*, 171–182.

Bögels, S. M., & Phares, V. (2008). Fathers' role in the etiology, prevention and treatment of child anxiety: A review and new model. *Clinical Psychology Review, 28*, 539–528.

Bögels, S. M., & Van Melick, M. (2004). The relationship between child-report, parent self-report, and partner report of perceived parental rearing behaviors and anxiety in children and parents. *Personality and Individual Differences, 37,* 1583–1596.

Bowlby, J. (1971). *Attachment and loss, vol. 1: Attachment.* Harmondsworth: Penguin Books.

Bowlby, J. (1977). The making and breaking of affectional bonds I. Aetiology and psychopathology in the light of attachment theory. *British Journal of Psychiatry, 130,* 201–210.

Bretherton, I. (1992). The origins of attachment theory: John Bowlby and Mary Ainsworth. *Development Psychology, 28*(5), 759–775.

Brody, G. H., & Forehand, R. (1985). The efficacy of parent training with martially distressed and nondistressed mothers: A multimethod assessment. *Behavior Research and Therapy, 23,* 291–296.

Burnett, R. (2009). Mindfulness in schools. Learning lessons from the adults—Secular and Buddhist Report.

Campbell-Sills, L., Barlow, D. H., Brown, T. A., & Hofmann, S. G. (2006). Effects of suppression and acceptance on emotional responses of individuals with anxiety and mood disorders. *behavior Research and Therapy, 44,* 1251–1263.

Carter, S. (1998). Neuroendorcine perspectives on social attachment and love. *Psychoneuroendocrinology, 23*(8), 779–818.

Carter, C. S. (2006). Biological perspectives on social attachment and bonding. In C. S. Carter, L. Ahnert, K. E. Grossmann, S. B. Hrdy, M. E. Lamb, S. W. Porges and N. Sachser, Eds.) Attachment and Bonding A New Synthesis. The MIT Press.

Chang, J. J., Halpern, C. T., & Kaufman, J. S. (2007). Maternal depressive symptoms, father's involvement, and the trajectories of child problem behaviors in a US national sample. *Archives of Pediatrics & Adolescent, 161*(7), 697–703.

Cheron, D. M., Eichenreich, J. T., & Pincus, D. B. (2009). Assessment of parental experiential avoidance in a clinical sample of children with anxiety disorders. *Child Psychiatry and Human Development, 40,* 383–403.

Chodron, P. (2000). *When things fall apart: Heart advice for difficult times* (p. 143). Boston: Shambala Publications.

Coatsworth, J. D., Duncan, L., Greenberg, M., & Nix, R. (2010). Changing parents mindfulness, child management skills and relationship quality with their youth: Results from a randomized pilot intervention trial. *Journal of Child and Family Studies, 19,* 203–217.

Cohen, J. (1988). *Statistical power analysis for the behavioral sciences.* Hillsdale, NJ: Erlbaum.

Cohen, S., Kessler, R. C., & Gordon, L. U. (Eds.). (1997). *Measuring stress: a guide for health and social scientists.* New York: Oxford University Press.

Coyne, L. W., & Wilson, K. G. (2004). The role of cognitive fusion in impaired parenting: An RFT analysis. *International Journal of Psychology and Psychological Therapy, 4,* 468–486.

Crane, R. S., Kuyken, W., Williams, J. M. G., Hastings, R. P., Cooper, L., & Fennell,

M. J. V. (2012). Competence in teaching mindfulness-based courses: concepts, development and assessment. *Mindfulness, 3*(1), 76–84.

Crnic, K. A., Gaze, C., & Hoffman, C. (2005). Cumulative parenting stress across the preschool period: Relations to maternal parenting and child behavior at 5 years. *Infant and Child Development, 14*, 117–132.

Cummings, E. M. (1994). Marital conflict and children's functioning. *Social Development, 3*, 16–36.

Cushman, A. (2001). Mothering as meditation practice. *Tricycle, The Buddhist Review*, Fall issue, p. 104.

Davidson, R. J., & Begley, S. (2012). *The emotional life of your brain*. New York: Hudson Street Press.

Davidson, R. J., Kabat-Zinn, J., Schumacher, J., Rosenkranz, M., Muller, D., Santorelli, S. F., et al. (2003). Alternations in brain and immune function produced by mindfulness meditation. *Psychosomatic Medicine, 65*, 564–570.

De Brock, A., Vermulst, A. A., Gerris, J. R. M., & Abidin, R. R. (1992). Nijmeegse Ouderlijke Stress Index. Handleiding experimentele versie [Nijmeegse Ouderlijke Stress Index. Manual]. Lisse: Swets & Zeitlinger.

De Bruin, E. I., Topper, M., Muskens, J. G. A. M., Bögels, S. M., & Kamphuis, J. H. (2012). Psychometric properties of the five facets mindfulness questionnaire (FFMQ) in a meditating and a non-meditating sample. *Assessment, 19*, 187–197.

De Bruin, E. I., Zijlstra, B. J. H., Geurtzen, N., Van Zundert, R. M. P., Van de Weijer-Bergsma, E., Hartman, E. E., Duncan, L. & Bögels, S. M. (2013). Mindful Parenting assessed further: Psychometric properties of the Dutch version of the Interpersonal Mindfulness in Parenting scale (IM-P). *Mindfulness*, doi: 10.1007/s12671-012-0160-4.

Deater-Deckard, K. (1998). Parenting stress and child adjustment: Some old hypotheses and new questions. *Clinical Psychology: Science and Practice, 5*, 314–32.

Diamond, G. S., & Liddle, H. A. (1999). Transforming negative parent-adolescent interactions: From impasse to dialogue. *Family Process, 38*, 5–26.

Diamond, G. S., Reis, B. F., Diamond, G. M., Siqueland, L., & Isaacs, L. (2002). Attachment-based family therapy for depressed adolescents: a treatment development study. *Journal of the American Academy of Child & Adolescent Psychiatry, 41*(10), 1190–1196.

Diamond, G. S., & Siqueland, L. (1998). Emotions, attachment and the relational reframe. *Journal of Structural and Strategic Therapy, 17*, 36–50.

Diamond, G. S., Wintersteen, M. B., Brown, G. K., Diamond, G. M., Gallop, R., Shelef, K., et al. (2010). Attachment-based family therapy for adolescents with suicidal ideation: A randomized controlled trial. *Journal of the American Academy of Child and Adolescent Psychiatry, 49*, 122–131.

Duncan, L. G. (2007). Assessment of mindful parenting among parents of early adolescents: Development and validation of the Interpersonal Mindfulness in Parenting Scale. Unpublished dissertation.

Duncan, L. G., Coatsworth, J. D., & Greenber, M. T. (2009). A model of mindful parenting: Implications for parent–child relationships and prevention research. *Clinical Child & Family Psychology Review, 12*, 255–270.

Egeland, B., Jacobvitz, D., & Sroufe, L. A. (1988). Breaking the cycle of abuse. *Child Development, 59*, 1080–1088.

Egeland, B., Jacobvitz, D., et al. (1987). Intergenerational continuity of abuse. In R. J. Gelles & J. B. Lancaster (Eds.), *Child abuse and neglect: Biosocial dimensions* (pp. 255–76). New York: Aldine de Gruyter.

Emmons, R. A. (2007). *Thanks!: How the new science of gratitude can make you happier.* New York: Houghton Mifflin.

Feinberg, M. E., Solmeyer, A. R., & MacHale, S. M. (2012). The third rail of family systems: Sibling relationships, mental and behavioral health, and preventive intervention in childhood and adolescence. *Clinical Child & Family Psychology Review, 14*, 43–57.

Feldman, C. (2001). *The Buddhist path to simplicity: Spiritual practice for everyday life.* London: HarperCollins.

Ferdinand, R. F., Verhulst, F. C., & Wiznitzer, M. (1995). Continuity and change of self-reported problem behaviors from adolescence into young adulthood. *Journal of the American Academy of Child and Adolescent Psychiatry, 34*, 680–690.

Figes, K., & Zimmerman, J. (1998). *Life after birth. What even your friends won't tell you about motherhood.* New York: St. Martin's Press.

Firestone, P., & Witt, J. E. (1982). Characteristics of families completing and prematurely discontinuing a behavioral parent-training program. *Journal of Pediatric Psychology, 7*, 209–222.

Forehand, R., Furey, W. M., & McMahon, R. J. (1984). The role of maternal distress in a parent training program to modify child non-compliance. *behavioral Psychotherapy, 12*, 93–108.

Germer, C. K. (2009). *The mindful path to self-compassion.* New York: Guilford.

Gerris, J. R. M., Vermulst, A. A., Boxtel, D. A. A. M. van, Janssens, J. M. A. M., Zutphen, R. A. H. van & Felling, A. J. A. (1993). *Parenting in Dutch families. A representative description of Dutch family life in terms of validated concepts representing characteristics of parents, children, the family as a system and parental socio-cultural value orientations.* Nijmegen: University of Nijmegen, Institute of Family Studies.

Gilbert, P., p.c., June 23, 2012.

Gilbert, P. (2009). *The compassionate mind. A new approach to life's challenges.* London: Constable and Robinson.

Ginott, H. G. (1965). *Between parent and child.* New York: Three Rivers Press.

Goetz, J. L., Keltner, D., & Simon-Thomas, E. (2010). Compassion: An evolutionary analysis and empirical review. *Psychological Bulletin, 136*(3), 351–374.

Hanson, R. (2009). *The practical neuroscience of Buddha's brain: Happiness, love, and wisdom.* Oakland: New Harbinger.

Hawkes, K., O'Connell, J. F., & Blurton Jones, N. G. (1989). Hardworking Hadza grandmothers. In V. Standen & R. A. Foley (Eds.), *Comparative sociology: The behavioral ecology of humans and other mammals.* London: Basil Blackwell.

Hawkes, K., O'Connell, J. F., & Blurton Jones, N. G. (2001). Hazda meat sharing. *Evolution and Behavior, 22*, 113–132.

Hawkes, K., O'Connell, J. F., Blurton Jones, N. G., Alvarez, H., & Charnov, E. L. (1998). Grandmothering, menopause, and the evolution of human life histories. *Proceedings of the National Academy of Sciences, 95*, 1336–1339.

Hewlett, B. S. (2004). Fathers in forager, farmer and pastoral cultures. In M. Lamb (Ed.), *The role of the father in child development* (4th ed.). New York: Wiley.

Hrdy, S. B. (1999). *Mother nature. Maternal instincts and how they shape the human species.* New York: Ballantine Books.

Hrdy, S. B. (2009). *Mothers and others. The evolutionary origins of mutual understanding.* Cambridge: Harvard University Press.

Johnson, S. (2008). *Hold me tight.* New York: Little, Brown, and Company.

Kabat-Zinn, J. (1990). *Full catastrophe living.* New York: Bantam Doubleday Dell.

Kabat-Zinn, J. (1994). *Wherever you go, there you are.* New York: Hyperion. 248 p.

Kabat-Zinn, M., & Kabat-Zinn, J. (1997). *Everyday blessings: The inner work of mindful parenting.* New York: Hyperion.

Kabat-Zinn, M. & Kabat-Zinn, J., p.c., September 2012.

Karreman, A., van Tuijl, C., van Aken, M. A. G., & Dekovic, M. (2008). Parenting, coparenting, and effortful control in preschoolers. *Journal of Family Psychology, 22*, 30–40.

Knausgard, K. O. (2012). *My struggle. Book one.* Brooklyn: Archipelago Books.

Konner, M. (2010). *The evolution of childhood: Relationships, emotion, mind.* Cambridge: Harvard University Press.

Kuyken, W., Watkins, E., Holden, E., White, K., Taylor, R. S., Byford, S., et al. (2010). How does mindfulness-based cognitive therapy work? *Behavior Research and Therapy, 48*, 1105–1112.

Lama, D., & Cutler, H. (1998). *The art of happiness: A handbook for living.* New York: Riverhead Books.

Lamb, M. (Ed.). (2003). *The role of the father in child development* (4th ed.). New York: Wiley.

Lane, R. (1957). The beginnings of the modern Japanese novel: Kana-zōshi. *Harvard Journal of Asiatic Studies, 20*, 644–701.

LeDoux, J. (1996). *The emotional brain: The mysterious underpinnings of emotional life.* New York: Simon and Schuster.

Majdandzic, M., Vente, W., Feinman, M., Aktar, E., & Bögels, S. M. (2012). Coparenting and parental and child anxiety: A review. *Clinical Child and Family Psychology Review, 15*, 28–42.

Margraf, J. (2012). Presentation at the *Conference of the German network of psychotherapy research*, Hannover, 12–14 April 2012.

Marlowe, F. (2000). Paternal investment and the human mating system. *behavioral processes, 51*, 45–61.

McHale, J. P. (1997). Overt and covert coparenting processes in the family. *Family Process, 36*, 183–201.

Meppelink, R., de Bruin, E.I., & Bögels, S.M. (in prep.). The effects of mindful parenting in child psychiatry on parental stress, parental experiential avoidance, parental mindfulness, and general mindfulness.

Miller, A. L., Rathus, J. H., Linehan, M. M., & Swenson, C. R. (2007). *Dialectical behavior therapy with suicidal adolescents.* New York: Guilford.

Möller, E., Majdandzic, M., de Vente, W., & Bögels, S. M. (2013). The evolutionary basis of sex differences in parenting and its relationship with child anxiety in Western societies. *Journal of Experimental Psychopathology, 4,* 88–117.

Mulkens, S., Bögels, S. M., De Jong, J., & Louwers, J. (2001). Fear of blushing: Effects of task concentration training versus exposure in vivo on fear and physiology. *Journal of Anxiety Disorders, 15,* 413–432.

Najman, J. M., Williams, G. M., Nikles, J., Spence, S., Bor, W., O'Callaghan, M., et al. (2001). Bias influencing maternal reports of child behavior and emotional state. *Social Psychiatry and Psychiatric Epidemiology, 36,* 186–194.

Napthali, S. (2003). *Buddhism for mothers: A calm approach to caring for yourself and your children.* Crow's Nest, NSW: Allen & Unwin.

Neff, K. (2011). *Self-compassion.* New York: William Morrow.

Neff, K. D., & Germer, C. K. (2013). A pilot study and randomized controlled trial of the mindful self-compassion program. *Journal of Clinical Psychology, 69,* 1, 28–44.

Nelson, P. (1977). *There's a hole in my sidewalk.* Los Angeles: Popular Library.

Nhat Hanh, T. *Anger: Wisdom for cooling the flames.* New York: Riverhead Books.

Nhat Hanh, T. (2009). *Happiness.* Berkeley, CA: Parallel Press.

Nhat Hanh, T. (2010). *Reconciliation: Healing the inner child.* Berkeley, CA: Parallax Press.

NICHD Early Child Care Research Network. (2003). Early child care and mother-child interaction from 36 months through first grade. *Infant Behavior and Development, 26,* 345–370.

Owens, E. B., Hinshaw, S. P., Kraemer, H. C., Arnold, L. E., Abikoff, H. B., Cantwell, D. P., et al. (2003). Which treatment for whom for ADHD? Moderators of treatment response in the MTA. *Journal of Consulting and Clinical Psychology, 71,* 540–552.

Paquette, D. (2004). Theorizing the father-child relationship: Mechanisms and developmental outcomes. *Human Development, 47,* 193–219.

Prinzie, P., Onghena, P., & Hellinckx, W. (2007). Reexamining the parenting scale. *European Journal of Psychological Assessment, 23,* 24–31.

Reisinger, J. J., Frangia, G. W., & Hoffman, E. H. (1976). Toddler management training: Generalization and marital status. *Journal of Behavior Therapy and Experimental Psychiatry, 7,* 335–340.

Restifo, K., & Bögels, S. M. (2009). Family risk factors for youth depression: A family systems integration and treatment model. *Clinical Psychology Review, 29,* 294–316.

Reyno, S. M., & McGrath, P. J. (2006). Predictors of parent training efficacy for child externalizing behavior problems—a meta-analytic review. *Journal of Child Psychology and Psychiatry, 47,* 99–111.

Salzberg, S. (2006). *Loving kindness: The revolutionary art of happiness.* Boston: Shambhala Classics.

Sapolsky, R. M. (1994). *Why zebras don't get ulcers.* New York: St. Martin's Griffin.

Segal, Z., Williams, J., & Teasdale, J. (2002; 2012). *Mindfulness-based cognitive therapy for depression. A new approach to preventing relapse.* New York: Guilford.

Siegel, D. J., & Hartzell, M. (2003). *Parenting from the inside out.* New York: Penguin.

Smyke, A. T., Zeanah, C. H., Fox, N. A., Nelson, C. A., & Guthrie, D. (2010). Placement in foster care enhances quality of attachment among young institutionalized children. *Child Development, 81*(1), 212–223.

Sonuga-Barke, E. J. (2010). Editorial: 'It's the environment stupid!' On epigenetics, programming and plasticity in child mental health. *Journal of Child Psychology and Psychiatry, 51*, 113–115.

Sonuga-Barke, E. J. S., Daley, D., & Thompson, M. (2002). Does maternal ADHD reduce the effectiveness of parent training for preschool children's ADHD? *Journal of the American Academy of Child and Adolescent Psychiatry, 41*, 696–702.

Sroufe, L. A., Carlson, E. A., Levy, A. K., & Egeland, B. (1999). Implications of attachment theory for developmental psychopathology. *Development & Psychopathology, 11*(1), 1–13.

Stams, G. J. M., Juffer, F., & van IJzendoorn, M. H. (2002). Maternal sensitivity, infant attachment, and temperament in early childhood predict adjustment in middle childhood: The case of adopted children and their biologically unrelated parents. *Developmental Psychology, 38*, 806–821.

Tanahashi, K. (1995). *Moon in a dewdrop. Writings of Zen Master Dogen.* New York: New Point Press.

Taylor, S. E., Cousino Klein, L., Lewis, B. P., Gruenewald, T. L., Gurung, R. A. R., & Updegraff, J. A. (2000). Biobehavioral responses to stress in Females: Tend-and-befriend, not fight-or-flight. *Psychological Review, 107*, 411–429.

Teasdale, J., Segal, Z., & Kabat-Zinn, J. (2007). *The mindful way through depression. Freeing yourself from chronic unhappiness.* New York: Guilford.

Theodoridou, A., Rowe, A. C., Penton-Voak, I. S., & Rogers, P. J. (2009). Oxytocin and social perception: Oxytocin increases perceived facial trustworthiness and attractiveness. *Hormones and Behavior, 56*, 128–132.

Tomasello, M. (2008). *Origins of human communication.* Cambridge, MA: MIT Press.

Van IJzendoorn, M. H. (1995). Adult attachment representations, parental responsiveness, and infant attachment: A meta-analysis on the predictive validity of the adult attachment interview. *Psychological Bulletin, 117*, 387–403.

Van Ijzedoorn, M., Sagi, A., & Lambermon, M. (1992). The multiple caretaker paradox: Data from Holland and Israel. In R. C. Pianta (ed), *Beyond the parents: The role of other adults in children's lives* (pp. 5–24). New Directions for Child Development 57. San Francisco: Jossey Bass.

Verhoeven, M., Bögels, S. M., & Van der Bruggen, C. (2011). Unique roles of mothering and fathering in child anxiety: Moderation by child's age and gender. *Journal of Child and Family Studies* (online).

Verhulst, F. C., Van der Ende, J., & Koot, H. M. (1996). *Dutch Manual for the CBCL/4–*

18. Rotterdam: Afdeling kinder-en Jeugdpsychiatrie, Sophia Kinderziekenhuis/ Academisch Ziekenhuis Rotterdam, Erasmus Universiteit Rotterdam. Video downloaded from www.youtube.com/watch?v=vJG698U2Mvo

Webster-Stratton, C. (1985). Predictors of treatment outcome in parent training for conduct disordered children. *Behavior Therapy, 16,* 223–243.

Webster-Stratton, C. (1990a). Stress: A potential disruptor of parent perceptions and family interactions. *Journal of Clinical Child Psychology, 19,* 302–312.

Webster-Stratton, C. (1990b). Long-term follow-up of families with young conduct problem children: from preschool to grade school. *Journal of Clinical Child Psychology, 19,* 144–149.

Williams, M., & Penham, D. (2011). *Mindfulness: A practical guide to finding peace in a frantic world.* London: Piatkus.

Williams, M., p.c., December 16, 2011.

Williams, M., Teasdale, J., Segal, Z., & Kabat-Zinn, J. (2007). *The mindful way through depression. Freeing yourself from chronic unhappiness.* New York: Guilford.

Wiznitzer, M., Verhulst, F. C., van den Brink, W., Koeter, M., van der Ende, J., Giel, R., et al. (1992). Detecting psychopathology in young adults: The young adult self report, the general health questionnaire and the symptom checklist as screening instruments. *Acta Psychiatric Scandinavia, 86,* 32–37.

Young, J. E. (1994). *Cognitive therapy for personality disorders: A schema-focused approach* (Practitioner's resource series). Sarasota, FL: Professional Resource Press/Professional Resource Exchange.

Young, J. E., Klosko, J. S., & Weishaar, M. E. (2003). *Schema therapy: A practitioner's guide.* New York: The Guildford Press.

Zahn-Waxler, C., Radke-Yarrow, M., Wagner, E., & Chapman, M. (1992). Development of concern for others. *Developmental Psychology, 28,* 126–136.

INDEX